Nurses Contributions to Quality Health Outcomes

Marianne Baernholdt · Diane K. Boyle
Editors

Nurses Contributions to Quality Health Outcomes

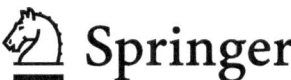 Springer

Editors
Marianne Baernholdt
School of Nursing
University of North Carolina at Chapel Hill
Chapel Hill, NC
USA

Diane K. Boyle
Fay W. Whitney School of Nursing
University of Wyoming
Laramie, WY
USA

ISBN 978-3-030-69062-5   ISBN 978-3-030-69063-2   (eBook)
https://doi.org/10.1007/978-3-030-69063-2

This Springer imprint is published by the registered company Springer Nature Switzerland AG
The registered company address is: Gewerbestrasse 11, 6330 Cham, Switzerland

So never lose an opportunity of urging a practical beginning, however small, for it is wonderful how often in such matters the mustard-seed germinates and roots itself.
– Florence Nightingale

Florence Nightingale Quotes. (n.d.) BrainyQuote.com. https://www.brainyquote. com/quotes/florence_nightingale_121022

In this year of the nurse, we dedicate this book to all nurses who tirelessly work to provide quality healthcare.

We would also like to acknowledge the two women whom set us on our research journey as our dissertation Chairs and long-term research mentors:

Norma M. Lang and Roma Lee Taunton

Foreword

Riveting headlines 20 years ago from the Institute of Medicine (IOM, now National Academy of Medicine, NAM) revealed healthcare errors were a leading cause of death, projecting upward of 100,000 preventable deaths annually. This transformational report, *To Err is Human: Building a Better Health System,* compelled healthcare professionals to embark on an aggressive quest to reduce harm by improving quality and safety across the system. Two decades later, nurses face a formidable foe in the COVID-19 pandemic, killing hundreds of thousands of Americans and almost 1.5 million people worldwide. Nurses are addressing multiple crises to keep themselves, their co-workers, and their patients safe while enduring moral distress in the face of inadequate personal protective equipment, broken supply chains, and woefully inadequate staffing. Nurses are fulfilling their duty to provide care by adopting crisis care standards while worrying about themselves and their loved ones. They are often confronted with the moral dilemma of deciding how much high-quality care they can provide in suboptimal conditions. In response, nurses continue to advocate for the supports they need to allow them to provide care in all situations, mitigate risks, and remain dedicated to assuring acceptable levels of care quality during this crisis and beyond.

Over the last half century, healthcare organizations and clinicians have re-engineered systems, implemented quality improvement tools, peer review, public reporting of outcomes, participated in programs that reward good versus penalizing poor performance, and redesigned our education of professionals. The initial conditions of participation implemented when Medicare legislation was enacted in 1965 to ensure beneficiaries' health and safety included a provision for 24-hour nursing services in hospitals. A primary focus was on determining the extent of underuse, overuse, and misuse of services, establishing a link between quality and reimbursement for necessary care but rarely, if ever, did measurement of nursing care enter into the assessment.

Consistent with the conceptualizations of Avedis Donabedien, who proposed structure, process, and outcomes as domains for evaluating the quality of care, the nursing profession had adopted a quality assurance model in the 1970s to address the outcomes, processes, and structure of standards and criteria of care. The model was predicated on nurses embracing professional accountability for the outcomes of their care.

The Quality Health Outcomes Model (QHOM) described in the pages that follow was developed and introduced in 1998 before the NAM report. It presented the need to generate, organize, and use evidence in the approach to find the linkage between nursing interventions and patient outcomes. At about the same time, the American Nurses Association established the National Database of Nursing Quality Indicators® (NDNQI®) in 1998, which ultimately became the roadmap for understanding and taking action to address conditions that threatened hospitalized patients' outcomes. It also helped establish the relationship of nurse staffing and other nurse characteristics to outcomes and demonstrate nurses' value in promoting quality patient care. Both the QHOM model and NDNQI reinforce the need for evidence to guide improvement in care and outcomes.

Initial quality measures developed by multi-stakeholder groups through the National Quality Forum (NQF) for implementation by the Centers for Medicare and Medicaid (CMS) focused primarily on physician processes. The introduction of a set of voluntary Consensus Standards for Nursing-Sensitive Care by NQF in 2004 provided an impetus to quantify and study the impact of nursing care on patient outcomes. Today the relationship of nursing care—both quantity and quality—to patient safety and outcomes is well established. However, what continues to be elusive is recognizing and valuing the evidence that supports more significant resourcing of nurses to make their maximum contribution to care delivery. Concomitantly nurses should occupy top leadership roles influencing policy, reimagining care delivery models that address team-based interprofessional practice, redesigning work environments and workflow, and commanding resources that allow the right dosing of nursing care to meet patient needs.

As care was re-envisioned for a twenty-first century healthcare system that would reduce the burden of injury, illness, and disability and provide safe, effective, patient-centered, timely, efficient, and equitable, nurses stepped up. But they were never the leaders of the band. Instead, nurses were the "functional doers" as described in the Future of Nursing Report. They became care coordinators, case managers, quality data entry clerks, quality monitors, black belts, green belts, the ones who forced teams to conduct time-outs for safety checks, filled out checklists, and populated countless other forms by hand or electronically to ensure organizations could have good report cards and satisfy compliance requirements to payers. Nurse scientists had to scramble for funding to study nurses' contributions to care and outcomes, as well as patient characteristics and conditions that increase vulnerability in the hospital setting.

In 2011, CMS launched the Partnership for Patients as a network of organizations to improve healthcare quality, safety, and affordability. The primary aims were to reduce hospital-acquired conditions and readmissions. The first 4 years' impressive results showed a reduction of more than 2 million hospital-acquired conditions, equating to an approximate 87,000 fewer associated deaths and savings of close to $20 billion. Nurses' innovation, vigilance, and commitment to actions that improved quality drove reductions in all the categories of harm. Those highly associated with preventing deaths, pressure ulcers, and catheter-associated urinary tract infections are clearly related to nurses' actions. Yet, in analyzing the successes, attributes such as financial incentives, public reporting, and investment in electronic health records were highlighted as major contributors to progress.

Similarly, despite two or more decades of data on the effects of nurse staffing on hospital-acquired conditions and patient outcomes, nurses still struggle to be recognized as the ones who provide vigilant surveillance of a patient's condition that could mean the difference between life and death, or the critical information that helps a family care for a loved one, or the insights to constantly problem-solve almost any challenging situation. Nursing's contributions can no longer remain invisible. It is widely recognized that nurses are fundamental to any healthcare system, but these must also translate into power and influence. Conveying the impact that nursing care has on improving the human experience, and ultimately quality, is priceless and without parallel.

This book tells the undeniable story of nursing's contributions at the individual, group, and systems levels. It spotlights the unrewarded reliance on nurses' brainpower, curiosity, and tenacity to ensure the practice environment and intellectual work of nurses support better care and outcomes. What will be essential is that every nurse who reads this book puts it in the hands of a powerbroker who can support nurses in any care delivery setting. Nothing should speak louder than our contributions to quality. The world has seen the inextricable dependence on nurses and survival in the pandemic. And as nurses have repeatedly vocalized, "don't call me a hero, give me what I need to do my job and protect myself and my patients," the expert authors have done just that throughout. They have produced evidence of what is needed for nurses to provide safe, effective, patient-centered, timely, efficient, and equitable care. They have staked out the space for nurses to influence policy for quality measurement. They have illuminated the rationale for supporting the workforce and work environment and the advances nurses have been making to deploy technology solutions better to improve and support clinical workflow. The case is made clear that nurses are implementing solutions to transform care delivery by improving care processes, interprofessional relationships, and communication, as well as implementing roles that address the holistic needs of patients and families in a complex system. Most compelling is the articulation of outcomes that help those we serve and the workforce and organizations at large. These outcomes come at the hands of nurses who bring to bear systems thinking, keen observations and critical reasoning, scientific inquiry and measurement, and a dedication to amplify this work so that nurses are recognized as the experts who have largely operated behind the scenes and must now emerge as the leaders they are and have been for some time.

Pamela F. Cipriano, PhD, RN, NEA-BC, FAAN
Dean and Sadie Heath Cabaniss Professor,
University of Virginia School of Nursing,
Charlottesville, Virginia
Past President, American Nurses Association

Contents

Part I Introduction

1 Overview of the Quality Health Outcomes Model   3
Diane K. Boyle and Marianne Baernholdt
Introduction   3
Background of the Quality Health Outcomes Model   4
The Quality Health Outcomes Model   5
Theoretical and Analytic Advantages of the QHOM   7
Use of the QHOM in the Literature   9
How This Book Is Organized 12
Summary 12
References 15

Part II Context

2 Healthcare Policy 21
Lauryn S. Walker and Deborah E. Trautman
Introduction 21
Healthcare Policy Linkages to QHOM 22
Access to Care 23
Healthcare Spending 27
Quality Measurement 31
Other Policy Interventions 31
Using Multilevel Policies to Manage the Opioid Crisis 34
Summary and Future Directions 36
References 36

3 The Nurse Workforce 39
Sean P. Clarke
Introduction 39
The Nurse Workforce: Context for the Quality Health
Outcomes Model 40
Interplay of Nursing Supply and Demand at Various Levels
of the Healthcare System 42

Managing Supply and Demand of the Nurse Workforce   50
The Future of the Nurse Workforce   55
References.   57

Part III System

4 The Nurse Work Environment.   63
Shelly A. Fischer and Diane K. Boyle
Introduction.   63
Nurse Work Environment: Specific Linkages with the QHOM   64
System.   66
System Interventions.   75
Implications and Future Directions.   77
References.   78

5 Workflow, Turbulence, and Cognitive Complexity   85
Bonnie Mowinski Jennings
Introduction.   85
Workflow, Turbulence, and Cognitive Complexity:
Specific Linkages with the QHOM.   86
System Characteristics   87
Client Characteristics   96
Client (Nurse) Outcomes   99
Implications and Future Directions. 100
References. 101

6 Health Information Technology and Electronic Health Records 109
Susan McBride and Mari Tietze
Introduction. 109
Health IT: Linkages to the QHOM 109
Environmental Context of Healthcare Regulation in the USA 111
System Characteristics that Influence Health IT Adoption. 113
Health IT Interventions. 115
Health IT Competencies 119
Client. 121
Outcomes 122
Summary. 123
References. 123

Part IV Client

7 Health Literacy and Social Determinants of Health 129
Terri Ann Parnell
Introduction. 129
Health Literacy: Specific Linkages to the QHOM 130
Client. 131
Interventions 132

System... 135
Outcomes: Health Literacy Impact Upon Quality and Safety 137
Implications and Future Directions............................ 139
References...................................... 140

8 Chronicity 143
Amy J. Barton
Introduction..................................... 143
Chronicity: Linkages to the QHOM 144
Client... 144
Interventions 147
Implications and Future Directions.......................... 151
References...................................... 152

Part V   Interventions

9 Nursing Care Processes 157
Terry L. Jones
Introduction..................................... 157
Nursing Care Processes: Linkages to QHOM 158
The Essence of Nursing Interventions 159
System Characteristics' Effect on Nursing Interventions............. 162
Examples of Nursing Interventions 163
Implications and Future Directions.......................... 170
References...................................... 172

10 Interprofessional Practice and Education 177
Alan W. Dow, Deborah DiazGranados, and Marianne Baernholdt
Introduction..................................... 177
Interprofessional Practice: Linkages with the QHOM 178
Interprofessional Practice and Education Within a Complex System.... 179
Characteristics Important for Interprofessional Practice 181
Interprofessional Practice Interventions 183
Example of an IPP Intervention in One Healthcare System........... 186
Summary and Future Directions............................ 187
References...................................... 189

11 Care Coordination 193
Beth Ann Swan
Introduction..................................... 193
Care Coordination: Linkages to the QHOM..................... 194
System Characteristics of Care Coordination.................... 194
Client... 196
Care Coordination Interventions........................... 199
Outcomes of Care Coordination 201
Summary....................................... 202
References...................................... 203

Part VI   Outcomes

12   Client and Family Outcomes: Experiences of Care............... 207
       Stefanie Bachnick and Michael Simon
       Introduction.. 207
       Person-Centered Care: Linkages with the QHOM................. 208
       Person-Centered Care Interventions.......................... 208
       Client and Family Characteristics........................... 210
       System Characteristics 211
       Outcomes Associated with Person-Centered Care Interventions 212
       Challenges Measuring Person-Centered Care 213
       Implications and Future Directions........................... 215
       References... 216

13   Nurse Outcomes: Burnout, Engagement, and Job Satisfaction 221
       Peter Van Bogaert and Erik Franck
       Introduction.. 221
       Nurse Outcomes: Linkages with the QHOM 222
       Nurse Outcomes 223
       Interventions: Client (Nurse) 226
       Interventions: System 230
       Example of Nurse Outcome Program of Research................. 231
       Implications and Future Directions........................... 233
       References... 234

14   Organizational Outcomes: Financial and Quality Measures 239
       Nancy Dunton and Amenda Fisher
       Introduction.. 239
       Healthcare Organizational Outcomes: Specific Linkages with the
       QHOM 240
       Evolution of Policies and Programs to Promote Safer Patient Care..... 242
       Hospital Organizational Outcomes............................ 248
       Implications and Future Directions........................... 251
       References... 252

Part VII   Closing

15   The Way Forward... 257
       Marianne Baernholdt and Diane K. Boyle
       Introduction.. 257
       The QHOM in the Context of Quality and Safety Reports........... 257
       Future Directions 261
       References... 262

Contributors

Stefanie Bachnick Department of Public Health, Institute of Nursing Science, University of Basel, Basel, Switzerland

Marianne Baernholdt School of Nursing, University of North Carolina at Chapel Hill, Chapel Hill, NC, USA

Amy J. Barton Professor and Daniel and Janet Mordecai Endowed Chair in Rural Health Nursing, College of Nursing, University of Colorado Anschutz Medical Campus, Aurora, CO, USA

Peter Van Bogaert Department of Nursing and Midwifery Science, Centre for Research and Innovation in Care (CRIC), University of Antwerp, Antwerpen, Belgium

Diane K. Boyle Fay W. Whitney School of Nursing, University of Wyoming, Laramie, WY, USA

Sean P. Clarke Rory Meyers College of Nursing, New York University, New York, NY, USA

Deborah DiazGranados Wright Center for Clinical and Translational Research, School of Medicine, Virginia Commonwealth University, Richmond, VA, USA

Alan W. Dow Medicine and Health Administration, Virginia Commonwealth University, Richmond, VA, USA

Nancy Dunton Center for Healthcare Quality Research, School of Nursing, University of Kansas, Kansas City, KS, USA

Shelly A. Fischer College of Nursing, University of Colorado Anschutz Medical Campus, Aurora, CO, USA

Amenda Fisher Health & Well-Being, Walmart Inc., Bentonville, AR, USA

Erik Franck Department of Nursing and Midwifery Science, Centre for Research and Innovation in Care (CRIC), University of Antwerp, Antwerpen, Belgium

Bonnie Mowinski Jennings Nell Hodgson Woodruff School of Nursing, Emory University, Atlanta, GA, USA

Terry L. Jones School of Nursing, Virginia Commonwealth University, Richmond, VA, USA

Susan McBride Nursing Informatics, School of Nursing, Texas Tech University Health Sciences Center, Lubbock, TX, USA

Terri Ann Parnell Health Literacy Partners, LLC, Garden City, NY, USA

Michael Simon Department of Public Health, Institute of Nursing Science, University of Basel, Basel, Switzerland

Nursing Research Unit, Inselspital University Hospital, Bern, Switzerland

Beth Ann Swan Nell Hodgson Woodruff School of Nursing, Emory University, Atlanta, GA, USA

Mari Tietze Texas Woman's University, T. Boone Pickens Institute of Health Sciences-Dallas Center, Dallas, TX, USA

Deborah E. Trautman American Association of Colleges of Nursing, Washington, DC, USA

Lauryn S. Walker Virginia Department of Medical Assistance Services, Richmond, VA, USA

Part I
Introduction

Overview of the Quality Health Outcomes Model

Diane K. Boyle and Marianne Baernholdt

Introduction

Twenty years ago, the release of the Quality Health Outcomes Model (QHOM) (Mitchell et al. 1998) by the Quality Healthcare Expert Panel of the American Academy of Nursing proved incredibly timely. Shortly after the QHOM release, the Institute of Medicine [IOM, now the National Academy of Medicine (NAM)] published *To Err is Human: Building a Better Health System* (2000), which revealed that healthcare errors were a leading cause of death in the USA. The report estimated up to 98,000 preventable deaths each year and hundreds of thousands of nonfatal injuries. Further, the IOM recommended a paradigm shift of making evidence-based changes at the systems level to improve quality and safety. At about the same time, the American Nurses Association established the National Database of Nursing Quality Indicators® (NDNQI®), which contains nursing-sensitive structure, process (intervention), and outcome measures for monitoring how nursing care affects outcomes (Press Ganey n.d.). NDNQI quickly became a mechanism for nurses to understand and address care delivery problems that endangered hospitalized patients' outcomes. Although progress has been made, today, the healthcare industry still faces significant and compelling challenges related to patient safety. In a 2016 analysis for the *BMJ*, Makary and Daniel (2016) found that the mean number of deaths from preventable medical errors was about 250,000 per year in the USA and, therefore, it was the third leading cause of death.

The healthcare environment in which nurses and other healthcare professionals practice is complex and rapidly changing. The need for evidence about which factors contribute to improved safety and quality has never been greater. Nurses

D. K. Boyle (✉)
Fay W. Whitney School of Nursing, University of Wyoming, Laramie, WY, USA

M. Baernholdt
School of Nursing, University of North Carolina at Chapel Hill, Chapel Hill, NC, USA
e-mail: marianne_baernholdt@unc.edu

© Springer Nature Switzerland AG 2021
M. Baernholdt, D. K. Boyle (eds.), *Nurses Contributions to Quality Health Outcomes*, https://doi.org/10.1007/978-3-030-69063-2_1

play a significant role in the delivery and coordination of care activities within and across healthcare teams. Consequently, few healthcare elements do not pass through nurses' hands and few outcomes are not influenced by nursing care.

The QHOM and its four primary constructs—system, client, interventions, and outcomes—organize quality and safety components within a nursing framework. Using the QHOM, nurses and other healthcare professionals can conceptualize and measure quality and safety components simultaneously at a single level or multiple levels, such as individual, family, community, and population levels (Mitchell et al. 1998; Mitchell and Shortell 1997). The flexibility of the QHOM makes it an ideal framework for solving some of today's compelling quality and safety challenges.

Background of the Quality Health Outcomes Model

Up to the late 1990s, researchers investigating factors contributing to quality healthcare and better patient outcomes primarily used Donabedian's (1966, 1988) linear structure, process, outcomes (S-P-O) framework. Structures of care were defined as setting attributes where patient care takes place, including provider characteristics, technology, specialty mix, patient volume, and financing. Processes of care were provider-client interactions and how episodes of illness are managed. Outcomes of care were the results of care—typically the "Five Ds" of death, disability, dissatisfaction, disease, and discomfort (Lohr 1988). In the traditional S-P-O framework, nursing structure components typically were buried in nonspecific features of organizational structure. Further, nursing processes were almost nonexistent, which did not advance the understanding of the nursing system and process factors that interacted with client factors to achieve optimal client outcomes (Michell et al. 1997a). Research that explicitly addressed the interactive effects of organizational and process factors in care delivery and client outcomes was lacking.

In the mid-1990s, the American Academy of Nursing's (AAN) Quality Healthcare Expert Panel (QEP) recognized a need for a more interactive conceptual framework for nursing and health services research. A taskforce within QEP developed the QHOM, incorporating dynamic and reciprocal interactions among system, client, process or interventions, and outcomes (Mitchell et al. 1998; Mitchell and Lang 2004). Interventions acted on the system or client, which in turn affected outcomes. The QHOM was derived from literature, QEP members' research, and expert opinion.

Developers of the QHOM also garnered input by hosting two invitational conferences in 1996 and 2002 sponsored by the Agency for Healthcare Research and Quality (AHRQ, formerly the Agency for Health Care Policy and Research), with additional support from a variety of other organizations. Both conferences brought together nurse scientists, health services researchers, healthcare purchasers, and policymakers. The 1996 conference, *Outcomes Measures and Care Delivery Systems* (see *Medical Care,* 1997, Vol. 35, November NS supplement for complete details on the conference and its outcomes), focused on (a) identifying outcome indicators shown to be sensitive to elements of nursing care delivery systems, (b) identifying promising indicators for measure development or incorporation into studies of care delivery systems, and (c) developing research and policy recommendations regarding measure development for incorporation into existing data sources (Michell et al. 1997a). The 2002 conference, *Measuring and Improving Healthcare Quality* (see *Medical Care,* 2004, Vol. 42, Number 2 supplement for complete details on the conference and its outcomes), built on the 1996 conference and focused on (a) linkages of nursing processes (interventions) and outcomes; (b) linkages of health outcomes, quality of nursing care, and nurse staffing; and (c) methodologies and challenges of quality indicators measured within large databases (Lang et al. 2004). The resultant QHOM was then published in 1998 in *Image: Journal of Nursing Scholarship* (Mitchell et al. 1998) and updated after the 2002 conference (Mitchell and Lang 2004).

The Quality Health Outcomes Model

The QHOM (Fig. 1.1) is a nonlinear model depicting interrelationships among the nursing metaparadigm constructs of person (client), environment (system), health (outcomes), and nursing care (interventions) (Mitchell et al. 1998; Mitchell and Lang 2004). The QHOM reimagines Donabedian's (1966) long-standing linear S-P-O framework to assess the quality of care by realigning the constructs to incorporate multiple, dynamic feedback loops among the healthcare delivery system, interventions, client, and outcomes, allowing more sensitivity to nursing care. The

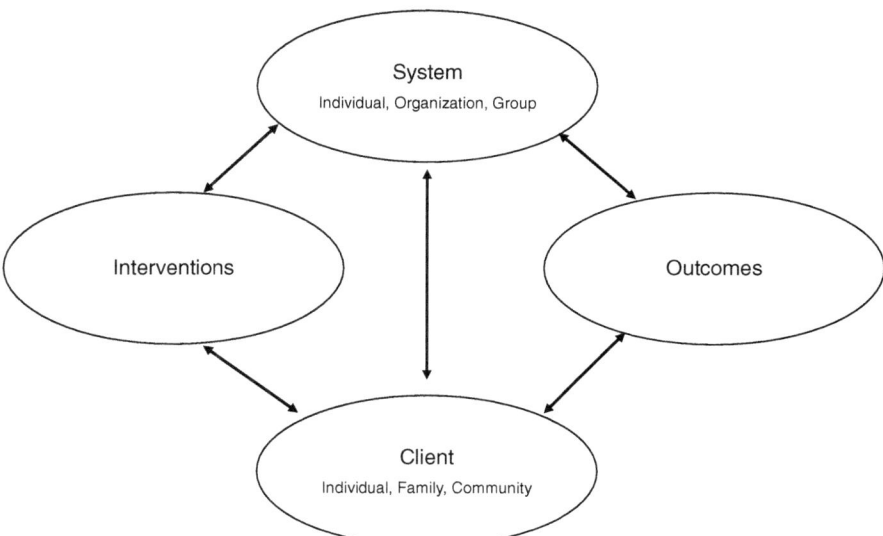

Fig. 1.1 Quality Health Outcomes Model (source: Mitchell, P.H., Ferketich, S., & Jennings, B.M. (1998). Quality Health Outcomes Model. Image: Journal of Nursing Scholarship, 30(1), 43–46. Reproduced with permission from Wiley)

QHOM contains no direct link between interventions and outcomes. Instead, an intervention's effect is mediated or moderated by client and system characteristics, rather than having independent effects on outcomes (Mitchell and Lang 2004). Although the QHOM includes nursing metaparadigm constructs (person, environment, health, and nursing care), it is intended for use in all health services research and quality improvement activities.

Components of the QHOM

System

The QHOM includes the S-P-O framework's traditional structure variables (Mitchell et al. 1998). For healthcare organizations these include attributes such as size, ownership, technology, population served, case mix index, and location. Additionally, specific nurse work environment characteristics (organizational or unit level) can be included to determine their effect on outcomes. Examples of nurse work environment characteristics are transformational leadership, practice autonomy, professional relationships, empowerment, shared decision-making, patient-centered culture, appropriate staffing structures, and professional development (Kramer et al. 2010).

Client

The client can be an individual, a group such as a family, a community, or a population. Client characteristics are broad and include differing states of client health, demographics (e.g., age, gender, income), disease risk factors, health habits, and preferences (Mitchell et al. 1998). The client can also be framed beyond the traditional patient. Clients can be nurses or other healthcare providers, a single organization, or a healthcare system.

Interventions

Interventions, in general terms, are the *activities of care* and *clinical processes*. These clinical care processes directly or indirectly target patients, families, and communities to achieve desired health outcomes. Interventions are the *mechanisms* through which clinicians impact health; thus, they are the key *active ingredients* of quality healthcare. Nursing surveillance, implementation of prevention protocols, and nurse cognitive processes are nursing intervention examples. Mutual exchange of time, expertise, and resources among the multiple health professions is an example of an interdisciplinary intervention (Mitchell and Shortell 1997).

Interventions can also be targeted at organizations or clinicians as a client. Two organizational intervention programs with demonstrated outcomes (e.g., improved nurse satisfaction, better retention of nursing staff and nursing leaders, higher quality interprofessional teamwork and nursing practice, better fiscal outcomes) are the Magnet Recognition Program® (ANCC n.d.-a) and the Pathway to Excellence (PWE) Recognition Program (ANCC n.d.-b). An example intervention targeted at clinicians is a training program to improve interprofessional collaboration.

Outcomes

To capture nursing's effect (individual, unit/group, or organization) on outcomes, Mitchell et al. (1998) added five client outcomes to the usual "Five Ds" (death, disability, dissatisfaction, disease, and discomfort.). These added outcomes incorporated psychosocial, physical, functional, and physiologic elements thought to be more directly related to client functioning in everyday life, capacity for self-care, and engagement in health-promoting behaviors, as well as client' perceptions of care. The five added outcomes are *achievement of appropriate self-care, demonstration of health-promoting behaviors, health-related quality of life, client's perception of being well cared for*, and *symptom management*. See Table 1.1 for descriptions of QHOM added outcomes.

Just as clients and interventions can be conceptualized beyond the patient, outcomes can be conceptualized for clinicians and organizations. Examples of clinician outcomes are engagement, job satisfaction, burnout, and retention or turnover. Examples of organizational outcomes are fiscal and reputational status.

Theoretical and Analytic Advantages of the QHOM

The four QHOM constructs can be conceptualized and measured simultaneously at a single level or multiple levels, such as individual, family, community, and population levels (Mitchell et al. 1998; Mitchell and Shortell 1997). Another way to stratify levels is through the lens of micro, meso, and macro factors (Serpa and Ferreira 2019). Microlevel factors are at the level of the individual (patient, clinician). These might include patient chronicity (Chap. 8) and health literacy (Chap. 7). For clinicians, microlevel factors might be job satisfaction (Chap. 13). Meso-level factors

Table 1.1 QHOM outcome definitions

Concept	Definition
Achievement of appropriate self-care	The capacity and performance of self-care appropriate to current health status, where both capacity and performance are necessary dimensions (Henry and Holzemer 1997). *Capacity* is the maximum potential for actions. *Performance* is the actual activity. Achievement of appropriate self-care is considered the best proxy measure for the effectiveness of nursing care (Michell et al. 1997b)
Demonstration of health-promoting behaviors	A wide-ranging array of behaviors that promote health such as exercise and smoking cessation (Mitchell and Lang 2004)
Health-related quality of life	An individual or group's perceived health status, such as physical, mental, functional, or social aspects or health or illness, or general quality of life (Michell et al. 1997b; Mitchell et al. 1998)
Patient's perception of being well cared for	Patient perceptions in assessing healthcare delivery systems—a broader construct than patient reports of satisfaction (Michell et al. 1997b)
Symptom management	Patient-defined outcomes of managing specific symptoms, for example pain or nausea (Mitchell and Lang 2004)

span from the unit and team level to the organizational level. These might include an organization's nurse work environment (Chap. 4) or the level of interprofessional practice (Chap. 10). Macro-level factors work at the regulatory, societal, and political levels (Chaps. 2 and 3). Examples include licensure requirements and regulations, accreditation requirements for the Magnet or Pathway to Excellence Programs or Joint Commission accreditation, federal hospital payment systems, and staffing regulations.

The QHOM allows for research and quality improvement aims to be constructed at the appropriate level. For example, because variations exist in organizational structures, processes, and outcomes among units in the same hospital, aims may need to be addressed at the unit level rather than the hospital as a whole. If aims are about primary care, home healthcare, and other out-of-hospital settings, the focus unit can be the individual clinic or home healthcare unit, rather than the entire health system or corporation. Simultaneously other aims can address the hospital or corporate level.

The QHOM directs the inclusion of intervention (process) variables in quality assessment and improvement initiatives. The QHOM does not, however, define or prescribe specific interventions for quality assessment. Instead, the selection of intervention variables is purpose driven and context dependent. For example, the selection might depend on the aspect of care evaluated (e.g., primary care vs. acute care), the discipline evaluated (e.g., nursing vs. pharmacy), and the outcome of care evaluated (e.g., patient satisfaction vs. morbidity or mortality). Moreover, the QHOM directs the concurrent measurement of relevant variables from all constructs. Assessment of any single construct in isolation does not provide a complete quality assessment and does not provide direction for improvement. Consequently, a measure's relevance is based on its relationship to other variables in the measure set. Characteristics of an ideal measure set for quality assessment and improvement initiatives include the following: (1) they provide a complete, evidence-based model of the intervention of interest; (2) they address the full continuum of outcomes expected to be influenced by the intervention of interest; and (3) they include measures that are sensitive to change in the care being evaluated (Donabedian 2003; Jones 2016; Needleman et al. 2007).

The QHOM also allows for flexibility in the specification of levels included in data analysis. One example is accounting for organizational structures common in healthcare. Nurses and other clinicians are nested in units or workgroups, units and workgroups are nested in organizations, organizations are often nested in corporate systems, and so forth. As individual nurses and clinicians in workgroups and organizations are exposed to common features, events, and processes over time, they may develop consensual views of the workgroup and organization through interacting and sharing (Kozlowski and Klein 2000). Consensual views of safety culture and morale are examples. Multilevel modeling and data analysis can account for these consensual views.

On the other hand, there is variation in individual-level (micro) performance by nurses and other healthcare professionals that is to be expected (Yakusheva et al. 2020). The QHOM allows for linking individual clinicians to individual patients under the clinician's care—and then studying, for example, variations in care and patient outcomes. The elegance of the QHOM allows for modeling that includes system factors' (e.g., staffing, professional autonomy) effect on individual variations in care and subsequent outcomes.

Use of the QHOM in the Literature

Since its development in the mid-1990s the QHOM has inspired the development of related models and served as a theoretical framework for studies and projects. A literature review spanning 1996–2003 (Mitchell and Lang 2004) found that the model had guided a handful of studies in different settings from labor and delivery to oncology inpatient care. More importantly, the QHOM had served as an impetus for developing other models that linked organizational features and outcomes and developing measures for the system, client characteristics, interventions, and quality outcomes, and has been used in national and international datasets.

A review of published literature from 2002 to 2018 was undertaken to determine if the QHOM remains valuable as a theoretical guideline for studies and projects. PubMed, Web of Science, CINAHL, and other EBSCO databases were searched using the keywords "quality health outcomes model." Also, manual searches of critical articles' references were done. The search revealed 25 citations, where 6 were reviews or discussion papers, and of the remaining 19, 1 was a DNP project and 3 were dissertation studies.

From the six review or discussion papers, some papers discussed frameworks or conceptual models. Brewer and colleagues (Brewer et al. 2008) adapted the QHOM to develop a System Research Organization Model (SROM) to guide evidence-based healthcare design. Another article evaluated frameworks pertinent to research on isolation precaution effectiveness and recommended the QHOM because of its reciprocal relationships and multilevel analyses (Cohen and Shang 2015). In a third paper, the QHOM was used to plan simulations for training aimed at increasing patient safety (Lassche and Wilson 2016). Finally, Swan and Boruch (2004) used the QHOM to identify gaps in the evidence base in nursing and presented recommendations for practice, research, and policy to increase nursing's contribution to quality healthcare. The last two papers were reviews that focused on acute care psychiatric patients and are included in the review of studies below.

Of the 19 studies, reviews, and projects, 1 study used the QHOM to examine current issues related to quality measures (Baernholdt et al. 2017) by conducting focus groups with developers, regulators/endorsers, data collectors, and consumers. The QHOM guided both the questions and later the analyses. Only one study took place outside of the USA, namely in China (Shang et al. 2014). The studies and projects took place in various healthcare continuum settings, including specific patient groups and interventions. Not all studies included all four of the QHOM constructs. For example, intervention was the least discussed construct.

System

The most common system studied was hospitals or nursing units (Altares 2015; Badger 2017; Effken et al. 2005; Gerolamo 2004, 2006; Gilmartin and Sousa 2016; Gilmartin et al. 2016; Hilleren-Listerud 2014; Jost 2016.; Lake et al. 2012; Malley et al. 2018; Mark and Harless 2009; McAlister et al. 2013; Rowland 2005; Shang et al. 2014; Wilson et al. 2010). Specialized nursing units included intensive care units (ICU) (Gilmartin and Sousa 2016; Gilmartin et al. 2016), neonatal intensive care units (NICU) (Hallowell et al. 2016; Lake et al. 2012), and inpatient psychiatric units (Gerolamo 2004, 2006). One study took place in a clinic (Berry et al. 2018), another in hospice (both inpatient units and at home) (Baernholdt et al. 2015), while two studies occurred in the community (Borglund 2008; Sin et al. 2005).

Client

There were several client and family groups included across studies. Surgical patients were the focus of four studies (Altares 2015; Badger 2017; Hilleren-Listerud 2014; Mark and Harless 2009), two studies focused on ICU patients (Gilmartin and Sousa 2016; Gilmartin et al. 2016), and two reviews focused on acute care psychiatric patients (Gerolamo 2004, 2006). Pregnant women were included in three studies (McAlister et al. 2013; Rowland 2005; Wilson et al. 2010) as were low-birth-weight infants (Hallowell et al. 2016; Lake et al. 2012; McAlister et al. 2013). On the other end of clients' life span, one study included hospice patients and their families (Baernholdt et al. 2015). Patients with specific diseases or procedures were the focus of two studies: patients with gastrointestinal cancer (Berry et al. 2018) and older adults with multiple chronic conditions hospitalized for elective hip or knee replacement and their caregivers (Malley et al. 2018). Community-dwelling adults were included in two studies: adults with a disability (Borglund 2008) and older Korean American adults (Sin et al. 2005). Finally, staff nurses were the client in one study (Jost 2016).

Interventions

The interventions targeted three broad categories: work environment and processes, patient and family, and pregnant women and new mothers. The studied work environment categories included hospitals recognized for nursing excellence (Lake et al. 2012), registered nurse (RN) skill mix (Altares 2015; Mark and Harless 2009) and education (Hallowell et al. 2016), and use of contract nurses (Shang et al. 2014). Three studies described health information technology interventions. One implemented a patient acuity software system that generated patient acuity scores, which then were used to guide staffing decisions (Badger 2017). The second study used virtual units to model fluctuations in patient complexity and staffing, including education and experience, to educate managers about potential nursing unit interventions to improve care quality (Effken et al. 2005). The third study described a clinical decision support system implementation (Jost 2016). Another four papers included processes for improving care such as comparing case management types (Borglund 2008), implementing a central line bundle intervention (Gilmartin and Sousa 2016; Gilmartin et al. 2016), and a daily delirium screening by RNs (Hilleren-Listerud 2014).

Interventions targeting patients and families encompassed information about patient's condition and emotional support (Baernholdt et al. 2015), an app as an adjunct to usual patient education regarding cancer symptoms and medication management (Berry et al. 2018), and an exercise program (Sin et al. 2005). Four studies included interventions targeting pregnant women and new mothers. Preventive and supportive services during pregnancy (Rowland 2005), elective induction or cesarean delivery (McAlister et al. 2013), and induction (Wilson et al. 2010) were the focus of three studies, whereas breastfeeding support (Hallowell et al. 2016) was included in one study.

Outcomes

As with the previous QHOM constructs, a wide variety of outcomes were included in the studies spanning patient safety, organization, patient-reported outcomes, pregnancy, and nursing process. Patient safety was the focus of seven studies and two reviews. Patient safety outcomes in surgical patients included mortality and failure to rescue (Altares 2015), and other complications such as pneumonia, septicemia, urinary tract infection, thrombophlebitis, fluid overload, and decubitus ulcer (Malley et al. 2018; Mark and Harless 2009). NICU mortality and nosocomial infections (Lake et al. 2012) and central line-associated bloodstream infections (CLABSIs) (Gilmartin and Sousa 2016; Gilmartin et al. 2016) were specific intensive care outcomes studied. Suicide and self-injury and physical restraint episodes in psychiatric units (Gerolamo 2004, 2006) and falls and medication errors across populations (Effken et al. 2005) were studied in other settings. Three organizational outcomes were addressed. Length of stay and patients' discharge disposition were included in two studies (Badger 2017; Malley et al. 2018) and readmission rates in another two (Gerolamo 2004; Malley et al. 2018). Patient-reported outcomes were included in six studies. These outcomes included patient satisfaction (Baernholdt et al. 2015; Effken et al. 2005; Gerolamo 2004; Shang et al. 2014), quality of life (Borglund 2008), and symptom management, including pain and functional improvement (i.e., ability for self-care, muscle strength, agility/balance) (Baernholdt et al. 2015; Effken et al. 2005; Gerolamo 2004; Sin et al. 2005). One study reported patients' acceptability and utilization rate of an app (Berry et al. 2018). Specific pregnancy outcomes included cesarean (Wilson et al. 2010) and early-term birth rates (McAlister et al. 2013). For the newborns, NICU admission rate (McAlister et al. 2013) and rate of low-birth-weight infants discharged home on human milk were studied (Hallowell et al. 2016). Three papers included nursing practice outcomes. One study examined specific elements of nursing practice such as communication, sharing of information, and workflow (Jost 2016); another one focused on clinician's acceptability working with a patient app (Berry et al. 2018); and another examined the implementation of multidisciplinary delirium intervention in a surgical unit (Hilleren-Listerud 2014).

The literature review provides evidence that the QHOM model remains relevant after more than 20 years. Since the QOM was last reviewed in 2004, the model has been used widely to inform theoretical papers, policy and review papers, and studies across the care continuum focused on a wide variety of clients, interventions, and outcomes. Thus, nurses' contribution to quality healthcare has been and can continue to be depicted using the QHOM.

How This Book Is Organized

This book provides a comprehensive exploration of the QHOM. The four primary QHOM constructs—system, client, interventions, and outcomes—are examined and expanded using a wide variety of contemporary nursing and healthcare topics. The importance of two contextual factors that influence the QHOM—healthcare policy and nurse workforce supply and demand—is explored. The topics covered in this book are those essential for nurses to be effective practitioners and leaders in quality healthcare. Chapter topics can be explored individually or as a whole in connection with all book topics. Topics were assigned to the most germane QHOM construct, recognizing that each topic has components of all four QHOM constructs. For example, health literacy was once thought only to affect individual clients. However, health literacy is also an essential component of the nursing profession and healthcare systems. Sections, specific chapters, and chapter content are provided in Table 1.2.

Summary

This book provides an outstanding in-depth resource for understanding how to use the QHOM in nursing research and quality improvement. The QHOM is a contemporary and essential mechanism for organizing quality and safety components within a nursing framework. The book is intended for use to guide education, research, and practice. The QHOM allows nurses and other healthcare professionals to use their best thinking and collaboration to meet the current quality and safety challenges. See Chap. 15 for future directions for the QHOM.

Table 1.2 Chapter contents

Chapters	Chapter content
Section I. Introduction	
Chapter 1: *Overview of the QHOM* Diane K. Boyle Marianne Baernholdt	Chapter 1 describes the constructs of the QHOM: system, client, interventions, and outcomes. Theoretic and analytic advantages of the QHOM are considered. Uses of the QHOM in previous research are reviewed. An overview of the book content is provided
Section II. Context	
Chapter 2: *Healthcare Policy* Lauryn S. Walker Deborah E. Trautman	Chapter 2 discusses how healthcare policy influences the constructs of the QHOM through legislation, regulation, professional standards of care, health insurance policy, or payment mechanisms
Chapter 3: *The Nurse Workforce* Sean P. Clarke	Chapter 3 focuses on workforce issues within the QHOM. Two forces at the heart of workforce analysis, supply and demand, are examined in various nursing practice areas. Ongoing and emerging trends influencing the nurse workforce are discussed
Section III. System	
Chapter 4: *The Nurse Work Environment* Shelly A. Fischer Diane K. Boyle	Chapter 4 places the system concept of the nurse work environment (NWE) within the context of the QHOM and explores the essential structures of NWEs. Four specific components of NWE are discussed: joy in work and clinician well-being, safety culture, incivility and bullying, and staffing. Two interventions to improve NWEs, the Magnet Recognition Program® and the Pathway to Excellence Recognition Program, are considered
Chapter 5: *Workflow, Turbulence, and Cognitive Complexity* Bonnie Mowinski Jennings	Chapter 5 focuses on the system characteristics of nursing workflow and turbulence. Extensive discussion is provided on how poor workflow and high turbulence tend to increase nurses' cognitive complexity and how poor workflow, high turbulence, and elevated cognitive complexity can contribute to work stress and cognitive failure, thereby adversely affecting patient safety and quality care
Chapter 6: *Health Information Technology and Electronic Health Records* Susan McBride Mari Tietze	Chapter 6 views health information technology (health IT) through the lens of the QHOM. The environmental context that propelled the rapid expansion of health IT is reviewed. The impact of health IT changes on clinical processes and outcomes is discussed. The QHOM model is used to describe methods to address the negatives and optimize technology by using fundamental quality improvement tools and methods. Advances in health IT competencies needed by healthcare professionals are discussed
Section IV. Client	
Chapter 7: *Health Literacy and the Social Determinants of Health* Terri Ann Parnell	Chapter 7 discusses health literacy's association with the social determinants of health and explores their essential relationship to the QHOM. Although health literacy was once thought only to affect individuals, the chapter depicts how health literacy is essential to the nursing profession and healthcare systems. Health literacy interventions are also reviewed

(continued)

Table 1.2 (continued)

Chapters	Chapter content
Chapter 8: *Chronicity* Amy J. Barton	Chapter 8 places the concept of client chronicity within the context of the QHOM and explores its relevance to nursing care and research. Four evidence-based models are described within the context of the QHOM: The Chronic Care Model, Innovative Care for Chronic Conditions, The Chronic Disease Self-Management Program, and The Transitional Care Model. Also, the co-occurrence of multiple chronic conditions or multimorbidity is discussed within the context of complex adaptive care
Section V. Interventions	
Chapter 9: *Nursing Care Processes/ Interventions* Terry L. Jones	Chapter 9 examines the complex nature of nursing processes known as nursing care interventions in the QHOM. Specifically, nursing interventions at the client and the system level are addressed, and two specific nursing interventions, nurse surveillance and symptom management, are examined as exemplars
Chapter 10: *Interprofessional Practice and Education* Alan W. Dow Deborah DiazGranados Marianne Baernholdt	Chapter 10 discusses how the QHOM helps understand the phenomenon of interprofessional practice (IPP) and interprofessional education (IPE) as interventions to improve outcomes in healthcare's complex environment. The chapter discusses what characteristics are essential for IPP at the micro, meso, and macro levels, focusing on organizational culture. IPP interventions are described, followed by an example of an IPP intervention in one healthcare system
Chapter 11: *Care Coordination* Beth Ann Swan	Chapter 11 explores the essential relationship of care coordination within the QHOM. Specifically, one key component is the significant role of registered nurses (RNs) in providing care coordination as an intervention for individuals, families, communities, and populations
Section VI. Outcomes	
Chapter 12: *Client and Family Outcomes: Experiences of Care* Stefanie Bachnick Michael Simon	Chapter 12 examines client and family experiences of care, i.e., person-centered care (PCC). By embedding PCC into the QHOM, characteristics and interventions influencing PCC outcomes are explored at the micro and macro levels. How client and family characteristics, as well as system characteristics, influence and affect outcomes are described. Finally, the chapter provides suggestions for tackling measurement and methodological challenges to improve PCC as one key element of quality of care
Chapter 13: *Nurse Outcomes: Burnout, Engagement, and Job Satisfaction* Peter Van Bogaert Erik Franck	Chapter 13 uses the QHOM to explain how nurses can be empowered to deal with the continuous challenges and healthcare organization changes. Empowerment interventions aimed at the system and the individual nurse levels are described. Nurse outcomes, such as engagement and job satisfaction, are discussed
Chapter 14: *Organizational Outcomes: Financial and Quality Measures* Nancy Dunton Amenda Fisher	Chapter 14 examines organizational outcomes through the lens of the QHOM. Financial and quality measures outcomes are discussed. Elements influencing organizational outcomes are considered, such as the healthcare environment, characteristics of the healthcare organization, and interventions designed to promote healthcare quality

Table 1.2 (continued)

Chapters	Chapter content
Section VII. Closing	
Chapter 15: *The Way Forward* Marianne Baernholdt Diane K. Boyle	The quality and safety reports guiding healthcare policy and practice since the late 1990s when the Quality Health Outcomes Model (QHOM) was developed are revisited, including reports focused on nurses. Aspects of these reports covered in this book's chapters, framed within the four constructs of the QHOM and the healthcare context, are highlighted. Finally, future directions are discussed

References

Altares SD (2015) The impact of nursing skill mix on the outcomes of hospitalized adult surgical patients. http://repository.upenn.edu/edissertations/1990

American Nurses Credentialing Center (n.d.-a) ANCC magnet recognition program. https://www.nursingworld.org/organizational-programs/magnet/

American Nurses Credentialing Center (n.d.-b) ANCC pathway to excellence program. https://www.nursingworld.org/organizational-programs/pathway/

Badger MK (2017) Patient acuity as a predictor of length of hospital stay and discharge disposition after open colorectal surgery. Doctoral Dissertation

Baernholdt M, Campbell CL, Hinton ID, Yan G, Lewis E (2015) Quality of hospice care: comparison between rural and urban residents. J Nurs Care Qual 30(3):247–253. https://doi.org/10.1097/NCQ.0000000000000108

Baernholdt M, Dunton N, Hughes RG, Stone PW, White KM (2017) Quality measures. J Nurs Care Qual 33(2):149–156. https://doi.org/10.1097/NCQ.0000000000000292

Berry D, Blonquist T, Nayak M, Grenon N, Momani T, McCleary N (2018) Self-care support for patients with gastrointestinal cancer: iCancerHealth. App Clin Informat 09(04):833–840. https://doi.org/10.1055/s-0038-1675810

Borglund ST (2008) Case management quality-of-life outcomes for adults with a disability. Rehabili Nurs 33(6):260–267. https://doi.org/10.1002/j.2048-7940.2008.tb00238.x

Brewer BB, Verran JA, Stichler JF (2008) The systems research organizing model: a conceptual perspective for facilities design. HERD 1(4):7–19. https://doi.org/10.1177/193758670800100402

Cohen CC, Shang J (2015) Evaluation of conceptual frameworks applicable to the study of isolation precautions effectiveness. J Adv Nurs 71(10):2279–2292. https://doi.org/10.1111/jan.12718

Donabedian A (1966) Evaluating the quality of medical care. Milbank Memorial Fund Quart 44(part 2):166–206

Donabedian A (1988) The quality of care: how can it be assessed? JAMA 260:1743–1748. https://doi.org/10.1001/jama.1988.03410120089033

Donabedian A (2003) An introduction to quality assessment in health care. Oxford University Press, New York, NY

Effken JA, Brewer BB, Patil A, Lamb GS, Verran JA, Carley K (2005) Using OrgAhead, a computational modeling program, to improve patient care unit safety and quality outcomes. Int J Med Inform 74(7–8):605–613. https://doi.org/10.1016/j.ijmedinf.2005.02.003

Gerolamo AM (2004) State of the science: outcomes of acute inpatient psychiatric care. Arch Psychiatr Nurs 18(6):203–214. https://doi.org/10.1016/j.apnu.2004.09.003

Gerolamo AM (2006) The conceptualization of physical restraint as a nursing-sensitive adverse outcome in acute care psychiatric treatment settings. Arch Psychiatr Nurs 20(4):175–185. https://doi.org/10.1016/j.apnu.2005.12.005

Gilmartin HM, Sousa KH (2016) Testing the quality health outcomes model applied to infection prevention in hospitals. Qual Manag Health Care 25(3):149–161. https://doi.org/10.1097/QMH.0000000000000102

Gilmartin HM, Sousa KH, Battaglia C (2016) Capturing the central line bundle infection prevention interventions. Nurs Res 65(5):397–407. https://doi.org/10.1097/NNR.0000000000000168

Hallowell SG, Rogowski JA, Spatz DL, Hanlon AL, Kenny M, Lake ET (2016) The associations between the work environment, nursing care and human milk use for very low birth weight infants discharged from NICUs. Nurs Res 65(2):E66–E67. https://doi.org/10.1016/j.ijnurstu.2015.09.016

Henry SB, Holzemer WL (1997) Achievement of appropriate self-care: does care delivery system make a difference? Med Care 35(11 suppl):NS33–NS40. https://doi.org/10.1097/00005650-199711001-00004

Hilleren-Listerud A (2014) Reducing postoperative delirium. Doctoral dissertation

Institute of Medicine (2000) To err is human: building a safer health system. The National Academies Press, Washington, DC

Jones TL (2016) What nurses do when time is scarce—and why. J Nurs Adm 46(9):449–454. https://doi.org/10.1097/NNA.0000000000000374

Jost SG (2016) Nurses as knowledge work agents: measuring the impact of a clinical decision support system on nurses' perceptions of their practice and the work environment. Doctoral dissertation

Kozlowski SWJ, Klein KJ (2000) A multilevel approach to theory and research in organizations: contextual, temporal, and emergent processes. Jossey-Bass, San Francisco

Kramer M, Schmalenberg C, Maguire P (2010) Nine structures and leadership practices essential for a magnetic (healthy) work environment. Nurs Adm Q 34(1):4–17. https://doi.org/10.1097/NAQ.0b013e3181c95ef4

Lake ET, Staiger D, Horbar J, Cheung R, Kenny MJ, Patrick T, Rogowski JA (2012) Association between hospital recognition for nursing excellence and outcomes of very low-birth-weight infants. JAMA 307(16):1709–1716. https://doi.org/10.1001/jama.2012.504

Lang NM, Mitchell PH, Hinshaw AS, Jennings BM, Lamb GS, Mark BA, Moritz P (2004) Measuring and improving healthcare quality. Med Care 42(2 Suppl):II-1–II-3

Lassche M, Wilson B (2016) Transcending competency testing in hospital-based simulation. AACN Adv Crit Care 27(1):96–102. https://doi.org/10.4037/aacnacc2016952

Lohr KN (1988) Outcomes measurement: concepts and questions. Inquiry 25(1):37–50

Makary MA, Daniel M (2016) Medical error—The third leading cause of death in the US. BMJ 353:i2139. https://doi.org/10.1136/bmj.i2139

Malley AM, Bourbonniere M, Naylor M (2018) A qualitative study of older adults' and family caregivers' perspectives regarding their preoperative care transitions. J Clin Nurs 27(15–16):2953–2962. https://doi.org/10.1111/jocn.14377

Mark BA, Harless DW (2009) Nurse staffing and post-surgical complications using the present on admission indicator. Res Nurs Health 33(1):35–47. https://doi.org/10.1002/nur.20361

McAlister BS, Tietze M, Northam S (2013) Early term birth. West J Nurs Res 35(8):1026–1042. https://doi.org/10.1177/0193945913484390

Michell PH, Heinrich J, Moritz P, Hinshaw AS (1997a) Outcome measures and care delivery systems: introduction and purposes of conference. Med Care 35(11 suppl):NS1–NS5

Michell PH, Heinrich J, Moritz P, Hinshaw AS (1997b) Measurement to practice: summary and recommendations. Med Care 35(11 suppl):NS124–NS127

Mitchell PH, Lang NM (2004) Framing the problem of measuring and improving healthcare quality: has the Quality Health Outcomes Model been useful? Med Care 42(2 suppl):II-4–II-11

Mitchell PH, Shortell SM (1997) Adverse outcomes and variations in organization of care delivery. Med Care 35(11 suppl):NS19–NS32

Mitchell PH, Ferketich S, Jennings BM (1998) Quality health outcomes model. Image J Nurs Scholar 30(1):43–46. https://doi.org/10.1111/j.1547-5069.1998.tb01234.x

Needleman J, Kurtzman ET, Kizer KW (2007) Performance measurement of nursing care. State of the science and the current consensus. Med Care Res Rev 64(2):10S–43S. https://doi. org/10.1177/1077558707299260

Press-Ganey (n.d.) Turn nursing quality insights into improved patient experiences. https://www. pressganey.com/docs/default-source/default-document-library/clinicalexcellence_ndnqi_ solution-summary.pdf?sfvrsn=0

Rowland C (2005) An exploration of variations in birth outcomes using PRAMS data guided by the quality health outcomes model. Doctoral dissertation

Serpa S, Ferreira CM (2019) Micro, meso, and macro levels of social analysis. Int J Soc Stud 7(3):120–124. https://doi.org/10.11114/ijsss.v7i3.4223

Shang J, You L, Ma C, Altares D, Sloane DM, Aiken LH (2014) Nurse employment contracts in Chinese hospitals: impact of inequitable benefit structures on nurse and patient satisfaction. Hum Resour Health 12(1):1–10. https://doi.org/10.1186/1478-4491-12-1

Sin MK, Belza B, LoGerfo J, Cunningham S (2005) Evaluation of a community-based exercise program for elderly Korean immigrants. Public Health Nurs 22(5):407–413. https://doi. org/10.1111/j.0737-1209.2005.220505.x

Swan BA, Boruch RF (2004) Quality of evidence. Med Care 42(Suppl):II-12–II-20. https://doi. org/10.1097/01.mlr.0000109123.10875.5c

Wilson BL, Effken J, Butler RJ (2010) The relationship between Cesarean section and labor induction. J Nurs Scholarsh 42(2):130–138. https://doi.org/10.1111/j.1547-5069.2010.01346.x

Yakusheva O, Needleman J, Bettencourt AP, Buerhaus P (2020) Is it time to peak under the hood of system-level approaches to safety and quality? Nurs Outlook 68:141–144. https://doi. org/10.1016/j.outlook.2019.11.004

Part II

Context

Healthcare Policy

Lauryn S. Walker and Deborah E. Trautman

Introduction

Health policy is the decisions, strategies, actions, and procedures through which an entity achieves specific healthcare goals. Policy may take many forms, including legislation; regulation; state-, federal-, or association-based standards of care; health insurance policies; payment mechanisms; and public health interventions (see Box 2.1 for definitions). Globally, healthcare systems differ by country based on the historical development of health policy legislation. Although some countries, such as Germany, have had state-based healthcare systems since the early 1800s, health policy became increasingly more popular as a mechanism to reduce healthcare costs and improve healthcare outcomes following World War II. Recognizing a need for a systematic approach to care, the United Kingdom enacted the National Health Service (NHS) in 1948, a federally sponsored program for medical training and care administration. The following year, in 1949, American President Harry Truman proposed the first significant healthcare legislation in the United States, the Fair Deal, beginning what would become a long history of systematic healthcare reform proposals.

L. S. Walker (✉)
Virginia Department of Medical Assistance Services, Richmond, VA, USA
e-mail: lauryn.walker@dmas.virginia.gov

D. E. Trautman
American Association of Colleges of Nursing, Washington, DC, USA
e-mail: dtrautman@aacnnursing.org

© Springer Nature Switzerland AG 2021
M. Baernholdt, D. K. Boyle (eds.), *Nurses Contributions to Quality Health Outcomes*, https://doi.org/10.1007/978-3-030-69063-2_2

Box 2.1 Definitions

Legislation: Healthcare requirements and guidance written in law.

Regulation: A rule or directive from a local, state, or federal authority. This includes federal interpretation of laws, such as requirements from the Centers for Medicare & Medicaid Services (CMS).

Standards of care: Professional guidelines determined by clinical experts and published to inform best practices and clinical standards.

Health insurance policies: Rules set by insurers determining who receives coverage, how it is received, what services are covered, cost of coverage for the individual, and amount of payment to providers.

Payment mechanisms: Payment may be used to incentivize use or reductions in the use of certain types of services. These policies may be set by federal or state entities, insurers, or employers aiming to achieve specific health outcomes.

Public health interventions: State-sponsored public health interventions are a form of policy aimed at targeting specific conditions or health concerns, such as immunization campaigns run through a health department.

Healthcare Policy Linkages to QHOM

In the QHOM (Mitchell et al. 1998), healthcare policy is in the environmental context that affects all components of the model (Fig. 2.1). As half of the global healthcare professional sector (World Health Organization 2020), nurses are vital stakeholders for health policy and play critical roles in policy development and implementation. At its core, policy is a tool or *intervention* that may influence healthcare quality and safety by either influencing and modifying *system* characteristics or even directly affecting clients. As policy may be developed and implemented at the national or local level, nurses will find health policy influences within each component of the QHOM.

Health policy is frequently considered a vehicle for large systemic change, such as creating the United Kingdom's National Health Service, which trains providers, determines medically necessary criteria, and sets payment standards for providers. In this scenario, the passage of health legislation creating the NHS was a significant intervention that influenced *system* characteristics by providing base funding to hospitals and consistent training for providers. It also influenced *clients* directly by ensuring that clients have access to care regardless of the ability to pay. However, health policy may also take the form of smaller, more specific *interventions*. For instance, some countries and states have established staffing ratio laws to restrict the number of patients a nurse may have at any given time. Such policies are state-based *interventions* that are intended to improve nurse and patient safety through changes in hospital workforce characteristics (Rothberg et al. 2005). Health policy is commonly used as an *intervention* to achieve better health outcomes. Common interventions that aim to improve outcomes through clients include policies that increase access to care, such as health insurance coverage. Other examples include direct

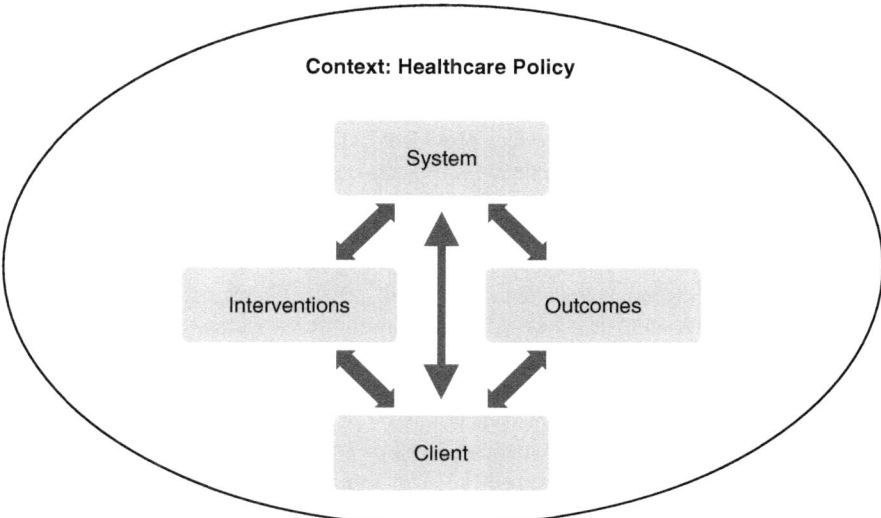

Fig. 2.1 Framework for healthcare policy context

care programs such as immunization campaigns or testing and treating communicable diseases through local health department clinics. Other policies may be used as interventions aimed at improving outcomes by generating *system* characteristic changes. Like the staffing ratios example, these policies may include workforce regulations or payment mechanisms to incentivize specific behaviors. These types of policies are described in more detail below.

Health policy is a key *intervention* that filters through every level of healthcare. It largely determines what services are reimbursed and how much, who has access to what services, and best practices for providing condition-specific care. For all these reasons, nurses aiming to improve healthcare quality or patient safety, even outside the spectrum of health policy, must consider how health policy influences their environment, creates or reduces barriers, or influences what clients they may reach. This chapter describes the types of policy interventions that nurses will need to consider when evaluating patient safety and quality initiatives and describes examples of how health policy has been used as an *intervention*.

Access to Care

Health insurance is one of the primary ways that health policy influences healthcare quality and safety. Health insurance can be defined as a contract with an organization (public or private) in which an individual agrees to pay a premium, or regular amount, in exchange for the insurer to pay for some or all healthcare expenses. Although some healthcare systems, such as the NHS in the United Kingdom, consider healthcare services to be public goods and therefore do not require health insurance, in many other countries, including the United States, health insurance is a key to accessing care. Individuals without health insurance may be unable to receive services or may be very limited in their selection of services due to care costs.

In the United States, health insurance generally is required to access healthcare services. Providers offer healthcare services in exchange for payment, typically based on the number and complexity of services provided. Individuals are expected to cover the cost of the care, whether through their own means or their insurer. Individuals without insurance coverage are more likely to forego needed care, with as many as 30% of the uninsured foregoing medical services due to costs and 20% forgoing needed prescriptions due to cost (Tolbert et al. 2020). In total, 8.5% of Americans, or 27.5 million individuals, report being uninsured (Berchick et al. 2019). Uninsured rates are highest among low-income adults aged 19–64, who may not have access to public insurance programs (Tolbert et al. 2020). The most common reason for not having health insurance is that the cost of purchasing insurance is too high (Tolbert et al. 2020).

In the United States, health insurance may be purchased or gained through three main avenues: (1) it may be provided at no or low cost by the government to eligible populations (public insurance program), (2) an employer may cover all or part of the cost, or (3) an individual may purchase their own coverage plan. Health policy may increase access to care by building new requirements for this public and private system. The Affordable Care Act (ACA; Patient Protection and Affordable Care Act 2010) affected all three mechanisms (see Box 2.2).

Box 2.2 Patient Protection and Affordable Care Act (2010)

In March of 2010, President Barack Obama signed the Patient Protection and Affordable Care Act, health reform, into law. The ACA included provisions aimed at reducing cost and improving care quality; however, much of the focus was on increasing access to health insurance. Since its passage, 20 million Americans have gained health insurance (Tolbert et al. 2020).

Major provisions include:

- Increasing eligibility to Medicaid (state-based public insurance) through expanded income limits.
- Creating a state-based Health Insurance Marketplace for individuals to purchase insurance with subsidies provided to low-income individuals.
- Requiring private insurers to offer coverage for dependent children until the child reaches 26 years old.
- Requiring health plans to offer essential health benefits, including preventive services, maternity and newborn care, behavioral health services, hospitalizations, prescriptions, and emergency services.
- Health insurers may not set a cap on the annual or lifetime dollar amount paid for essential benefits, nor may they refuse coverage or increase cost of coverage for an individual based on their medical history.
- Expansion of Medicaid eligibility.
- Medicare pay-for-performance programs including Hospital Readmissions Reduction Program, Hospital Value-Based Purchasing Program, and Hospital-Acquired Condition Reduction Program.

Public Insurance Programs

Medicare

In 1965, President Lyndon Johnson signed the Social Security Act into law, establishing the Medicare program (Cubanski et al. 2015). The program provides social insurance to the elderly and persons with disabilities. Medicare is funded through federal taxes and is federally administered, resulting in consistent rules and regulations across all 50 states. Medicare currently covers most Americans over the age of 65, people receiving social security disability insurance (SSDI), people with end-stage renal disease (ESRD), and people with amyotrophic lateral sclerosis (ALS). Medicare is administered by the Centers for Medicare and Medicaid Services (CMS), a federal agency responsible for setting reimbursement methodologies, rates, program requirements, and data collection. CMS is part of the US Government's executive branch and the Department of Health and Human Services.

In total, Medicare covers nearly 60 million Americans (Henry J Kaiser Family Foundation 2020). There are two potential avenues for receiving Medicare services. The first is through the fee-for-service program operated by the federal government with a set premium structure based on beneficiary income. The second avenue is through the Medicare Advantage program, in which a person may opt to receive benefits through a private insurance plan. Medicare coverage is divided into parts A–D (Cubanski et al. 2015).

Upon turning 65, most Americans will automatically receive Part A covering costs associated with inpatient hospitalizations. Part A coverage is funded primarily through income taxes, and there is no additional cost to the participant. Benefits in Part A coverage include costs associated with inpatient hospitalizations, skilled nursing facilities, and some home health and hospice services. In some circumstances, there could be cost sharing required for an inpatient stay; however, no monthly premiums are required.

Part B pays for services such as physician outpatient services and preventive care. Part B is funded in part through premiums paid by the beneficiary and set based on the individual's income and ability to pay. Beneficiaries who want additional coverage for doctor's office visits may opt to enroll in Part B. However, enrollment is not automatic as it is in Part A. Beneficiaries may also be required to pay copayments for provider visits.

Part C, also known as Medicare Advantage, is a substitute option for Parts A and B, and sometimes Part D (see below). As opposed to enrolling in Parts A and B for hospital and physician services, beneficiaries may opt to enroll in a private insurance plan, referred to as Medicare Advantage plans. These plans have the flexibility to offer additional services above those provided through Parts A and B but may also require higher premiums. In addition to offering inpatient, outpatient, and preventive care, many Part C plans will offer prescription medication coverage. The popularity of Part C plans has increased in recent years, with 34% of Medicare enrollees currently enrolled in a Medicare Advantage plan (Henry J Kaiser Family Foundation 2020).

Part D coverage was added as part of the Medicare Modernization Act of 2003 to include prescription drug coverage for Medicare enrollees. Coverage for prescription drugs is a voluntary component of Medicare, so members are not automatically enrolled. The benefit is administered through private plans that contract with the Medicare program. Members are required to pay a premium, which varies by plan, as do other cost-sharing arrangements.

Medicaid

Medicaid is the largest single insurer in the United States, covering more than 71 million Americans (Medicaid and CHIP Payment and Access Commission 2020). Medicaid is a safety net program, with coverage guaranteed to people in greatest need based on income and complex disability status. It is also the primary payer for long-term care services (Congresional Research Services 2018) and mental health services (Medicaid.Gov n.d.). Unlike Medicare, which is a federally administered program, Medicaid is a state-federal partnership. Although specific base criteria must be met, each state has the flexibility to determine who is eligible for the program and what services are covered. Additionally, Medicaid is funded through both state and federal dollars. The proportion of state and federal dollars varies by state and is based on the wealth of the respective state's population.

Before the ACA, most states only covered low-income children and pregnant women, with minimal coverage, if any, offered to childless adults. However, as part of the ACA, 37 states have expanded coverage to all adults up to 138% of the federal poverty level (FPL). Pregnant women and children may be covered with higher incomes at the state's discretion through the Children's Health Insurance Program. As a result, Medicaid enrollment has increased by 25% following the ACA's passage (Medicaid and CHIP Payment and Access Commission 2020). See Box 2.2 for other ACA policies.

Employer-Sponsored Coverage

The most common method of gaining insurance in the United States is through one's employer as part of a benefits package. In total, 153 million, or 49% of Americans, gain insurance through this method (Henry J Kaiser Family Foundation 2019). Employer-sponsored plans are typically provided through a private insurance company with premiums negotiated between the employer and the plan. Employers will generally cover a portion of the monthly premium payments for an employee. On average, employees contribute 18% of the plan's cost for a single individual (Henry J Kaiser Family Foundation 2019). Some employers may offer health insurance to retired employees in addition to current employees. Not all employers offer health insurance as a benefit. Healthcare is generally provided by large employers, with nearly all employers with at least 1000 enrollees offering coverage. However less than half of employers with fewer than nine employees offer coverage. However, firms may not provide healthcare coverage to all employees. For instance, part-time employees may not be eligible for benefits. Still, the employers of 90% of all workers offer health coverage to at least some workers (Henry J Kaiser Family Foundation 2019).

Marketplace

The Health Insurance Marketplace, also called the Exchange, was established as part of the ACA to provide uninsured Americans affordable coverage (see Box 2.1). The Marketplace is a website (HealthCare.Gov) that assembles various private plans, organized by level of coverage that individuals can purchase for themselves if they are not offered insurance through their employer or that coverage is unaffordable. Although the federal government runs a Marketplace, some states have set up their own Marketplace with state-specific plans. Whether state or federally run, all Marketplaces provide subsidies to individuals based on their income level to cover part or all of a plan's premium costs. The plans included in the Marketplace are private plans, similar to those that may be offered to employees as an employer-sponsored plan. In 2020, 11.4 million individuals were enrolled in health coverage through a Marketplace plan (CMS 2020a).

Before the passage of the ACA, covered services varied greatly by insurer, and therefore, access to services significantly varied depending on the plans an employer offered to its employees. To ensure access to a minimum set of services, the ACA included a requirement that health plans offered on the Marketplaces, with few exceptions, offer ten essential health benefits. These benefits include (What Marketplace Health Insurance Plans Cover n.d.):

- Outpatient services
- Emergency services
- Hospitalizations
- Pregnancy, newborn, birth control, and breastfeeding services and devices
- Mental health and substance-use disorder services
- Prescription drugs
- Rehabilitative and habilitative services and devices
- Laboratory services
- Preventive services
- Pediatric service, including dental and vision services for children (adult dental and vision are not required)

Healthcare Spending

Prospective Payment Systems and Managed Care

With the expansion of health insurance coverage, such as Medicare and Medicaid in the 1960s and 1970s, US healthcare expenditures on average grew by 6.5% per year, adjusted for inflation. By the 1980s, healthcare prices quickly escalated, and utilization of services also increased (Catlin and Cowan 2015). Healthcare services were paid on a fee-for-service basis, meaning that each service had a specific cost. For each service provided, the practitioner would be paid that given amount. The incentive inherent in this payment policy is that the more services provided, the more a practitioner is paid. This incentive resulted in providers offering unnecessary services and escalating care costs (Levit et al. 1996). Escalating cost placed pressure on states and employers who covered the cost of healthcare services and put many services out of reach financially for those who remained uninsured. In recognition of escalating healthcare costs, new policies were introduced to control spending. In 1982, the US Congress capped hospital payments for services provided to Medicare beneficiaries and began developing a payment methodology based on diagnoses instead of services. The change meant that a provider treating any Medicare patient admitted for a given diagnosis, such as uncomplicated diabetes, would be paid the same amount for the admission, regardless of the number of services provided. This payment methodology, called diagnosis-related groups (DRGs), was fully implemented in 1997 with the adoption of the Balanced Budget Act (National Council on Disability n.d.). The use of DRGs for payment is referred to as a prospective payment system (PPS) as opposed to fee-for-service, because it anticipates and sets a payment in advance of when an individual presents with a healthcare need, thus controlling costs by reducing the incentive to provide unnecessary services.

In addition to legislation targeting hospital payments, the Health Maintenance Organization Act of 1973 provided funds to incentivize health insurers to implement managed care plans, where small groups of providers paid a set fee, or capitated rate, for each patient they managed. By the 1990s, managed care plans had become increasingly popular, with more than half of insured Americans insured through a managed care plan (National Council on Disability n.d.). Although credited with slowing the growth in healthcare spending, these payment policies were not without consequences. The Balanced Budget Act and the implementation of PPS, as well as managed care programs, are associated with cuts to staffing, especially registered nurses (RNs) and licensed practical/vocational nurses (LPNs/LVNs) (Lindrooth et al. 2006). As staffing levels decreased, external entities, including Leapfrog and the American Nurses Association, voiced concerns that the policies may negatively affect health outcomes (American Nurses Association 1995; Huntington 1997).

Pay-for-Performance Policies

Future iterations of health policies aimed at controlling healthcare spending more directly targeted quality of care and patient safety and shifted incentives to align with quality and safety goals (What is Pay for Performance in Healthcare? 2018). These policies, frequently called pay-for-performance policies, directly tie payments to quality metrics through bonus payments for high performers or penalties for low performers.

Hospital-Acquired Conditions (HACs)

In 2008, as part of the inpatient PPS update, CMS implemented the first pay-for-performance (P4P) program. This program, called the Hospital-Acquired Condition (HAC) program, identifies events that "could reasonably have been prevented through the application of evidence-based guidelines," and withholds payment from poor-performing hospitals. As of 2020, CMS had identified 14 hospital-acquired adverse events, such as air embolisms and pressure injuries (CMS 2020b). As part of the ACA, three additional reimbursement incentive programs were implemented by CMS between 2012 and 2014 to promote a higher quality of care for Medicare beneficiaries: Hospital Readmissions Reduction Program (HRRP), Hospital Value-Based Purchasing Program (HVBP), and Hospital-Acquired Condition Reduction Program (HACRP).

Hospital Readmissions Reduction Program (HRRP)

The Hospital Readmissions Reduction Program (HRRP), implemented in 2012, financially penalizes hospitals with higher-than-expected 30-day readmission rates for myocardial infarctions, heart failure, pneumonia, chronic obstructive pulmonary disease (COPD), elective hip or knee replacement, and coronary artery bypass graft (CABG) surgery (CMS 2020c). The policy's intent, or intervention, is to reduce the number of patients who are discharged following a hospital stay for one of the six diagnoses and then readmitted to the hospital for the same diagnosis within 30 days of discharge. This policy was based on a study by the Medicare Payment Advisory Commission (MedPAC) that found that 12% of readmissions within 30 days were potentially preventable (McIlvennan et al. 2015). Hospital performance is based on historical performance, risk-adjusted case mix to account for acuity, case volume, and diagnosis. Penalties are capped at 3% of Medicare PPS payment (CMS 2020c). In the federal fiscal year 2017, CMS estimated that hospitals would pay $528 million in penalties related to readmissions (Boccuti and Casillas 2017). The policy has been shown to reduce the targeted readmissions effectively. In the first 2 years alone, there were 150,000 fewer hospital readmissions than the years prior (McIlvennan et al. 2015).

Medicare Hospital Value-Based Purchasing Program (HVBP)

The Hospital Value-Based Purchasing Program (HVBP) was also established as part of the ACA and implemented in 2012. Unlike HRRP, which is focused on a single outcome—readmissions—HVBP includes measures for multiple quality measures. Each year, CMS selects a series of quality metrics in these specific domains: patient safety, patient experience or person and community engagement, cost efficiency, and clinical outcomes. Both the domains and specific quality metrics vary by year. Recent quality measures included potentially preventable infections, such as central line-associated bloodstream infections, 30-day mortality rates for pneumonia, heart failure and acute myocardial infarctions, and patient responses on satisfaction surveys (CMS 2017). Performance on each measure is used to calculate an annual Total Performance Score (TPS) for a hospital. The TPS for each hospital determines the hospital's financial reimbursement level for the forthcoming federal fiscal year.

CMS holds hospitals accountable for their performance on these measures by withholding 2% of their total payments until the performance on metrics is determined. The total funds resulting from the 2% withheld are then dispersed among all hospitals based on performance. Hospital performance is measured as the amount a hospital improved compared to its own performance the year prior and compared to a national benchmark attainment level. Therefore, based on their performance and their peers, a hospital may earn more funds than were withheld, the same amount, or less than were withheld. Since the HVBP's implementation, healthcare-acquired infections have declined; however, the degree to which the HVBP is responsible for that decline is unclear. Generally, research has supported the view that outcomes have been improving due to general trends in higher quality care, but likely not as a direct result of the HVBP (AHRQ 2014; Figueroa et al. 2016; Walker 2019).

Hospital-Acquired Condition Reduction Program (HACRP)

The final Medicare hospital pay-for-performance program, the Hospital-Acquired Condition Reduction Program (HACRP), established as part of the ACA, was implemented in 2015. HACRP was implemented to incentivize quality care further and reduce hospital-acquired conditions (HACs), leading to patient morbidity and costly care. Hospital performance is evaluated using six quality measures from the Agency for Healthcare Research and Quality's (AHRQ) Patient Safety Indicators (PSI) and the Centers for Disease Control and Prevention's (CDC) National Healthcare Safety Network's healthcare-associated infection (HAI) measures (NEJM Catalyst 2018). The measures are categorized into two weighted domains. The weightings and measures are used to generate the total, risk-adjusted HAC reduction score for a hospital. Hospitals receiving scores in the bottom quartile of performers will have their payments reduced by 1%, generating a savings of approximately $350 million for the Medicare program (NEJM Catalyst 2018).

Other payers, including Medicaid and commercial insurers, are also developing pay-for-performance or value-based payment policies. By 2017, a survey of commercial insurers found that nearly half of all insurance reimbursement was in the form of a value-based care model, meaning that payment was based on quality metrics (NEJM Catalyst 2018). A growing body of literature suggests that pay-for-performance policies have contributed to lower costs and higher quality care (Mathes et al. 2019). However, not all P4P programs are equally effective, and P4P programs are not without consequences. Some providers have criticized programs for inadequate risk adjustment, leading to penalties for providers that care for more vulnerable or acute patients. Additionally, there is some evidence that healthcare provider job satisfaction may be impacted.

Besides the payment policies and programs, there are other initiatives to improve healthcare quality and cost. For example, AHRQ set a national goal to reduce HACs by 20%. The goal is connected to the CMS Hospital Improvement Innovation Networks, a collaborative group of federal and private partners dedicated to improving healthcare quality by reducing HACs (AHRQ 2018a). To improve tracking and reduce HACs and adverse events, AHRQ is developing and testing the Quality and Safety Review System (AHRQ 2018b). The surveillance system automatically pulls data from electronic health records to generate HAC event rates and measure organizational performance over time. However, payment policies based on incentivizing quality measures and improving accurate reporting on these measures can only be as good as the quality measure itself. While there has been a significant effort undertaken at the federal level to measure quality adequately, refining quality measures with new evidence will continue to be a necessary policy tool.

Quality Measurement

The concerns related to the unintended consequences of the shifts in payment policies, e.g., reductions in nurse staffing, led to the formation of a coalition of public and private leaders who began to develop healthcare quality and safety measures to be used in quality improvement programs. Early on, measure use was voluntary, and comparison data typically were not available. By 1999, hundreds of measures existed, and the National Quality Forum (NQF) was established to promote the adoption of standardized measures to facilitate comparisons across healthcare organizations (National Quality Forum 2020). NQF remains a key nonpartisan not-for-profit organization tasked with developing and endorsing evidence-based quality metrics to be used across all healthcare measurement programs, whether public or private.

In 2001, the AHRQ implemented three measurement programs: Inpatient Quality Indicators, Patient Safety Indicators, and Prevention Quality Indicators (AHRQ 2018c). AHRQ produced national comparison data for organizations to target and track quality improvement initiatives. These data provided a basis for researchers and policymakers to determine standards and goals for future healthcare initiatives, including those pay-for-performance programs established as part of the ACA. In 2005 CMS implemented public reporting of a set of inpatient measures from their payment programs (e.g., the HVBP) in the Hospital Compare program to promote further improvements in healthcare quality. Hospital Compare is a publicly available website (https://www.medicare.gov/hospitalcompare/search.html) that compares hospitals on their performance on specific quality measures, including patient experience surveys, timeliness of care, and mortality and complication rates. Prospective Medicare patients are encouraged to visit the site and select hospitals based on quality and safety outcomes. See Table 2.1 for major public and private initiatives and policies that influenced the development of measures and measurement programs.

Other Policy Interventions

Professional Guidelines and Standards of Care

In addition to legislation and regulations, healthcare policy may take the form of professional guidelines and standards of care. Published standards and guidelines have

Table 2.1 Chronology of major public and private healthcare quality initiatives and policies

Year	Responsible organization	Title	Quality incentive
1997	American Nurses Association	National database of nursing quality indicators	Performance reports using standardized unit-level nursing quality indicators to support quality improvement initiatives
1999	National Quality Forum	National consensus standards	Standardized quality measures to support cross-organizational comparisons
2000	Leapfrog Group	Performance measurement and public reporting Awards programs: Top Hospitals, Hospital Safety Grade, and the Value-Based Purchasing Program	Influences purchasing decisions of employers and insurers Publicly recognizes high-performing hospitals
2001	Agency for Healthcare Research and Quality	Prevention quality indicators, inpatient quality indicators, and patient safety indicators	Provides national standards and benchmarks for numerous quality measures
Established in 2002 Data first published in 2005	CMS in collaboration with the Hospital Quality Alliance	Hospital Compare	Public reporting of hospital quality and safety measures
2006	Centers for Disease Control and Prevention	Healthcare-associated infections reporting program	Surveillance reports to be used by hospitals in quality improvement initiatives
Legislated in 2005 Implemented in 2008	CMS	Hospital-acquired condition present on admission indicator program	Nonpayment for treatment of 14 hospital-acquired conditions (HACs)
2009	Office of the National Coordinator for Health Information Technology (ONC)	Health Information Technology for Economic and Clinical Health Act (HITECH)	Provides funding for adoption of electronic health records
Legislated in 2010 as part of ACA Implemented in 2012	CMS	Hospital Readmissions Reduction Program	Hospital Medicare payment based partially on rate of readmissions for specific conditions
Legislated in 2010 as part of ACA Implemented in 2012	CMS	Hospital Value-Based Purchasing Program	Withholds 2% of Medicare payments and distributes funds based on performance on a variety of metrics in clinical outcomes, patient and community engagement, cost efficiency, and patient safety

Table 2.1 (continued)

Year	Responsible organization	Title	Quality incentive
Legislated in 2010 as part of ACA Implemented in 2014	CMS	Hospital-Acquired Condition Reduction Program	Reduces hospitals with high rates of HACs by 1% of base Medicare payments
Legislated in 2015 Implemented in 2018	ONC	Merit-Based Incentive Payment System (MIPS)	Began as a Quality Reporting Program, then implemented with financial accountability. Provides bonus payments to providers with high scores on quality measures, electronic interoperability, and cost efficiency

been used by clinicians for decades to promote effective care as evidence for specific treatments and services. Standards of care and guidelines are interventions intended to inform both clinical practice and policymakers on how to provide optimal care for a condition or population, consequently changing systems of care. Guidelines may be published by governmental agencies such as the CDC (n.d.-a), nongovernmental agencies such as the WHO, or professional organizations such as the American College of Obstetricians and Gynecologists (ACOG) (ACOG 2020; CDC n.d.-b; WHO n.d.).

The US Preventive Services Task Force (USPSTF), for instance, is an independent panel of expert clinicians and researchers who regularly publish recommendations on standards of care regarding preventive services such as screenings, medications, and counseling services. The panel must submit recommendations to Congress annually based on the collection of current evidence. Examples of USPSTF recommendations include criteria for lung cancer screening, timing and criteria for Papanicolaou (Pap) smears, and when to use aspirin as a preventive medication for heart disease and colorectal cancer (U.S. Preventive Services Task Force n.d.). Recommendations are then used to inform clinical practice or may be tied to future reimbursement policies through quality metrics.

Health Information Technology

As discussed in Chap. 6, there have been three CMS initiatives to improve health information technology that support improvement in patient care quality and safety through electronic health records (EHRs). In 2009, the Health Information Technology for Economic and Clinical Health Act (HITECH) was enacted as part of the American Recovery and Reinvestment Act of 2009 (see Table 2.1). The legislation included more than $30 billion for providers, states, and the Department of Health and Human Services to support the implementation of EHRs, enabling the exchange of patient data (Medicare.Gov 2020). In 2015, the Medicare Access and CHIP Reauthorization Act (MACRA) established the Quality Payment Program, a pay-for-performance program for physicians and other professionals. One method of meeting the requirements set forth through the Quality Payment Program is participating in the Merit-Based Incentive Payment System (MIPS). Providers participating in MIPS may earn bonus payments through quality improvement activities, advancing interoperability of EHRs, or earning high marks on cost efficiency measures.

Workforce Development

Policies may also be used in a targeted manner to support workforce development. Such policies may include specific state licensure requirements or be broader in scope. For instance, in the United States, Title VIII Nursing Workforce Development Programs are one of the primary sources of federal financial support for nursing education, recruitment, and retention. Title VIII funds include support for student loan repayment programs, diversity grants, and the Nurse Corps, which has been deployed during the COVID-19 public health emergency to areas experiencing care provider shortages (Nursing Community Coalition 2019). Similar policies support other healthcare providers, including graduate medical education (GME) funds to support physician training residency positions. Unlike Title VIII, GME is supported through several policies that support both the direct costs of training a resident and indirect costs to the hospital (CMS n.d.). See Chap. 3 for more information on the nursing workforce.

Using Multilevel Policies to Manage the Opioid Crisis

A recent illustration of how policies can be used at many levels is the response to the opioid crisis. As clinicians, the public, and the economy grapple with addressing the opioid epidemic, various forms of policy have been implemented to deal with this crisis: legislation has been passed, standards of care have been created, coverage and payment mechanisms have been used, and direct policy interventions have been implemented. Beginning in the 2010s, the United States, especially the Appalachian areas of the country, began to see significant increases in the number of deaths associated with opioid overdoses. The epidemic of overdose deaths appeared to be stemming from abuse and dependence of opioid prescription medications, often obtained legally through overprescribing of opioids by providers. With mixed and sometimes misinformation about the addictive nature of opioids, many providers were prescribing opioids to control chronic and minor pain (National Institute on Drug Abuse 2020).

By 2013, the economic burden associated with prescription opioid abuse and dependence totaled over $78.5 billion, with nearly $30 billion in direct healthcare costs for treatment of addiction management and overdoses (Florence et al. 2016). As the number of people affected grew, health insurance coverage policy was one avenue used to slow down the poor outcomes associated with opioid-use disorder

(OUD) and opioid abuse, such as overdose and high utilization of emergency services. With states selecting to expand Medicaid coverage for low-income adults following the ACA passage, coverage enabled more residents to gain access to OUD services. Through expanded eligibility, Medicaid quickly became the largest payer of OUD treatment (Center on Budget and Policy Priorities 2018). In addition to adding populations eligible to receive services, Medicaid programs changed policy to further influence the system of care to improve OUD treatment quality. Although states are required to cover OUD services, states can establish their own policies around which treatment to cover and how much to pay for a given treatment. Many states used this opportunity to increase medication-assisted treatment rates, which is considered the standard of care for OUD. By focusing on policies aimed at increasing medication-assisted treatment, Medicaid agencies increased the number of people able to access OUD and increased adherence to professional guidelines (Center on Budget and Policy Priorities 2018).

However, the opioid crisis changing nature was evident in 2018, wherein synthetic opioids, such as fentanyl, had entered the market and increased the number of opioid-related overdoses to 67,000 from 29,000 in 2014 (CDC 2020; Rudd et al. 2016). Synthetic opioids tend to be more potent than traditional opioids. As death tolls increased, a number of policy responses developed. One such policy was the establishment of the Guidelines for Prescribing Opioids for Chronic Pain by the CDC. These clinical guidelines provided a policy framework for clinicians and insurers to improve their care quality for individuals with chronic pain. By describing an appropriate indication and dose for opioids, the CDC guidelines synthesized evidence to counter the misinformation that had resulted in the overprescription of opioids. With the establishment of these guidelines, other policy interventions became possible too, for example, the requirement of prior authorizations for new opioid prescriptions, especially those for higher dosages or uses outside of CDC's recommendation, before it may be filled or paid.

As the access to recommended treatment increased and opioid prescribing decreased, policies aimed at improving OUD care quality began to develop. These types of policies are still in their infancy and may follow various models. For instance, Vermont Medicaid had developed a "hub-and-spoke" model, which identifies the primary provider to initiate treatment (hub) in a region, and then connects the patient with other resources, e.g., other providers (spokes). Pennsylvania Medicaid has developed a "Centers of Excellence" program where patients can see one provider and receive comprehensive OUD treatment and medical care for other conditions. This program is similar to the Virginia Medicaid model, which uses credentialing policy to identify "preferred" OUD providers, referred to as Office-Based Opioid Treatment programs, who have met specific criteria to meet patients' comprehensive needs, including medical and behavioral (OUD) health needs.

In this scenario, policies were used as an intervention to influence the system characteristics, such as services covered, administrative burden, structure of the delivery system, and guidelines to establish standards of care. Policy was also used to impact clients through expanding eligibility for Medicaid to include more individuals.

Summary and Future Directions

In summary, health policy is a powerful tool to influence healthcare quality and safety. Health policy may be used to set the standard for high-quality care and provide more granular interventions to modify and structurally change systems. Major interventions include the use of health insurance to improve access to high-value care or reduce access to low-value care if services are not covered. Health policy may also be used to control spending and promote specific outcomes through payment mechanisms, such as reducing payment for iatrogenic conditions. Finally, through targeted funding, health policy may promote specific initiatives of interest, such as funding provided to increase the use of EHRs among hospitals and outpatient providers.

The future of health policy is reliant on evidence-based quality metrics that meaningfully improve patient outcomes. As quality measures continue to improve and increase in number, pay-for-performance policies will need to be developed and honed to incentivize high-quality care properly while maintaining staffing morale. The measures may require additional risk-adjustment criteria to ensure that providers continue to reach vulnerable patients. Additionally, to date, most pay-for-performance policies are single-payer programs. Although both public and private insurers use these policies, they often do not align, leading to providers that must react to numerous policies in a less focused manner.

To date, most quality measures are at the individual patient level. However, health policy tends to deal with populations, regulating thousands of providers and millions of individuals at a time. Health policy will need to move towards population-based measures in order to promote health equity. With nearly 9% of the US population still uninsured, continued focus on increasing access to healthcare services remains a critical component of the future of health policy (Berchick et al. 2019).

References

Agency for Healthcare Research and Quality (2014) Interim update on 2013 annual hospital-acquired condition rate and estimates of cost savings and deaths averted. https://www.ahrq.gov/sites/default/files/publications/files/interimhacrate2013_0.pdf

Agency for Healthcare Research and Quality (2018a) AHRQ national scorecard on hospital-acquired conditions: updated baseline rates and preliminary results 2014–2016. https://www.ahrq.gov/sites/default/files/wysiwyg/professionals/quality-patient-safety/pfp/natlhacratereport-rebaselining2014-2016_0.pdf

Agency for Healthcare Research and Quality (2018b) AHRQ quality and safety review system. https://www.ahrq.gov/professionals/quality-patient-safety/qsrs/index.html.

Agency for Healthcare Research and Quality (2018c) AHR quality indicators™. https://www.ahrq.gov/cpi/about/otherwebsites/qualityindicators.ahrq.gov/qualityindicators.html.

American College of Obstetricians and Gynecologists (2020) Home Page. https://www.acog.org/

American Nurses Association (1995) Nursing report card for acute care. American Nurses Publishing, Washington, DC

American Recovery and Reinvestment Act of 2009, Pub. L. No. 111-5, 123 Stat. 115 (2009)

Balanced Budget Act of 1997, Pub L. No. 105-33, 111 Stat 251 (1997)

Berchick E, Barnett J, Upton R (2019, November) Health Insurance Coverage in the United States: 2018. Current Population Reports. US Census Bureau. https://www.census.gov/content/dam/Census/library/publications/2019/demo/p60-267.pdf

Boccuti C, Casillas G (2017) Aiming for Fewer Hospital U-turns: The Medicare Hospital Readmission Reduction Program. Henry J Kaiser Family Foundation. https://www.kff.org/medicare/issue-brief/aiming-for-fewer-hospital-u-turns-the-medicare-hospital-readmission-reduction-program/

Catlin A, Cowan C (2015) History of health spending in the United States, 1960–2013. Centers for Medicare and Medicaid Services. https://www.cms.gov/Research-Statistics-Data-and-Systems/Statistics-Trends-and-Reports/NationalHealthExpendData/Downloads/HistoricalN-HEPaper.pdf

Center for Medicare and Medicaid Services (2017) Hospital value-based purchasing. https://www.cms.gov/Outreach-and-Education/Medicare-Learning-Network-MLN/MLNProducts/downloads/Hospital_VBPurchasing_Fact_Sheet_ICN907664.pdf

Center on Budget and Policy Priorities (2018) Medicaid works for people with substance use disorder. https://www.cbpp.org/research/health/medicaid-works-for-people-with-substance-use-disorders

Centers for Disease Control and Prevention (2020) Drug overdose deaths. https://www.cdc.gov/drugoverdose/data/statedeaths.html

Centers for Disease Control and Prevention (n.d.-a) Guidelines for prescribing opioids for chronic pain. https://www.cdc.gov/drugoverdose/pdf/prescribing/Guidelines_Factsheet-a.pdf

Centers for Disease Control and Prevention (n.d.-b) Home page. https://www.cdc.gov/

Centers for Medicare and Medicaid Services (2020a) Health insurance exchanges 2020 open enrollment report. https://www.cms.gov/files/document/4120-health-insurance-exchanges-2020-open-enrollment-report-final.pdf

Centers for Medicare and Medicaid Services (2020b) Hospital-acquired conditions. CMS.gov: https://www.cms.gov/Medicare/Medicare-Fee-for-Service-Payment/HospitalAcqCond/Hospital-Acquired_Conditions

Centers for Medicare and Medicaid Services (2020c) Hospital readmissions reduction program. CMS.gov: https://www.cms.gov/Medicare/Medicare-Fee-for-Service-Payment/AcuteInpatientPPS/Readmissions-Reduction-Program

Centers for Medicare and Medicaid Services (n.d.) Direct graduate Medicare education. CMS.Gov: https://www.cms.gov/Medicare/Medicare-Fee-for-Service-Payment/AcuteInpatientPPS/DGME

Congressional Research Services (2018) Who pays for long-term services and supports? https://fas.org/sgp/crs/misc/IF10343.pdf

Cubanski J, Swoope C, Boccuti C, Jacobson G, Casillas G, Griffin S, Neuman T (2015) A primer on Medicare: key facts about the Medicare program and the people it covers. Henry J Kaiser Family Foundation. http://files.kff.org/attachment/report-a-primer-on-medicare-key-facts-about-the-medicare-program-and-the-people-it-covers

Figueroa J, Tsugawa Y, Zheng J, Orav E, Jha A (2016) Association between the Value Based Purchasing pay for performance program and patient mortality in US hospitals: observational study. BMJ 353:i2214. https://doi.org/10.1136/bmj.i2214

Florence C, Luo F, Xu L, Zhou C (2016) The economic burden of prescription opioid overdose, abuse and dependence in the United States, 2013. Med Care 50(10):901–906

Health Maintenance Organization Act of 1973, Pub. L. No. 93-222, 87 Stat. 914 (1973)

Henry J Kaiser Family Foundation (2019) 2019 Employer health benefits survey. https://www.kff.org/report-section/ehbs-2019-summary-of-findings/

Henry J Kaiser Family Foundation (2020) Total number of Medicare beneficiaries: 2018. https://www.kff.org/medicare/state-indicator/total-medicare-beneficiaries/?currentTimeframe=0&sortModel=%7B%22colId%22:%22Location%22,%22sort%22:%22asc%22%7D

Huntington J (1997) Health care in chaos: will we ever see real managed care? Online J Issues Nurs 2(1):1. Manuscript 1. www.nursingworld.org/MainMenuCategories/ANAMarketplace/ANAPeriodicals/OJIN/TableofContents/Vol21997/No1Jan97/HealthCareinChaos.aspx

Levit K, Lazenby H, Braden B, Cowan C, McDonnell P, Sivarajan L et al (1996) DataView: National Health Expenditures, 1995. Health Care Finan Rev 18(1):175–214

Lindrooth R, Bazzoli G, Needleman J, Hasnain-Wynia R (2006) The effect of changes in hospital reimbursement on nurse staffing decisions at safety net and nonsafety net hospitals. Health Serv Res 41(3):701–720. https://doi.org/10.1111/j.1475-6773.2006.00514.x

Mathes T, Pieper D, Morche J, Polus S, Jaschinski T, Eikermann M (2019) Pay for performance for hospitals. Cochrane Datab Syst Rev 7(7):CD011156. https://doi.org/10.1002/14651858. CD011156.pub2

McIlvennan C, Eapen Z, Allen L (2015) Hospital Readmissions Reduction Program. *Circulation* 131(20):1796–1803. https://doi.org/10.1161/CIRCULATIONAHA.114.010270

Medicaid and CHIP Payment and Access Commission (2020) Medicaid enrollment changes following the ACA. https://www.macpac.gov/subtopic/medicaid-enrollment-changes-following-the-aca/

Medicaid.Gov (2020) Federal financial participation for HIT and HIE. Medicaid.gov: https://www.medicaid.gov/medicaid/data-systems/health-information-exchange/federal-financial-participation-for-hit-and-hie/index.html

Medicaid.Gov (n.d.) Behavioral Health Services. Medicaid.Gov. https://www.medicaid.gov/medicaid/benefits/behavioral-health-services/index.html

Medicare Access and CHIP Reauthorization Act of 2015, Pub. L. No. 114-10, 129 Stat. 87 (2015)

Medicare Prescription Drug, Improvement, and Modernization Act of 2003, Pub. L. No. 108-174, 117 Stat. 2066 (2003)

Mitchell PH, Ferketich S, Jennings BM (1998) Quality health outcomes model. Image J Nurs Sch 30(1):43–46

National Council on Disability (n.d.) A brief history of managed care. https://ncd.gov/policy/appendix-b-brief-history-managed-care

National Institute on Drug Abuse (2020) Opioid overdose crisis. https://www.drugabuse.gov/drug-topics/opioids/opioid-overdose-crisis#two

National Quality Forum (2020) Home page. http://www.qualityforum.org/Home.aspx

NEJM Catalyst. What is Pay for Performance in Healthcare? (2018) New England Journal of Medicine, Catalyst. https://catalyst.nejm.org/doi/full/10.1056/CAT.18.0245

Nursing Community Coalition (2019) Promoting America's Health through nursing care: priorities for the 116th congress. http://dnanurse.org/docs/advocacy/TitleVIII2019Brochure.pdf

Patient Protection and Affordable Care Act of 2010, Pub. L. No. 111–148, 124 Stat. 119 (2010)

Rothberg M, Abraham I, Lindenauer P, Rose D (2005) Improving nurse-to-patient staffing ratios as a cost-effective safety intervention. Med Care 43(8):785–791

Rudd R, Aleshire N, Zibbell J, Gladden M (2016) Increases in drug and opioid overdose deaths—United States, 2000–2014. Morb Mortal Wkly Rep 64(50):1378–1382. https://www.cdc.gov/mmwr/preview/mmwrhtml/mm6450a3.htm

Tolbert J, Orgera K, Damico A (2020) Key facts about the uninsured population. Henry J Kaiser Family Foundation. https://www.kff.org/uninsured/issue-brief/key-facts-about-the-uninsured-population/#:~:text=In%202019%2C%2028.9%20million%20nonelderly,Hispanic%20people%20and%20for%20children

US Preventive Services Task Force (n.d.) Recommendations. https://www.uspreventiveservicestaskforce.org/uspstf/topic_search_results?topic_status=P

Walker L (2019) Patient-centered medical homes and hospital value-based. VCU Scholars Compass. https://scholarscompass.vcu.edu/cgi/viewcontent.cgi?article=6892&context=etd

What is Pay for Performance in Healthcare? (2018) New England Journal of Medicine, Catalyst. https://catalyst.nejm.org/doi/full/10.1056/CAT.18.0245

What Marketplace Health Insurance Plans Cover (n.d.) HealthCare.Gov: https://www.healthcare.gov/coverage/what-marketplace-plans-cover/

World Health Organization (2020) Nursing and midwifery. Health workforce: https://www.who.int/hrh/nursing_midwifery/en/

World Health Organization (n.d.) Home page. https://www.who.int/

The Nurse Workforce

Sean P. Clarke

Introduction

The term "nurse workforce" refers to the workers available at a local, regional, or even national level to deliver nursing care to a group of patients, clients, or citizens. The workforce has clear consequences for the quantity and nature of nursing services available and the conditions encountered by caregivers and patients in various settings. In workforce research and policy, many assumptions are made about the mix of nursing personnel who provide nursing services. The assumptions merit clarification. A set of supply and demand factors drive whether shortages, surpluses, or balances are observed in the nurse workforce at various healthcare system levels. These factors operate somewhat differently across countries, regions, organizations, and specialties. Local and higher level policy approaches address challenges in recruiting and retaining nurses, such as nurse workforce diversity, educational composition, and broad age differences. Policy regulating nurse staffing levels has potentially significant influences on the demand for nursing services. To date, experience with such policies, notably mandatory staffing ratios, has been limited. Moving forward, economic and technological changes will influence the nature of nursing services within care delivery systems and thus the demand for nurses. These changes may provide opportunities to preserve and even surpass the safety and quality outcomes that nurses and their interventions facilitate for the profession's clients but may require changes in the nurse workforce to drive a brighter future for the profession and its clients.

S. P. Clarke (✉)
Rory Meyers College of Nursing, New York University, New York, NY, USA
e-mail: sc7372@nyu.edu

© Springer Nature Switzerland AG 2021
M. Baernholdt, D. K. Boyle (eds.), *Nurses Contributions to Quality Health Outcomes*, https://doi.org/10.1007/978-3-030-69063-2_3

The Nurse Workforce: Context for the Quality Health Outcomes Model

The nurse workforce is an element of context (macro-level) influencing the inter-play of constructs within the QHOM (Mitchell et al. 1998) (Fig. 3.1), notably by influencing the characteristics of nurses delivering various interventions and the environment in which these interventions are delivered. In the model, system ele-ments (macro and meso) shape the characteristics of the individual workers (micro-level; nurses or nursing workers) providing interventions to specific clients and the conditions under which they deliver them to clients. In turn, clients then experience outcomes. The nurse workforce and its relationship to other contextual factors and QHOM constructs could easily be applied to health professionals and workers out-side nursing whose services could be complementary (even essential) in providing care to a specific population.

Workforce issues play two critical roles in the quality of nursing care. First, the presence of enough providers of service who have appropriate preparation and ade-quate experience to carry out necessary work and function as part of smoothly func-tioning teams can be considered a precondition for providing safe care. Second, initiatives intended to shape either the workforce or the quality of care are closely related to each other and have reciprocal influences. For instance, policy initiatives to regulate staffing levels can influence the demand for nurses and nursing workers. Further, attention or inattention to quality of work-life and diversity issues in the workforce influences recruitment and retention, staffing levels, and ultimately the quality of care.

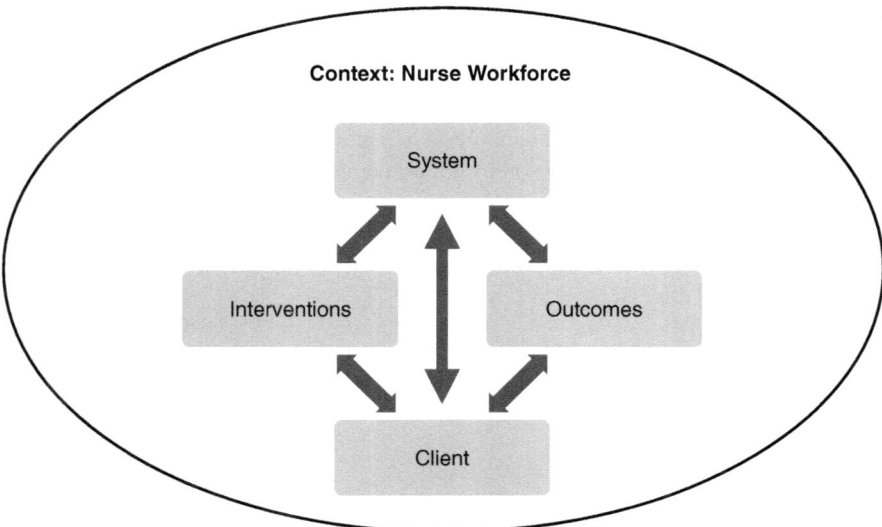

Fig. 3.1 Framework for the nurse workforce context

Arguably, a workforce composed of appropriately qualified nurses or nursing workers provides the foundation for delivering high-quality nursing care. Words such as "appropriately qualified" are used purposefully, as are broad terms like "high quality" and even "nursing care," but leave much room for interpretation. It is challenging, if not impossible, to find consensus on what constitutes enough personnel with the correct training (and further, a sufficiently stable and experienced workforce) in a specific healthcare setting. It is also challenging to establish, empirically, or by consensus, what the needs might be for nurses across a whole society or even the ideal prerequisite training for nursing work. Furthermore, "sufficiently large" and "appropriately qualified" are subjective terms that imply a common understanding of the work to be done and how it should be organized. There are many tacit assumptions about where and how care is to be delivered and the types and numbers of workers required to perform it.

The extensive practical concerns of deploying nurses and nursing personnel to deliver healthcare have generally relied on tradition, rather than a careful review or even empirical research findings, to drive most local and societal level decisions about the nurse workforce. Nonetheless, common sense would suggest that high-quality nursing care cannot easily be delivered with thin staff coverage or with coverage by staff with minimal preparation to deal with the more complex and rapidly changing patient needs in a specific setting.

Most discussion and research on workforce-related topics emphasize professional (registered) nurses (RNs). However, nursing care is provided by a mix of professional nurses, practical (or vocational) nurses, and unregulated workers. The nature of the nurse workforce varies across settings, regions, and countries. Many jurisdictions consider RNs, regardless of the type of education they have received, to be "professional" (as opposed to "practical") nurses. However, many have drawn a distinction between "technical" nurses (RNs holding associate degrees from junior/community colleges where the original intent of the type of education was an emphasis on technique and procedure) and "professional" nurses (those holding bachelor's degrees and having a broader education more thoroughly grounded in the liberal arts and sciences) (Montag 1963). Use of the term "technical" in contrast to "professional" and reference to the notion of different job descriptions and role expectations for RNs holding different levels of degrees or "differentiated practice" (Koerner 1992) have faded considerably in the past 20 years. However, for over a century, a vocal minority within the profession has pressed the case for the bachelor's degree as the entry point and has won it in some countries and jurisdictions. In places where the entry point issue has not been resolved, advocates have continued to argue for restricting RN licensure to those holding bachelor's and higher degrees (see the discussion of education and entry to practice towards the end of the chapter).

Historically, nurses have undertaken extensive ranges of activities that encompass clients' psychological and physiological needs across the life span and across settings. An assumption is that nurses (particularly professional nurses) do the visible and invisible work that put their time and skills to best use. It is rare to consider whether some proportion of nurses' work may be dedicated to tasks and actions that have minimal impacts on patient well-being or do not require a nurse's (or an RN's, or perhaps a bachelor's educated RN's) education. What complicates such discussions is that within the scope of nursing work, many functions that might require hands-on training but arguably little formal education, at least on the surface, would seem able to be assigned to workers other than RNs in at least some circumstances. At times, the scope of nursing practice has been a very emotional subject, loaded with overtones touching on both economics and professional identity. In different settings, and indeed in some jurisdictions and countries, practical nurses, unregulated personnel, and even family caregivers can and do take on some nursing "tasks." Yet, it has been argued that some nursing work (i.e., having high stakes in terms of safety or skill, or the expectation that work will be executed with judgment and ongoing assessment of the client's health status) constitutes the practice of registered nursing and requires the education and credentialing of an RN. To the extent that RNs are the predominant type of nursing staff in North American acute care hospitals, one could argue that this has been more or less settled in many regions and settings. However, the determination that an RN is always the "correct" type of worker to fill a given patient care role has been questioned, especially by some outside the profession.

Most nurse workforce discussions imply that there are firm boundaries around the activities that nurses can perform, should be involved in, and actually perform. The exact nature of nurses' work, and indeed all health professionals and professional and skilled workers in general, has been a topic of intense discussion and debate. In reality, of course, in some contexts, other types of professional and nonprofessional workers carry out work done by nurses, and nurses (often with additional training) either potentially could or do act as replacements for other types of healthcare workers. Economists refer to this as "substitution" and it has potentially important impacts on demand for nurses. As will be discussed at the end of the chapter, reconsidering these boundaries and opportunities for substitution may become more prominent, moving forward in a changing healthcare system. A full exploration of debates regarding nursing care's nature and scope is beyond this chapter's scope. From this point forward in the chapter, although many of the ideas have relevance for discussions about other types of nursing workers, the emphasis will be on RNs (rather than on practical nurses, unlicensed care providers/patient care technicians, or advanced practice nurses).

Interplay of Nursing Supply and Demand at Various Levels of the Healthcare System

Discussions and analyses of the nurse workforce typically begin with concepts from labor economics applied to one or more healthcare system levels or an organization delivering nursing services—the notions of supply and demand. In addition to considering whether the nursing supply is adequate to meet demand, another important distinction is the difference between reviewing the state of a nurse workforce in the present or at a point in the past and projecting what might happen in the future. Although estimating future supply and demand is of apparent interest to managers, human resources specialists, government officials, and those considering careers in nursing and has been the focus of energy for researchers and leaders, it is a considerably challenging exercise. Currently, there are about four million RNs in the United States (AACN 2019), not necessarily all of whom are working in nursing jobs, over 400,000 licensed nurses in Canada (CIHI 2020), and almost 650,000 in the United Kingdom (RCN 2020). A recent World Health Organization report places the worldwide number of nurses at 28 million, 19 million of whom are "professional" nurses (WHO 2020). The scale of these workforces and the range of geographic regions within these countries and work settings where nurses work render estimates and projections of supply and demand all the more challenging.

Supply

The supply of workers is the number of people who are able and willing to be employed in a field at a point in time. Ultimately, the supply of nurses is influenced by a relatively small number of factors. One of the significant determinants is the output of educational programs preparing students for entry to the profession. At many points in the history of nursing, including the present time (November 2020), the supply of available nursing education slots has been smaller than the number of applicants (a result of either high demand with or without low numbers of educators, clinical placements, or space in colleges and universities). However, over some periods and in some regions, the number of qualified applicants has been less than the number of slots in nursing education programs and the demand for new graduates. The second major determinant of supply has been personal choices leading to exit from the profession or its specialties (or decisions not to enroll in nursing education). The third determinant has been migration in or out of a country or region.

Nursing Education Programs

Preparation for professional nursing in industrialized countries generally requires at least 2 years of higher education after secondary school graduation (12th grade in most societies). The baccalaureate degree typically represents a minimum of 4 academic years of schooling after secondary school graduation. Accelerated (shortened) nursing programs were developed for students with previous postsecondary education. In either a traditional or an accelerated path, students and their families and schools of nursing commit to multiple years of prelicensure education. In addition to qualified faculty in specific content areas and physical space in classrooms (or electronic infrastructure to substitute for physical space), the finite number of students an area's healthcare organizations or other settings can accommodate at any one time also places constraints on admissions to and graduations from nursing school. Further, retention is imperfect in nursing education; students may fail to complete prerequisites or basic courses in a program before beginning their clinical educations. Also, failures and student decisions not to continue in their programs occur routinely in nursing programs. A relatively small number of graduates do not pass the licensure examinations at the end of their programs.

It is notable that for more than a decade as of the time of this writing (November 2020), interest in education for registered nursing practice and numbers of graduations have been at their highest levels in the history of the profession in the United States. The COVID-19 pandemic has placed nurses and other frontline health workers and the importance of their work in the spotlight and has highlighted the demands and risks nurses face. Further, the long-term economic impact of the COVID-19 crisis on healthcare delivery and the job market for nurses is unclear. All of these factors could have a strong influence on nursing's desirability as a career over the coming years.

Personal Choices Influencing Entry and Exit from the Profession and Specialties

A host of personal and economic factors affect nurses' decisions to work in nursing and particular specialties in hospitals and healthcare at large. Put simply, even if they do not always express it in such terms, nurses, like all types of workers, will make choices about how they spend their time and will attempt to find the most rewarding use of their time. Choices include the most congenial or best remunerated work in nursing, another field, or not working at all.

Economic conditions in society at large can have a significant impact on nurses' willingness to work or to accept specific types of jobs. In leaner financial times, especially when families might need income, more nurses tend to be willing to work and to work longer hours. Some seek out the best paying work or consider less well-paying or less prestigious nursing work when no other positions are available. In contrast, in more prosperous economic times, considerations about the desirability of different workplaces and specialties or even the attractiveness of work and workplaces outside nursing can change, as can perceptions about whether it is necessary to work at all.

Increasing gender and age diversity have been characteristics of nursing for some years. However, in the past, the substantial number of women of childbearing age in the nurse workforce and the accompanying challenges in securing good childcare led to patterns of departures and trends towards part-time employment linked to maternity leaves and childrearing. With the aging population in the United States and other countries and accompanying aging of the nurse workforce, age-related decisions around retirement timing, sometimes connected with family caregiving responsibilities for spouses, partners, and older relatives, appear to more commonly influence decisions about when to stop work.

Gender balance in the field may serve as either an incentive or a disincentive for entering or staying in the field. Several wage-related structural inequalities may play a role for working women. Blau and Kahn (2017) offer a partial explanation that nurses' compensation has often been below that of people doing work of comparable complexity in fields where there is a more even gender balance. Wage compression in nursing is well documented (entry salaries may be attractive but increases throughout a career may tend to be small) (Greipp 2003), which might serve as a disincentive for entering or staying in nursing over the long run.

Other difficult-to-quantify forces influence nurses' personal choices about entry and exit from nursing. The nursing profession's public image as noble but selfless, unintellectual, "dirty work" may influence nurses' compensation and ultimately pose a challenge in recruiting and retaining nurses (Girvin et al. 2016). The physical and emotional demands of nurses' work and a perception that employers and the public expect nurses to overextend themselves may affect nurses' decisions to leave particular jobs or to abandon the profession altogether. Nursing work safety can play a role in individuals' decisions regarding continuing in the field or retiring. Examples of work safety issues include the stresses and risks highlighted by emerging infectious diseases such as COVID-19 or particularly difficult times in healthcare when there are cuts in positions.

Geographical Mobility Regionally, Nationally, Internationally

In general, except for those entering the profession with the specific intent of emigrating to other regions or countries, nurse labor markets tend to be local in the sense that prospective members of the profession are likely to attend nursing school in the same communities where they hope to live and work. Barring somewhat unusual circumstances, they tend not to leave. However, where salary differentials between urban and rural areas are large, nurses may choose to keep their homes in rural areas while commuting to work in regions where they can earn more (see, for instance, Skillman et al. 2006). Over the years, in the United States, nurses' movement to areas of opportunity and away from regions seen as having fewer or lower paying positions has been responsible for the workforce's shape and distribution. In the coming decades, population will shift away from current nurse-dense regions of the United States and towards areas where nursing education programs are less plentiful, and lower salaries (the Southeast and Southwest) are projected. These shifts could potentially lead to significant nurse shortages (Auerbach et al. 2017).

Nurse migration from lower to higher income countries has been a long-standing phenomenon that has played a significant role in smoothing out imperfect balances between local needs for nursing and domestic nursing education outputs in the United States. Impacts on migrating nurses' home countries and their healthcare systems are mixed. Concerns about "brain drain" from societies that invest heavily in nurses' education are offset somewhat by economic benefits to these nurses, their families, and their larger societies (Kingma 2006).

Demand

Demand for nurse labor has a technical sense and meaning quite different from generally understood or intuitive "need" for nursing services. In workforce analysis, demand is the number of work hours an employer is willing to hire based primarily on wage levels and the expected revenues the employer expects to generate; it is often thought of in terms of *unmet* demand rather than perceptions of the adequacy of the number of nurses in practice in the eyes of nurses, patients, other healthcare system stakeholders, or society at large (US DHHS 2017). Open positions are, of course, very different from the level of confidence of clients and those working in healthcare organizations where a sufficient number of nurses are working, and from unaddressed needs for nursing services in the population (as defined by numbers of people experiencing specific health problems or needs for healthcare services). The size and qualifications of a workforce that would be in a position to deliver tested and validated nursing interventions to the public at levels and in a manner that would foster optimal patient outcomes have never been determined. Open unfilled positions for nurses in healthcare organizations are thus used as a proxy for societal needs.

The creation and maintenance of nursing positions result from management decisions that consider local and higher level health system forces. The population characteristics of a particular region in terms of age, gender, and similar factors influence health needs and the resources and insurance coverage of the population for paying for care. The proportion of patients in a region served by a particular healthcare organization (market share) and the models of care being used also drive decisions about the numbers and types of nurses or nursing workers to be hired. "Models of care" is a broad term that refers to the formal and informal principles regarding which types of nurses and related workers provide care and how they work together to provide services in particular settings (Dubois et al. 2013). For instance, some institutions and settings predominantly or exclusively employ RNs (and prefer bachelor's educated RNs). Additionally, regulatory forces (such as legislated mandatory minimum staffing ratios), agency and unit leaders' visions of care, historical patterns of staffing and models of care, and financial considerations (budget limits) will influence demand.

Supply, Demand, Shortage, and Surplus at Various Levels of the Healthcare System

In simplest terms, a labor shortage occurs when the supply of workers is insufficient to meet demand. A surplus (which translates to underemployment or unemployment of some proportion of a group of workers) is the reverse—it occurs when supply exceeds demand (Greenlaw and Shapiro 2018). Both supply and demand can vary enormously and show dramatic differences even across units or specialties in the same healthcare organization. One unit can experience a very different situation relative to a shortage or surplus than another unit. Pronouncements about supply and demand (shortages, surpluses, or balances of supply and demand) should be normally accompanied by careful qualifiers about where and in what specialties the statements are being made.

Workforce conditions in agencies and organizations tend to be heavily influenced by geographical location. Geography will influence whether multiple employers compete for nurses and new graduates and whether a concentration of multiple employers in a region serves as a draw to attract nurses to that area (Skillman et al. 2006). Where there are variations in compensation and other management practices, differences may be seen in nurse supply across agencies within a single community. However, a limited supply of new nursing graduates coming into a local employment market in a region and the attractiveness of an area for nurses and their families can lead to community-wide shortages. The desirability of working in a particular specialty and the history and reputation of the particular unit or clinic within a facility can play important roles in whether there are an adequate number of qualified individuals available to fill open positions. States, provinces, and territories (and of course entire countries) are often affected by common economic conditions that can influence the supply of new nurse graduates and the ease of recruiting and retaining nurses. Compared to the local cost of living, nurse compensation can have important influences on nurses' recruitment and retention. Navigating immigration and employment arrangements as well as laws and regulations surrounding licensure, even though nurses can seek licensure in new jurisdictions when they migrate, can be complicated and time consuming (Shaffer et al. 2020). As for all professions, it is common to think of national and state/provincial/territory boundaries as imposing important constraints on nurse workforce supply.

Global or worldwide nurse shortages—defined as poor working conditions and the inability of nursing education programs in all countries to keep up with demand—lead to shortfalls of nurses in relation to population health needs (WHO 2020). However, because there are many differences across countries in the titling and preparation of nurses, how nurses are used in delivering services, and the multiple barriers to nurses' extensive international mobility, a truly international market for nurses and their labor does not exist. Instead, similarities in the general forces affecting nurse workforces across countries make sharing experiences across world regions informative and point to advocacy opportunities at a global level.

Supply, Demand, Shortage, and Surplus in Specific Settings

Acute Care Hospitals and Hospital Specialties

In inpatient acute care hospital settings, nursing care requires a large nurse workforce tailored to the delivery of intense and complex interventions and close monitoring for potentially life-threatening complications of illnesses and treatments. Nonetheless, only approximately 60% of American RNs are currently employed in hospitals (US DHHS 2019)—the downward trend in hospitals as an employment setting has been observed for several decades (US DHHS 2010, 2019). Hospitals and specific settings within them employ large numbers of nurses around the clock. The need for night shift and weekend coverage creates unique pressures on nurses and managers. It can drive nurses at specific points in their lives to consider settings or roles that do not require varying work hours and schedules or working at times that are at odds with their friends and family's off-hours. Hospital practice is characterized by bureaucratic control, including extensive procedures, systems, rules, and hierarchical relationships between nurses and nursing workers with other health disciplines and professions and across different patient care specialties. Concerns have been raised that hospitals may not be employers of choice relative to nonhospital settings for better educated healthcare workers who value autonomy (AHA Strategic Planning Committee 2001).

The general principle of local conditions being fundamental in nurse workforce analyses holds true even within a single type of hospital (for instance, pediatric hospitals generally have much less difficulty recruiting and retaining staff than general hospitals). There can be significant variations in supply and demand factors across specialties and units, even within the same institution. Certain specialties may be particularly attractive by virtue of pride in serving a specific population (for instance, children, newborn babies, patients undergoing cardiac surgery, or veterans). Many specialties come to feel like "tribes" of like-minded or similarly motivated nurses and other healthcare workers. However, it can be difficult to separate "personalities" and rhythms of work in different specialties from the benefits of working under strong and supportive managers and feeling colleagueship with a team of nurses and other workers and professionals. Even though nurses working in a new setting (even in the same specialty) generally require onboarding training and orientation, nurses often change specialties over their professional lives without further formal education, which is not common in the other health professions and occupations. This phenomenon might be a cause for optimism as needs for hospital care and demands for nursing services within hospitals shift in the coming years.

Considerable speculation, assumptions, and debate surround particular nursing specialties' desirability from a recruiting and retention perspective. Intuitively, in critical care units and emergency departments, where nurse-to-patient ratios are low to permit close monitoring and rapid response to patients at the highest risk of death, the work is most likely to exhaust and overwhelm nurses physically and emotionally of any of the hospital specialties. However, empirical research suggests that critical care units and emergency departments are not necessarily high-stress, high-turnover settings for nurses to the extent that might be assumed (Hooper et al. 2010; Mallidou et al. 2011). The most stressed, burned-out, and dissatisfied hospital nurses tend to be those working in less technologically intensive areas and are seen as less prestigious or desirable, such as gerontology or general medical and surgical units. Patient volumes on these units may be quite high, and the workload involved in caring for each patient may be quite heavy as well. These units sometimes serve as the usual first entry point of nurses (particularly new graduates) into a particular hospital workforce. Furthermore, nurses on medical-surgical or general units may work with many different medical trainees and physicians and surgeons creating stressors, instead of a small and stable team of physicians who form high-quality working relationships with the nursing staff. Various initiatives over the years, for instance the Robert Wood Johnson Foundation's Transforming Care at the Bedside (TCAB) project, recognized the specific challenges of these nurses and specifically targeted work conditions for nurses on medical-surgical units (Needleman et al. 2016).

Hospital nurse workforces, especially in major metropolitan areas, are characterized by a sizable segment of workers interested in career mobility. The goal of these nurses is often to work for a specific amount of time on a particular type of unit on a path towards more advanced training or other specialties (or work roles other than frontline hospital staff), or to experience city life or work in a large hospital immediately after graduation. There is a tradition of this career path in American nursing and other English-speaking or European countries. For instance, several years of critical care experience are typically required for admission to nurse anesthesia graduate programs, leading to work in American nurses' best paid specialty. Therefore, a certain degree of turnover appears to be built into positions in particular specialties, which has various implications in terms of supply, demand, and composition of the nurse workforce in these areas. Like the United States, a certain level of turnover related to career mobility influences workforce supply and demand in other countries.

Subacute and Rehabilitation Settings

Care in subacute and rehabilitation settings is characterized by decreased patient intensity and risk of deterioration relative to hospitals. However, there is a need for nurse-delivered treatments and nursing services that are too risky or burdensome for patients to receive in their own homes. Patient needs can be extremely variable in these settings and include the need for specialized physical and psychological healthcare needs (for instance, rehabilitation following spinal cord or brain injuries). There is also the possibility of rapid intervention in the event of life-threatening complications (Dombrowski et al. 2012; Neatherlin and Prater 2003). Generally, these settings are characterized by heavier RN patient loads than acute care hospitals and greater involvement of nursing personnel other than RNs in care delivery. The increased regionalization of the highest intensity acute care settings and financial considerations have led to expansion of rehabilitation and subacute facilities and nurses' roles within them.

Long-Term Care

A majority of individuals (elderly or not) living with serious chronic physical and mental health conditions reside in their own homes and receive services in institutions and clinics or less commonly receive home visits from providers. However, a certain proportion is admitted to residential settings. The broad term for such facilities is "long-term care," including many subtypes of institutions within this category of agencies. Certain features are common to these facilities: they are staffed predominantly by unlicensed/unregulated workers, with licensed practical and registered nurses overseeing the care provided by unlicensed workers or aides (Reinhard and Young 2009). The licensed nurses also deliver treatments unlicensed workers are not permitted to perform. Financial pressures on these facilities are often high, and salaries tend to be lower than in acute care and other settings. Baccalaureate-educated RNs tend to be less common in long-term care (US DHHS 2010; Jones et al. 2019). The technological intensity of care can vary widely, as can the patient populations' age ranges and the types of underlying health conditions that have led to their admission. Stressors for the nurses and nursing workers in these settings include heavy demands in physical care giving. Many residents have limited mobility and a limited likelihood of regaining independence (and in fact high likelihood of deterioration). Stressors in practice include low satisfaction of residents and their families with residents' conditions and/or the care being received.

Community-Based Care

Many healthcare services are provided on an episodic rather than a continuous basis to individuals who live in their own homes (or otherwise phrased, who are "community dwelling"). Depending on definitions and classifications being used, outpatient clinics where nurses may or may not work in cooperation with other types of health professions (and that may or may not physically or organizationally be part of a hospital) may be considered as community settings along with settings such as home health and public health services. Community settings are often characterized by independence—in many cases, nurses have minimal contact with other nurses as peers or managers, and nurses see patients alone for the most part. There can also be high demands for productivity and sometimes less favorable pay and quite variable working conditions and safety risks (De Groot et al. 2018; Friedberg et al. 2017; Markkanen et al. 2017).

In anticipation of some of the shifts in the US healthcare system described in the last sections of this chapter, experts have advocated for many years that students should spend more clinical education time in community environments (Wojnar and Whelan 2017). To this end, the Health Resources and Services Administration has funded demonstration projects to universities for developing educational models that provide baccalaureate students with more clinical experience in community settings (Vanhook et al. 2018). With these evolving community roles, it is hoped that better population health outcomes and more meaningful and satisfying work for nurses will emerge.

Other Settings

For many generations, nurses have practiced outside settings that are traditionally thought of as healthcare settings. These include clinical research, various roles in health insurance, sales and marketing of healthcare-related products, and community settings that do not operate specifically or primarily as healthcare delivery sites. In the past, all of these settings have been seen as competitors for hospitals in recruiting nurses. As the healthcare system continues to evolve, the nontraditional settings may increasingly become more common employers of nurses. Further, in the future, some of these practice areas may become venues for delivering patient interventions.

Managing Supply and Demand of the Nurse Workforce

Recruitment Efforts

Bringing nurses into jobs in a region or a specific setting generally involves offering sufficiently attractive working conditions and compensation (salary and benefits packages) to qualified applicants. Considerable debate regarding nurses' motivations has surrounded the importance of salaries over a positive work environment. Historically, nursing has followed a pattern where there are times of supply-demand equilibrium with relatively flat or stable salaries. These stable periods are followed by periods of shortage where salaries increase sharply to expand supply by bringing people into the field or encouraging them to come back to work. Various agencies' compensation strategies to recruit new staff have to be balanced against potential impacts on the morale of experienced staff who may watch newcomers earn comparable or even higher salaries on hire despite being recent arrivals to the field or an organization. Non-salary-related factors may also play a role in recruiting. For example, when advertising positions or speaking to prospects it is prudent to call attention to specific potentially desirable aspects of a particular city or community or offer benefits that compensate for less desirable aspects of a setting or position (e.g., housing subsidies for expensive real estate markets or salary differentials for offshifts). Among the non-salary benefits that may be attractive to recruits are subsidies for pursuing educational opportunities in line with their career ambitions (Gooch 2016; Marshall et al. 2017). Nurse residency programs to facilitate the education-to-work transition for new graduates can be a draw, and advancement pathways or career tracks ("career ladders") can be appealing to both new graduate nurses and experienced ones.

Retention Efforts

When nurses stay in place, it is generally assumed that various conditions in their current positions make departure less attractive than staying. A collective bargaining agreement or human resources policies, salary advantages, job security, and preferential scheduling may be associated with longevity in a particular institution, especially for longer term employees. Furthermore, "social capital" that nurses accrue over time—familiarity and friendship with fellow staff members, as well as fluency with policies, procedures, and routines—can encourage nurses to remain in their positions. Compensation on a par with that offered by other institutions within comparable commuting distance for nurses may also play a role in retention. Opportunities to transfer to other roles or work in other practice areas within a larger organization can also influence willingness to stay. A large body of literature and commonly held wisdom speak to the impact of organizational unit-level working conditions on retention (Lake et al. 2019; Petit Dit Dariel and Regnaux 2015; Wei et al. 2018), especially factors linked to manager competence and relationships with staff. Examples include manager provision of meaningful feedback, fairness, and equity in the treatment of staff, presence and attention to working conditions and interpersonal relations among staff, as well as a sense that the manager seeks to bring out the best in their setting's staff (Roche et al. 2015). Some go so far as to speak of nurse managers as the "chief retention officers" in their facilities (Anthony et al. 2005). Chapters 4 and 13 provide a more in-depth discussion of unit and organizational level working conditions.

Diversity Considerations

Addressing diversity challenges in the workforce involves seeking out and hiring workers who represent the communities that a healthcare organization serves (inclusion) and setting up environments where people of various backgrounds feel a sense of belonging to the healthcare organization's community. Although chapter space limitations preclude a full discussion of diversity considerations, many resources are available, including works specific to healthcare (Dreachslin et al. 2013). Several points bear mention here. In nursing, there is an underrepresentation of men and racial and ethnic minority groups. Relatively small but striking increases in male nurses and nurses from nonwhite and Hispanic backgrounds have been documented in recent decades by several researchers and organizations (US DHHS 2019; Zangaro et al. 2018). Similar trends have been seen in many but not necessarily in all countries. However, beyond gender, race, and ethnicity, efforts to recruit and retain staff showing a diversity of gender identity, sexual orientation, religious and spiritual beliefs, disability and ability, socioeconomic status, and national and regional origin have received attention recently.

After promoting entry to nursing education programs across individuals with varying backgrounds, enhancing the experience of members of underrepresented groups in training, and when entering the practice field after graduation, as well as offering high-quality, welcoming onboarding to nursing positions and ensuring positive ongoing experiences within positions are all considered critical. Strategies can include efforts to make sure about the opportunities to discuss both positive and negative experiences with peers of similar backgrounds and engaging individuals from underrepresented groups in planning outreach, recruitment, and retention efforts.

Arguments for efforts to increase diversity in the nurse workforce generally relate to the importance of having the workforce reflect the populations served by nursing, in a manner that spans specialties and roles (and including education, management, and staff development). Above and beyond wanting to spread opportunities for stable and well-paying nursing work across various groups, patients, families, and trainees need to see themselves and the groups they identify with represented among those providing care to have confidence that they will be treated with fairness and respect. Furthermore, workforce diversity enhances the likelihood that the full range of points of view, needs, and experiences of various groups are incorporated into care decisions regarding specific patients and families, as well as policies at institutional and higher levels in the healthcare system.

Inevitably, nurses will routinely work with individuals, families, and communities with different characteristics and experiences from their own, even if efforts to recruit and retain nursing staff from a diversity of backgrounds are successful. In addition to the inclusion of relevant prelicensure and specialty education programs, continuing professional development can also address cultural awareness and humility (Foronda et al. 2016). Sometimes, contrasted with "cultural competence," avoiding stereotypes and having awareness and humility are often understood as sensitivity to issues that might arise for people of different backgrounds within the healthcare system. Realizing that missteps are an important part of working with differences and can be handled respectfully and non-defensively is essential. Language training adapted to local needs and formal and informal methods for building cultural fluency or familiarity with customs and realities in groups that nurses come into frequent contact with can also be helpful. Building self-awareness of the influence of a nurses' background and history with encountering differences and offering communication strategies for building trust and helping relationships with people from different backgrounds are also crucial. Together, efforts to address diversity issues will likely prove increasingly important with increasing awareness of historical and current injustices and demographic trends worldwide.

Age and Generational Differences

Age or generation is not always included in diversity factors in discussions of the nurse workforce. However, currently, in many countries, the nurse workforce spans a wide range of ages (from early 20s to 70s or older). It includes at least four different generations (i.e. distinct groups of individuals who were born within similar timeframes and who therefore experienced major life milestones alongside a common set of historical events) (Christensen et al. 2018). The experiences of passing from kindergarten through high school and higher education and nursing education have been quite different across generations, as well as many aspects of personal, family, and work-life. Conflicts can and do arise in the workplace as members of these generations interact, especially when experiences with coworkers contrast with expectations. The technology used in practice settings has increased markedly. Nursing work's relationship to health information technology, including medical devices with digital interfaces, has created challenges for nurses from older generations (see Chap. 6). Younger nurses enter healthcare with different socialization and much different preparation for their work and expectations of the workplace than their older colleagues. They may find formality and deference in interactions that peers, superiors, and patients from older age groups are accustomed to clashes with their habits and inclinations. Attention to possible struggles and challenges nurses of different age groups can encounter, the potential for conflict in work relationships, and the need for continued professional development will continue to be essential elements for ensuring that nurses can meet the clients' needs and adapt to accelerating changes ahead (Wolff et al. 2010).

Nurse Education and the Entry to Practice Debate

Nursing history in the United States is marked by (a) shifts in the institutions where education to enter practice occurred (away from hospital diploma schools to junior colleges and more recently from junior colleges to institutions offering 4-year and higher degrees) and (b) progressive expansion of career opportunities for nurses that require baccalaureate or higher degrees. It is beyond this chapter's scope to explain the forces, the debates, and the implications of these movements in detail. However, the continued move towards 4-year (baccalaureate) education as the preferred credential for entry to practice and considerable pressure on nurses educated at other levels to earn a bachelor's degree in nursing after initial licensure have been driven by the quest to increase the nursing's social standing and position in the healthcare system (Goode et al. 2001; IOM 2011; Zittel et al. 2016). In the United States this move has taken the form of changing licensure requirements through state-level legislation, for instance, in New York (Menzik 2017). More commonly, formal or informal policies for preferentially hiring RNs with bachelor's degrees at particular institutions have been seen for quite some time. In other countries, moves to reform preparation for nursing have addressed educational programs themselves (Clarke and Patrician 2001). Whether the elevation of educational credentials required for entry to nursing practice has been a positive force in promoting equality of opportunity and achieving a diverse workforce is a complicated question. The geographical distribution of bricks-and-mortar bachelor's and higher level nursing education is not uniform across the United States. Thus, inequities in higher education opportunities can influence the shape of the nurse workforce, even in an increasingly digital era of program delivery. Financial, physical, and digital access remain of concern. Also, questions remain regarding elevating education requirements for generalist and advanced nursing practice. Will higher requirements meet the public's needs in a new era of healthcare? Or is the move towards higher degree preparation a form of credential inflation that primarily benefits higher education institutions rather than students and their families or society (Clarke 2016)? Suppose the practice field underuses the knowledge and skills of nurses educated at the bachelor's degree or higher levels. What implications does this underutilization have for future jobs (numbers and position types) and management strategies in the practice setting? The questions merit consideration in designing educational programs moving forward.

Dealing with Impacts of Workforce-Related Regulatory Efforts Such as Minimum Staffing Ratios

At a time of widespread nurse shortages, health system turbulence, and a refocusing of attention on patient safety, policy advocacy in California led to the passage of minimum staffing ratio legislation (AB 394) in 1999 that took effect in 2004 (Health Facilities 1999). This legislation mandated the development of a set of staffing guidelines for various hospital specialties through a negotiation process between labor and management representatives, and ultimately led to implementing minimum nurse-to-patient ratios in hospitals to be maintained at all times (Chapman et al. 2009). There are two fundamental stances on staffing ratios. One stance is that government regulation is essential to prevent managers and executives in hospitals and other healthcare institutions from putting dangerously low staffing levels in place that jeopardize patient and nurse safety. This argument draws on the mostly correlational and cross-sectional research literature linking nurse staffing with patient outcomes (Griffiths et al. 2016). The opposing stance is that staffing ratios are a blunt tool that constrains managers, executives, and staff unnecessarily while creating needless expense. Staffing ratios can create unintended consequences like the closure of units and even entire institutions and worsen working conditions for nurses (Buerhaus 2010). The anti-ratio stance commonly references the subtleties of the operations of different hospitals and units. There is no direct evidence of the effectiveness of minimum ratios on patient safety in jurisdictions that have implemented them (Serratt 2013).

In terms of the impact on the workforce, a few general statements can be made about staffing regulations. The drafters of such regulations assume that a sufficient number of nurses are available and willing to work for the wages on offer and that healthcare organizations can afford these wages but need some inducement to do so through the imposition of mandatory ratios (Gordon et al. 2008). Depending on the gap between staffing levels in place and the levels required to meet ratios or conditions, there is certainly the possibility that ratio legislation or requirements can increase demand for nursing staff in a particular institution, region, or country (and thus create shortages) (Buerhaus 2009; Douglas 2010). Also, adopting and enforcing minimum staffing ratios might render specific regions more attractive and help address recruitment and retention problems. If this turned out to be accurate, arguably, ratio legislation could worsen shortages in non-ratio-regulated regions. It is important to note that staffing ratios represent an understanding of healthcare facilities' operation, including models of care, at a particular point in time by those drafting them. Ratios may force nurses and managers to adhere to staffing patterns that are not practical or relevant for patient care in alternative settings or when technology is used to guide or enhance the provision of services.

The Future of the Nurse Workforce

Despite many nursing practice traditions that have endured across time and countries, enormous and seemingly ever more rapid social, economic, and technological changes continue to shape how nurses deliver interventions to patients. With these changes have come shifts in both the nature of nursing work and the demand for nurses as employees of healthcare organizations that are expected to continue into the next years.

The various stakeholders in healthcare systems are faced with a nearly constant set of dilemmas involving balancing costs against care quality and access to services. Meeting public expectations regarding the availability of high-quality and affordable services has been a growing challenge. Organizing healthcare workers and resources in ways that address the complex nature of health is another challenge. For 50 years, there have been repeated calls for an increased emphasis on enhancing health enhancement and disease prevention, as opposed to curative treatments for preventable illnesses and long-term support for chronic diseases. There have also been calls for a return to community-based (over institution-based) delivery of services. Indeed, over recent decades greater numbers of nurses have come to work outside hospitals and inpatient institutions in special roles. In industrialized countries, many of these nurses also have graduate training (such as nurse practitioners). They have taken on the provision of more and more services to promote wellness, prevent disease, and manage chronic illness complications.

Moving forward, as care affordability continues to be of great concern, governments and insurance carriers will look to care providers to take a more purposeful and focused role in reducing illness burden and improving the efficiency of resource use. Therefore, they will likely either expect or insist on greater use of technology and changes in delivery methods. Nurses and the interventions they provide may well have an expanded role in the healthcare system. The numbers of nursing positions may either grow or diminish, but the roles they perform will undoubtedly change. Perhaps nurses will increasingly collaborate with lesser trained workers and technicians (often in an arrangement involving delegation of responsibility for tasks to non-nurses), as well as rely more heavily on technology and devote more time to activities that require the full breadth and depth of their training. Collaboration between professionals and nonprofessionals, at one time discussed chiefly in connection with expanding access to care in emerging economies, may become increasingly common across health professions and result in further task shifting of work from other health professions to nursing and shifting work from nursing to technicians and unlicensed workers of various types (WHO 2007; WHPA 2008).

Technology has already played an unquestionable part in the evolution of nursing roles over time. For instance, at one time, blood pressure measurement using a cuff and stethoscope was restricted to physicians (Sandelowski 2000). Likewise, the drawing of blood and insertion of IV catheters were off-limits to nurses—it is now a standard part of US hospital nursing practice (although not necessarily internationally). In general, as new technologies emerge, professions tend to loosen their hold on some older ones. Various types of point-of-care technologies have increasingly made a wide array of assessments and therapeutic interventions possible and affordable on a large scale and with great consistency (see Chap. 6 for an example of intravenous pump integration into the electronic health record to improve care and decrease errors). In recent years nurses have also been playing prominent roles in helping individuals and families incorporate technologies in their daily lives as they manage their health at home.

Over the years, various commentators have mused that nursing and other health professions were likely immune from significant changes in demand related to technology or automation because of the need for direct observation, judgment, or face-to-face human contact. Of course, robotic technology to assist with repetitive tasks and improve precise manipulations in surgical settings has broken down some of these assumptions. While not widespread in healthcare yet, the use of robots or avatars to provide companionship or emotional support is no longer alien—it has been operationalized in limited contexts (for example, see Chi et al. 2017). For decades experts discussed the promise of information technology to improve the quality and consistency of expert judgments; now, artificial intelligence (AI) approaches are increasingly automating what had previously been seen as work reserved for live humans acting in real time. Technology is changing the nature of work performed by live humans across many fields, including healthcare (Jesuthasan and Boudreau 2018; Susskind and Susskind 2015). Reconsideration of the work of nurses in light of these developments has only just begun.

An example of emerging technology, telehealth, was once assumed to be a fallback strategy for situations where limited numbers of trained professionals or unworkable distances for face-to-face contacts rendered it impossible to provide services any other way. Many assumptions about the safety or privacy of interactions occurring at a distance have either been addressed or have faded. Telehealth was already growing in 2018 (US DHHS 2019) before the COVID-19 crisis, with one in three nurses indicating that telehealth technologies were in use in their workplaces. Telehealth has advanced rapidly as a healthcare delivery strategy in the current COVID-19 pandemic (as of the writing of this chapter in 2020) (Brody 2020), with cost considerations and patient preferences as well as practical constraints driving its adoption.

In the next years, nurses may increasingly serve as initiators of service, troubleshooters of problems, and even designers of systems in which patients receive most care in their own homes. The majority of services may be primarily delivered with technology assistance or by nonprofessionals and technicians. Given that nursing education emphasizes the delivery of direct care in institutional settings, rather than the management and coordination of care in community settings, without significant changes in nursing education and a willingness of clinicians and managers to engage with the evolution of services and changing patient and health system expectations, the deployment of individual nurses or nurses as a collective could decrease significantly in the next years without action. Perhaps the most significant losses patients and families would feel with a decreased presence of nurses in the healthcare system would be reduced expertise in and sensitivity to patients' and families' experience that nursing as a profession has historically brought to the delivery of health services. A preferred future would see an evolution of nurses' roles in line with the patient and health system outcomes. The involvement of nurses in care aims to foster healthcare system changes in the coming years to improve access, affordability, and quality of care. Policy decisions at multiple levels regarding the nurse workforce supported by data indicating which types of nursing involvement are essential to patients will be necessary to ensure enough nurses with the proper preparation to carry out their roles in a renewed system.

References

American Association of Colleges of Nursing (2019) Nursing fact sheet. https://www.aacnnursing.org/news-Information/fact-sheets/nursing-fact-sheet

American Hospital Association (AHA) Strategic Policy Planning Committee (2001) Workforce supply for hospitals and health systems. Trustee 54(6):suppl 4 p. following 6

Anthony MK, Standing TS, Glick J, Duffy M, Paschall F, Sauer MR, Kosty Sweeney D, Modic MB, Dumpe ML (2005) Leadership and nurse retention: the pivotal role of nurse managers. J Nurs Adm 35(3):146–155

Auerbach DI, Buerhaus PI, Staiger DO (2017) How fast will the registered nurse workforce grow through 2030? Projections in nine regions of the country. Nurs Outlook 65(1):116–122

Blau FD, Kahn LM (2017) The gender wage gap: extent, trends, and explanations. J Econ Lit 55(3):789–865

Brody J (2020) A pandemic benefit: the expansion of telemedicine. The New York Times. https://www.nytimes.com/2020/05/11/well/live/coronavirus-telemedicine-telehealth.html

Buerhaus PI (2009) Avoiding mandatory hospital nurse staffing ratios: an economic commentary. Nurs Outlook 57(2):107–112

Buerhaus PI (2010) It's time to stop the regulation of hospital nurse staffing dead in its tracks. Nurs Econ 28(2):110

Canadian Institute for Health Information (CIHI) (2020) Nursing in Canada, 2019: a lens on supply and workforce. CIHI, Ottawa. https://www.cihi.ca/sites/default/files/document/nursing-report-2019-en-web.pdf

Chapman SA, Spetz J, Seago JA, Kaiser J, Dower C, Herrera C (2009) How have mandated nurse staffing ratios affected hospitals? Perspectives from California hospital leaders. J Healthc Manag 54(5):321–335

Chi NC, Sparks O, Lin SY, Lazar A, Thompson HJ, Demiris G (2017) Pilot testing a digital pet avatar for older adults. Geriatr Nurs 38(6):542–547

Christensen SS, Wilson BL, Edelman LS (2018) Can I relate? A review and guide for nurse managers in leading generations. J Nurs Manag 26(6):689–695

Clarke SP (2016) The BSN entry to practice debate. **Nurs Manag** 47(11):17–19

Clarke S, Patrician P (2001) Entry to practice in Ontario. Am J Nurs 101(2):73–75

De Groot K, Maurits EEM, Francke AL (2018) Attractiveness of working in home care: an online focus group study among nurses. Health Soc Care Commun 26(1):e94–e101

Dombrowski W, Yoos JL, Neufeld R, Tarshish CY (2012) Factors predicting rehospitalization of elderly patients in a postacute skilled nursing facility rehabilitation program. Arch Phys Med Rehabil 93(10):1808–1813

Douglas K (2010) Ratios—if it were only that easy. Nurs Econ 28(2):119–125

Dreachslin JL, Gilbert MJ, Malone B (2013) Diversity and cultural competence in health care: a systems approach. Jossey-Bass, San Francisco

Dubois CA, D'Amour D, Tchouaket E, Clarke S, Rivard M, Blais R (2013) Associations of patient safety outcomes with models of nursing care organization at unit level in hospitals. Int J Qual Health Care 25(2):110–117

Foronda C, Baptiste DL, Reinholdt MM, Ousman K (2016) Cultural humility: a concept analysis. J Transcult Nurs 27(3):210–217

Friedberg MW, Reid RO, Timbie JW, Setodji C, Kofner A, Weidmer B, Kahn K (2017) Federally qualified health center clinicians and staff increasingly dissatisfied with workplace conditions. Health Aff 36(8):1469–1475

Girvin J, Jackson D, Hutchinson M (2016) Contemporary public perceptions of nursing: a systematic review and narrative synthesis of the international research evidence. J Nurs Manag 24(8):994–1006

Gooch K (2016) How 5 health systems are recruiting, retaining nurses during an RN shortage. https://www.beckershospitalreview.com/hr/how-5-health-systems-are-recruiting-retaining-nurses-during-an-rn-shortage.html

Goode CJ, Pinkerton S, McCausland MP, Southard P, Graham R, Krsek C (2001) Documenting chief nursing officers' preference for BSN-prepared nurses. J Nurs Adm 31(2):55–59

Gordon S, Buchanan J, Bretherton T (2008) Safety in numbers: nurse-to-patient ratios and the future of health care. Cornell University Press, Ithaca, NY

Greenlaw SA, Shapiro D (2018) Demand and supply at work in labor markets. In: Principles of microeconomics, 2nd edn. OpenStax, Houston, pp 84–92. https://openstax.org/details/books/principles-microeconomics-2e

Greipp ME (2003) Salary compression: its effect on nurse recruitment and retention. J Nurs Adm 33(6):321–323

Griffiths P, Ball J, Drennan J, Dall'Ora C, Jones J, Maruotti A, Pope C, Recio Saucedo A, Simon M (2016) Nurse staffing and patient outcomes: strengths and limitations of the evidence to inform policy and practice. Int J Nurs Stud 63:213–225

Health Facilities: Nurse staffing. California AB-394 (1999). http://leginfo.legislature.ca.gov/faces/billNavClient.xhtml?bill_id=199920000AB394

Hooper C, Craig J, Janvrin DR, Wetsel MA, Reimels E (2010) Compassion satisfaction, burnout, and compassion fatigue among emergency nurses compared with nurses in other selected inpatient specialties. J Emerg Nurs 36(5):420–427

Institute of Medicine (2011) The future of nursing: leading change, advancing health. National Academies Press, Washington, DC. https://www.nap.edu/catalog/12956/the-future-of-nursing-leading-change-advancing-health

Jesuthasan R, Boudreau JW (2018) Reinventing jobs. Harvard Business School Press, Boston

Jones TL, Yoder LH, Baernholdt M (2019) Variation in academic preparation and progression of nurses across the continuum of care. Nurs Outlook 67:381–392

Kingma M (2006) Nurses on the move: migration and the global health care economy. Cornell University Press, Ithaca, NY

Koerner J (1992) Differentiated practice: the evolution of professional nursing. J Prof Nurs 8:335–341

Lake ET, Sanders J, Duan R, Riman KA, Schoenauer KM, Chen Y (2019) A meta-analysis of the associations between the nurse work environment in hospitals and 4 sets of outcomes. Med Care 57:353–361

Mallidou AA, Cummings GG, Estabrooks CA, Giovannetti PB (2011) Nurse specialty subcultures and patient outcomes in acute care hospitals: a multiple-group structural equation modeling. Int J Nurs Stud 48(1):81–93

Markkanen P, Galligan C, Quinn M (2017) Safety risks among home infusion nurses and other home health care providers. J Infus Nurs 40(4):215–223

Marshall J, Edmonson C, England V (2017) Nurse manager's guide to recruitment and retention. HCPro, Middleton, MA

Menzik J (2017) New York governor signs BSN in 10 into law for nurses. https://www.nurse.com/blog/2017/12/20/new-york-governor-signs-bsn-in-10-into-law-for-nurses/

Mitchell PH, Ferketich S, Jennings BM (1998) Quality health outcomes model. Image J Nurs Sch 30(1):43–46

Montag ML (1963) Technical education in nursing? Am J Nurs 63(5):100–103

Neatherlin JS, Prater L (2003) Nursing time and work in an acute rehabilitation setting. Rehabilit Nurs 28:186–190

Needleman J, Pearson ML, Upenieks VV, Yee T, Wolstein J, Parkerton M (2016) Engaging front-line staff in performance improvement: the American Organization of Nurse Executives implementation of Transforming Care at the Bedside Collaborative. Jt Comm J Qual Patient Saf 42(2):61–69

Petit Dit Dariel O, Regnaux JP (2015) Do Magnet®-accredited hospitals show improvements in nurse and patient outcomes compared to non-Magnet hospitals: a systematic review. JBI Database System Rev Implement Rep 13(6):168–219

Reinhard SC, Young HM (2009) The nursing workforce in long-term care. Nurs Clin N Am 44(2):161–168

Roche M, Duffield C, Dimitrelis S, Frew B (2015) Leadership skills for nursing unit managers to decrease intention to leave. Nurs Res Rev 5:57–64

Royal College of Nursing (RCN) (2020) The UK nursing labour market review 2019. Author, London. https://www.rcn.org.uk/-/media/royal-college-of-nursing/documents/publications/2020/april/009-135.pdf?la=en

Sandelowski M (2000) Devices and desires: gender, technology, and American nursing. University of North Carolina Press, Chapel Hill, NC

Serratt T (2013) California's nurse-to-patient ratios, part 3: eight years later, what do we know about patient level outcomes? J Nurs Adm 43(11):581–585

Shaffer FA, Bakhshi MA, Farrell N, Álvarez TD (2020) Original research: the recruitment experience of foreign-educated health professionals to the United States. Am J Nurs 120(1):28–38

Skillman SM, Palazzo L, Keepnews D, Hart LG (2006) Characteristics of registered nurses in rural versus urban areas: implications for strategies to alleviate nursing shortages in the United States. J Rural Health 22:151–157

Susskind R, Susskind D (2015) The future of the professions. Oxford University Press, New York
U.S. Department of Health and Human Services, Health Resources and Services Administration (2010) The registered nurse population: findings from the 2008 National Sample Survey of Registered Nurses. U.S. Department of Health and Human Services, Health Resources and Services Administration, Rockville, MD. https://data.hrsa.gov/DataDownload/NSSRN/GeneralPUF08/rnsurveyfinal.pdf
U.S. Department of Health and Human Services, Health Resources and Services Administration (2017) National and regional supply and demand projections of the nursing workforce: 2014–2030. U.S. Department of Health and Human Services, Health Resources and Services Administration, Rockville, MD. https://bhw.hrsa.gov/sites/default/files/bhw/nchwa/projections/NCHWA_HRSA_Nursing_Report.pdf
U.S. Department of Health and Human Services, Health Resources and Services Administration (2019) Brief summary results from the 2018 national sample survey of registered nurses. U.S. Department of Health and Human Services, Health Resources and Services Administration, Rockville, MD. https://bhw.hrsa.gov/sites/default/files/bhw/health-workforce-analysis/nssrn-summary-report.pdf
Vanhook P, Bosse J, Flinter M, Poghosyan L, Dunphy L, Barksdale D (2018) The American Academy of Nursing on policy: emerging role of baccalaureate registered nurses in primary care (August 20, 2018). Nurs Outlook 66(5):512–517
Wei H, Sewell KA, Woody G, Rose MA (2018) The state of the science of nurse work environments in the United States: a systematic review. Int J Nurs Sci 5:287–300
Wojnar DM, Whelan EM (2017) Preparing nursing students for enhanced roles in primary care: the current state of prelicensure and RN-to-BSN education. Nurs Outlook 65(2):222–232
Wolff AC, Ratner PA, Robinson SL, Oliffe JL, McGillis-Hall L (2010) Beyond generational differences: a literature review of the impact of relational diversity on nurses' attitudes and work. J Nurs Manag 18(8):948–969
World Health Organization (WHO) (2007) Task shifting to tackle health worker shortages. https://www.who.int/healthsystems/task_shifting_booklet.pdf
World Health Organization (WHO) (2020) State of the world's nursing 2020: investing in education, jobs and leadership. https://www.who.int/publications/i/item/9789240003279
World Health Professions Alliance (2008) Joint health professions statement on task shifting. https://www.whpa.org/news-resources/statements/joint-health-professions-statement-task-shifting
Zangaro GA, Streeter R, Li T (2018) Trends in racial and ethnic demographics of the nursing workforce: 2000 to 2015. Nurs Outlook 66(4):365–371
Zittel B, Moss E, O'Sullivan A, Siek T (2016) Registered Nurses as professionals: accountability for education and practice. Online J Issues Nurs 21(3). http://ojin.nursingworld.org/MainMenuCategories/ANAMarketplace/ANAPeriodicals/OJIN/TableofContents/Vol-21-2016/No3-Sept-2016/Registered-Nurses-as-Professionals.html

Part III

System

The Nurse Work Environment

Shelly A. Fischer and Diane K. Boyle

Introduction

A healthy and safe nurse work environment (NWE) is "one in which leaders provide the *structures,* practices, systems, and policies that enable clinical nurses to engage in the work *processes* and relationships essential to safe and quality patient care *outcomes*" (Kramer et al. 2010, p. 4). Healthy NWEs possess good professional relationships, professional autonomy, a strong safety culture, structural empowerment and engagement, appropriate staffing and resources, a balanced work schedule, professional advancement opportunities, transformational leadership, and joy in work (Copanitsanou et al. 2017; Kramer et al. 2010; Perlo et al. 2017; Wei et al. 2018). Safe and healthy NWEs are essential to achieving the Quadruple Aim of enhancing the patient experience, improving population health, reducing costs, and improving clinician well-being (Boyle et al. 2019; Grant et al. 2020).

Over 20 years of research provides evidence of an association between healthy and safe work environments and better outcomes for nurses and patients. Patient outcomes most consistently associated with better NWEs are lower 30-day mortality rates, overall mortality rate, and failure to rescue; lower odds or rate of adverse events such as falls, pressure injuries, medication errors, and central line-associated bloodstream infections (CLABSI); and higher nurse-reported quality of care or safety ratings (Copanitsanou et al. 2017; DiCuccio 2015; Halm 2019; Lake et al. 2019; Lee and Scott 2018; Nascimento and Jesus 2020; Petit Dit Dariel and Regnaux 2015; Stalpers et al. 2015; Wei et al. 2018). Nurse outcomes most consistently associated with better hospital NWEs are lower burnout, lower emotional strains, or better psychological health; higher job satisfaction or lower job dissatisfaction; and

S. A. Fischer (✉)
College of Nursing, University of Colorado Anschutz Medical Campus, Aurora, CO, USA

D. K. Boyle
Fay W. Whitney School of Nursing, University of Wyoming, Laramie, WY, USA

© Springer Nature Switzerland AG 2021
M. Baernholdt, D. K. Boyle (eds.), *Nurses Contributions to Quality Health Outcomes*, https://doi.org/10.1007/978-3-030-69063-2_4

higher intent to stay or lower turnover (Copanitsanou et al. 2017; Halm 2019; Lake et al. 2019; Petit Dit Dariel and Regnaux 2015; Wei et al. 2018).

Consequently, initiatives such as the American Nurses Credentialing Center (ANCC) accreditation programs of Magnet Recognition and Pathway to Excellence Recognition (ANCC n.d.-a, n.d.-b) have played a central role in elevating the importance of work environments as an integral component of patient-centered care, improved patient outcomes, improved nurse outcomes, and lower cost. This chapter discusses how the QHOM frames the relationship between the system's characteristics of NWEs and interventions to improve NWEs.

Nurse Work Environment: Specific Linkages with the QHOM

The QHOM (Mitchell et al. 1998) serves as an efficient organizing framework to describe the concepts intrinsic to NWEs and the inevitable interactions and relationships (see Fig. 4.1). The primary construct within the QHOM showcased in this chapter is the system, specifically the essential structures of the NWE. Four specific aspects of NWEs—joy in work and clinician well-being, safety culture, bullying and incivility, and staffing—are given special consideration due to their

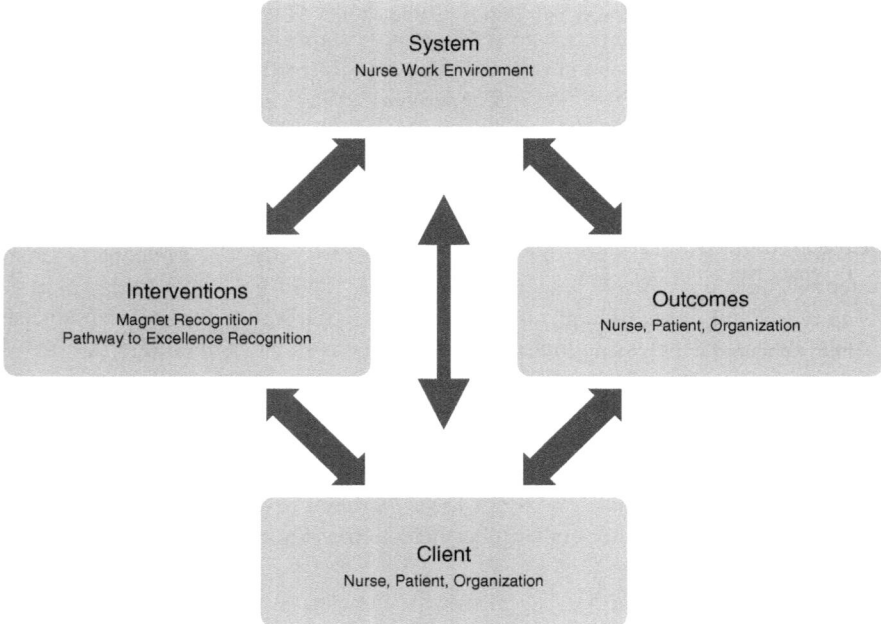

Fig. 4.1 Framework for the nurse work environment

contemporary significance. Successful system-level performance-driven interventions, the ANCC Magnet and Pathway to Excellence Recognition Programs, serve as road maps to nursing excellence and acknowledge healthcare organizations with healthy and safe NWEs. The Magnet Recognition Program also recognizes quality patient outcomes. The QHOM constructs of client and outcome are not discussed in this chapter.

NWEs are embedded in the complex adaptive healthcare system characterized by constant, nonlinear patterns of emerging change with multiple feedback loops (Marshall and Broome 2017; Plsek 2001). Therefore, the QHOM is an ideal lens for understanding the complex interdependent relationships among the system, client, interventions, and outcomes produced by these relationships. Outcomes are not static but rather provide inputs as feedback to the system and client. Importantly, unlike the linear Donabedian (1988) model, the QHOM defines the role of interventions, for example, applying for Magnet accreditation to improve the NWE. A broad range of activities are employed during the application process. These activities, in turn, work through the system and client to impact a variety of outcomes.

An advantage of the QHOM in relation to the NWE is the ability to examine and understand micro-, meso-, and macro-level factors (Serpa and Ferreira 2019). For purposes of this chapter, micro-level factors are at the individual level, for instance, psychological states such as attitudes toward empowerment and engagement and safety culture. See Chap. 13 for examples of interventions targeting the micro-level. Meso-level factors span from the unit and team level to the organizational level. Such factors might include how an organization's staffing resources are structured and deployed or how much professional autonomy is afforded to nurses in providing optimal patient care. NWE interventions at the meso-level are often focused on unit and organizational level changes such as improving collaboration between nurses and physicians, nursing participation in governance, and staffing and resources. Chapters 9 and 10 speak about processes or interventions at the unit or organizational level. Macro-level factors work at the regulatory, societal, and political levels. For example, accreditation requirements for the Magnet or Pathway to Excellence Programs or Joint Commission accreditation can impact NWEs. Hospital payment systems such as Medicare's Hospital Value-Based Purchasing Program (Medicare. gov n.d.) are also examples of macro-level approaches that can positively or negatively impact NWE (Chap. 2).

The QHOM helps consider how an intervention might be applied through these levels of impact. A macro-level intervention may have unanticipated effects at the micro or meso-level for nurses or patients, such as dictating staffing levels through state legislation (Chap. 3). Conversely, macro-level changes in staffing through legislation generally stem from problems identified at the micro and meso-levels in providing optimal care to patients. This complexity and interdependence are characteristics of the QHOM.

System

The Nurse Work Environment

Over the past 40 years, nurse leaders and researchers have emphasized the importance of understanding and improving NWE. In the early 1980s, nursing leaders and researchers began devoting considerable effort to understanding what makes a good place for nurses to work, rather than conceptualizing the organization and environment through the lens of other disciplines (e.g., sociology of work, workgroups, and organizations). Among the first of these initiatives was the American Academy of Nursing Task Force on Nursing Practice's study of 155 institutions to determine the NWE attributes that attract and retain nurses who provide quality patient care (McClure et al. 2002). Forty-one such institutions were identified and were given the moniker of "magnet" hospitals. Magnetic hospitals were characterized as having participative management with open communication; strong, supportive, and visible nurse leadership; recognition of the importance of nurse managers; adequate staffing levels; professional nursing practice; flexible scheduling; good relationships with physicians; and professional development and career advancement opportunities, among others (McClure et al. 2002). In 1990, the American Nurses Credentialing Center (ANCC) instituted the Magnet Hospital Recognition Program as an accreditation process. The Magnet program requires resources that not all hospitals have, so in 2007, the Pathway to Excellence Program was initiated (ANCC n.d.-b) to assure accessibility to an NWE recognition program for all hospitals, regardless of resources. For more details, see the system interventions section below about ANCC Accreditation Programs.

In response to the growing awareness and evidence base of the importance of the NWE, the Magnet and Pathway to Excellence Recognition Programs grew. Further, various other national entities released recommendations, principles, standards, and hallmarks for healthy and professional NWEs. Figure 4.2 provides a timeline of selected critical initiatives targeting NWE. In 2001, among the first of these initiatives was the American Nurses Association's (ANA) *Nurses Bill of Rights* (ANA n.d.). The *Bill of Rights* set forth seven principles of the NWE that the ANA believed every nurse had a fundamental right to see fulfilled. These included the right to an NWE that is safe, allows practice according to professional standards, and facilitates ethical practice. Simultaneously, The Joint Commission (2001) issued a call to action to address the USA's growing nursing shortage, *Healthcare at the Crossroads: Strategies for Addressing the Evolving Nursing Crisis.* The Joint Commission's recommendations focused on creating a culture that values nurse retention by transforming nurses' workplaces to empower and respect the nursing staff. The *Bill of Rights* and The Joint Commission's call to action were followed by the release of NWE standards from various nursing organizations. Prominent among these were the

- American Organization of Nurse Executives (now the American Organization of Nurse Leaders): *Elements of a Healthy Practice Environment* (AONL 2019), original release 2003.

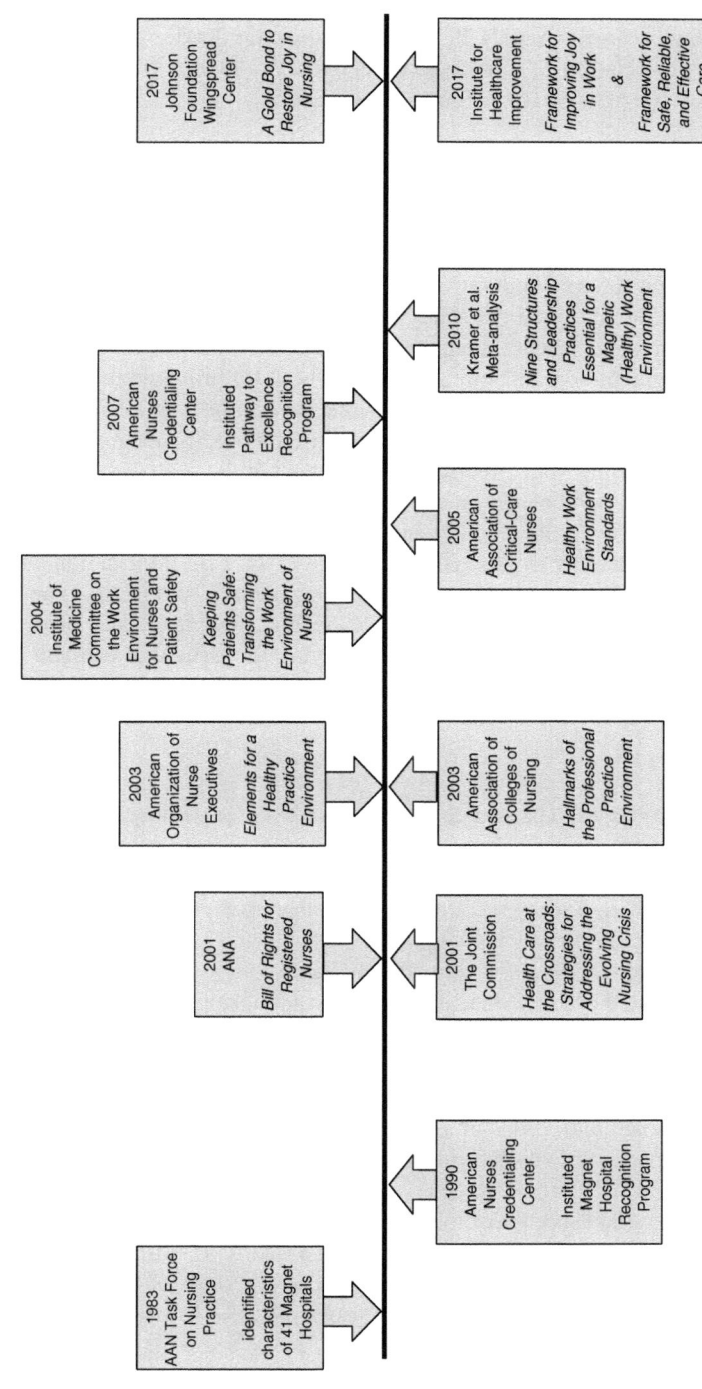

Fig. 4.2 Timeline of selected major national nurse work environment initiatives

- American Association of Colleges of Nursing: *Hallmarks of the Professional Practice Environment* (AACN 2020), original release 2003.
- American Association of Critical-Care Nurses: *Standards for a Healthy Work Environment* (AACN 2016), original release 2005.

Meanwhile, the Institute of Medicine Committee on the Work Environment for Nurses and Patient Safety released the 2004 landmark report, *Keeping Patients Safe: Transforming the Work Environment of Nurses (IOM 2004)*. The report was a call to action for healthcare organizations to recognize the crucial connection between NWEs and patient safety. The report found that the typical NWE was characterized by many serious threats to patient safety in four essential components of healthcare organizations: organizational management practices, workforce deployment practices, work design, and organizational culture. The IOM provided overarching and specific recommendations to improve the work environment in all four areas. For instance, they advocated for organizational culture and work design that promotes safety, adequate staffing, and effective nurse leadership.

In 2010, Kramer, Schmalenberg, and Maguire used a structure-process-outcome (S-P-O) framework to conduct a meta-analysis for purposes of distilling the essential structures for a healthy work environment (see Chap. 1 for information on S-P-O frameworks such as Donabedian 1966, 1988). They included publications and documents from various agencies that described healthy, magnetic, and professional NWEs and a series of published papers identifying the structural elements of the Essentials of Magnetism. The meta-analysis findings were nine categories of organizational structures essential to a healthy NWE (see Box 4.1).

Box 4.1 Structures/Best Leadership Practices Essential for Healthy Work Environments

1. Quality leadership at all levels in the organization
2. Availability of and support for education, career, performance, and competence development
3. Administrative sanction for autonomous and collaborative practice
4. Evidence-based practice education and operational supports
5. Culture, practice, and opportunity to learn interdisciplinary collaboration
6. Empowered, shared decision-making structures for control of the context of nursing practice
7. Generation and nurturance of a patient-centered culture
8. Staffing structures that take into account RN competence, patient acuity, and teamwork
9. Development and support of intradisciplinary teamwork

Source: Kramer, M., Schmalenberg, C., & Maguire, P. (2010). Nine structures and leadership practices essential for a magnetic (healthy) work environment. *Nursing Administration Quarterly, 34*(1), 4–17. Reprinted with permission from Wolters Kluwer Health, Inc.

Joy in Work

Joy in work and clinician well-being are aspects of the work environment that have evolved from the recently introduced fourth aim of the new Quadruple Aim (Bodenheimer and Sinsky 2014; Sikka et al. 2015). Besides the fourth aim of improving the work-life of healthcare clinicians and staff, the original Triple Aim was improving the health of populations, enhancing the patient experience of care, and reducing the per capita cost of health care. Joy in work is the feeling of accomplishment and fulfillment resulting from meaningful work (Sikka et al. 2015). Joy and meaning in work are integral to a healthy work environment for the individual and the collective. Bodenheimer and Sinsky introduced the fourth aim due to the multiple workplace stressors inhibiting optimal patient care. Among these stressors are increasing time pressures, poorly designed systems of care, staff shortages and overwhelming patient loads, demanding electronic medical record systems, government regulations, a general feeling of powerlessness, lack of authentic leadership, and hostile work cultures (Grant et al. 2020; Perlo et al. 2017; Johnson Foundation 2017). The consequences of these workplace stressors on clinicians are compassion fatigue, burnout, and, subsequently, turnover (Dyrbye et al. 2017; Perlo et al. 2017; McBride et al. 2018; Zhang et al. 2018). The Institute for Healthcare Improvement (IHI) (Perlo et al. 2017) and the Johnson Foundation at Wingspread Center (2017) recommended focusing on restoring joy and meaning in work rather than treating burnout.

Joy in work is a system property (Perlo et al. 2017). "It is generated (or not) by the system and occurs (or not) organization-wide. Joy in work—or lack thereof—impacts not only individual staff engagement and satisfaction, but also patient experience, quality of care, patient safety, and organizational performance" (Perlo et al. 2017, p. 5). The system components of joy in work are physical and psychological safety, meaning and purpose, choice and autonomy, recognition and reward, participative management, real-time measurement, wellness and resilience, and daily improvement (Perlo et al.). Focusing on joy in work is crucial for three reasons. First, healthcare professions regularly have the opportunity to improve others' lives. Caring and healing should be naturally joyful and rewarding activities. The compassion and commitment of healthcare staff are vital assets that, if nurtured and not hindered, can lead to joy as well as to effective and empathetic care. This asset-based approach often leads to designing more innovative and effective care processes (Perlo et al.). Second, joy in work is more than the absence of burnout. Joy is about the connection to meaning and purpose. Focusing on joy can reduce compassion fatigue and burnout while simultaneously bolstering resilience in healthcare workers (Perlo et al.). Third, organizational success can be contingent upon the level of joy experienced in the workplace. Joy and worker engagement dovetail. Greater worker engagement is associated with better performance and improved organizational clinical and financial outcomes. Ensuring joy is a crucial component of the psychology of change (Perlo et al.). Because joy in work is a system property, the IHI recommends identifying specific opportunities for improvement and implementing tests of change using Plan-Do-Study-Act (PDSA) cycles (see Chap. 6 for an overview of PDSA cycles) (Perlo et al. 2017).

Similarly, the multidisciplinary National Academy of Medicine (NAM) Action Collaborative on Clinician Well-Being and Resilience developed the NAM Conceptual Model of Factors Affecting Clinician Well-Being and Resilience. The model depicts patient well-being, clinician-patient relationships, and clinician well-being as the nucleus of a concentric model (Brigham et al. 2018). The nucleus is enclosed by individual and external factors affecting clinician well-being and resilience. The phenomenon of clinician well-being is having a personal state of fulfillment and engagement that leads to joy in practice and a connection to why one went into health care to begin with (Brigham et al.). Resilience is the ability to adapt to difficult conditions while sustaining purpose, balance, and mental and physical well-being (Padesky and Mooney 2012). The broader focus of the model is to improve clinician well-being and alleviate fatigue, moral distress, suffering, and burnout (Brigham et al. 2018).

Resilience is a term applied to the individual (micro-level), while "agility" is applied to the same concept at a collective or group level (meso-level) (Pipe et al. 2012). Resilience is a trait that can be learned and acquired (McAllister 2013; Mealer et al. 2017; Pipe et al. 2012). The return on investment made to improve resilience and build collective agility in nurses is well documented. Patients experience improved outcomes and better satisfaction with care (Cimiotti et al. 2012; Manomenidis et al. 2019; Mealer et al. 2017). Employees experience greater job engagement and increased levels of health, optimism, and self-care (Larrabee et al. 2010; Pipe et al. 2012). Administrators have better fiscal outcomes and increased staff retention (McAllister 2013; Mealer et al. 2017; Stagman-Tyrer 2014). This deeper understanding reinforces the NWE's conceptual linkages with well-being, joy in the workplace, and nurse resilience.

Safety Culture

Like joy in work, safety culture is an important contemporary aspect of the NWE and overall organization. Safety culture is "the product of individual and group values, attitudes, perceptions, competencies, and patterns of behavior that determine the commitment to, and the style and proficiency of, an organization's health and safety management" (AHRQ n.d., p. 1). The way organizations view the importance of safety has a significant impact on workers' perception of their safety. In turn, worker safety and patient safety are inextricably linked. Therefore, it stands to reason that a strong safety culture is an integral part of a healthy work environment.

The IHI and Safe and Reliable Healthcare collaborated for over 15 years to develop a safety culture framework (Frankel et al. 2017). The collaboration was in response to the Institute of Medicine's landmark report *To Err is Human: Building a Better Health System* (IOM 2000), which revealed that healthcare errors were a leading cause of death in the USA. The *Framework for Safe, Reliable, and Effective Care* (Frankel et al. 2017) contains two foundational and overlapping domains. The first domain is *culture* which is the product of individual and group values, attitudes, competencies, and behaviors that form a strong footing on which to build a learning system (Frankel et al. 2017). Culture has four components, psychological safety, accountability, teamwork and communication, and negotiation. The second domain is a *learning system* that can self-reflect and recognize strengths and weaknesses, both in real time and in intermittent review intervals (Frankel et al. 2017). A learning system has four components, transparency, reliability, improvement and measurement, and continuous learning.

Subsequent to the *Framework for Safe, Reliable, and Effective Care*, the IHI released the report *Safer Together: A National Plan to Advance Patient Safety* (National Steering Committee for Patient Safety 2020). The National Steering Committee for Patient Safety—a collaboration of 27 organizations representing federal agencies, healthcare delivery organizations and associations, patient and family advocates, and industry experts—developed a plan to improve patient safety while reducing harm to patients and healthcare providers. The plan contains a set of actionable and effective recommendations centered on four foundational and interdependent areas: culture, leadership, and governance; patient and family engagement; workforce safety; and learning system.

Incivility, Bullying, and Violence

Acts of workplace incivility, bullying, and violence undermine a safe and healthy work environment. These acts are part of a broader complex phenomenon that includes the acts, as well as failing to take action, when necessary, to address the acts (ANA 2015). Incivility, bullying, and violence occur on a continuum, may be physical or verbal, and may include assault, bullying, intimidation, harassment, and threats. Workplace incivility has been defined as low-intensity milder forms of negative behaviors. The perpetrator's purpose and uncivil behaviors are ambiguous (Anusiewicz et al. 2019). Incivility forms include rude and discourteous actions, gossiping and spreading rumors, refusing to assist a coworker, and using a condescending tone (ANA 2015). In contrast, bullying is a high-intensity form of negative behavior.

> Bullying at work means harassing, offending, or socially excluding someone or negatively affecting someone's work. For the label bullying (or mobbing) to be applied to a particular activity, interaction, or process, the bullying behavior has to occur repeatedly and regularly (e.g., weekly) and over some time (e.g., about 6 months). Bullying is an escalating process in which the person confronted ends up in an inferior position and becomes the target of systematic negative social acts. A conflict cannot be called bullying if the incident is an isolated event or if two parties of equal strengths are in conflict (Einarsen et al. 2011, p. 22).

Bullying behaviors are toward a clear target, present serious safety and health concerns, and often involve an abuse of power (ANA 2015; Anusiewicz et al. 2019).

Workplace violence involves instances where staff are abused, threatened, or assaulted in situations related to their work, including commuting to and from work (ICN 2017). It can involve explicit or implicit challenges to worker safety, well-being, or health. Nursing ranks among the riskiest occupations for violence and occupational injury. According to the United States Bureau of Labor Statistics (2017), nurses have the highest rate of nonfatal occupational injuries in all US occupations. Further, 12% of these injuries come from violence toward nurses, compared to only 4% for other occupations.

Edward et al. (2014) conducted a systematic review of 53 studies on aggression and violence in the nursing workplace. The studies included a broad range of practice settings in 14 different countries, pointing to workplace violence's international nature. Verbal abuse was the most frequent form of aggression experienced by nurses, with verbal abuse rates ranging from 17% to 94%. The rate of verbal abuse compared to physical abuse was about 3 to 1. Physician-to-nurse verbal abuse comprised about 42% of occurrences and nurse-to-nurse verbal abuse about 32% of occurrences. Edward et al. characterized these hostile actions between colleagues as repeated and persistent over time. The abuse comprised personal and professional aspects of the victim and was mainly related to insults, incivility, and rumors about their personal lives. Physical abuse instances ranged from 20.8% to 82% and were more prevalent in mental health, geriatric, long-term care, nursing homes, and emergency departments. More male nurses experienced physical abuse than females, as well as nurses on night and weekend shifts. The most common physical abuse acts were being spat upon, hit, pushed/shoved, scratched, and kicked, and were usually perpetrated by patients receiving direct care (Edward et al. 2014).

In a recent study of critical care nurse environments, Ulrich et al. (2019) found that in the past year, 80% of nurse participants reported verbal abuse at least once, 47% reported physical abuse at least once, 46% experienced discrimination, and 40% experienced sexual harassment. Further, 86% of participants reported at least one of the negative incidents in the past year. Of the participants experiencing these abuses in the past year (n = 6017), a total of 198,340 instances were reported. Although the source of verbal abuse was mainly from patients or families (73% and 64%, respectively), RNs reported verbal abuse from physicians (41%), other RNs (34%), and management staff (14%). Newly licensed nurses may be particularly vulnerable to workplace bullying (Anusiewicz et al. 2019).

Staffing

Of all the elements of NWEs, staffing has been researched most extensively; therefore, it deserves special attention. Lulat et al. (2018) conducted a scoping review of over 600 studies focused on the relationship between RN staffing levels and staff mix and patient, organizational, nurse, and financial outcomes. The studies' abstracts are contained in a database located on the Registered Nurses' Association of Ontario (Canada) website (https://rnao.ca/bpg/initiatives/RNEffectiveness). For patients, better staffing was associated with decreased mortality, increased quality of care, fewer pressure injuries and infections, and decreased length of stay, among other positive outcomes. Nurses working in environments with better staffing experienced higher job satisfaction and decreased turnover. Organizations experienced positive financial outcomes.

The American Nurses Association's (2020) Principles for Nurse Staffing provide an overarching framework to achieve appropriate nurse staffing, which is the match of registered nurse expertise with the needs of clients of nursing services in the context of the practice setting and situation (ANA 2020). Nurse characteristics to be considered in determining appropriate staffing are type of licensure, experience with patient population served, organizational experience, overall professional nursing experience, professional certifications, educational preparation, competence with technologies and specific clinical interventions, and language capabilities (ANA 2019, 2020; Halm 2019). Additional factors that influence staffing are turnover (admissions, discharges, and transfers), availability of technical support and other resources, interprofessional team composition and level of teamwork, unit physical space and layout, culture of the organization, population/client characteristics, and cost (ANA 2019; Halm 2019).

Measures of Components of the Nurse Work Environment

Valid and reliable measurement instruments are essential to rigorous research and quality improvement projects about the NWE. Extensive work has been done over the years to this end. Multiple tools are available to effectively test and analyze relationships of variables embedded within the QHOM framework for NWEs. Examples of both general and specific measures of the NWE are presented below.

Measures of the General Nurse Work Environment
The three most widely used instruments to quantify the NWEs are the Practice Environment Scale of the Nursing Work Index Revised (PES-NWI), Essentials of Magnetism II (EOMII), and the Healthy Work Environments Assessment Tool (Wei et al. 2018). The PES-NWI is based theoretically on the construct nurse practice environment, defined as the organizational characteristics of a work environment that facilitate or constrain professional practice (Lake 2002). Dimensions measured by the PES-NWI are nurse participation in hospital affairs; nursing foundations for quality of care; nurse manager ability, leadership, and support for nurses; staffing and resource adequacy; and collegial nurse-physician relationships. The PES-NWI has been endorsed continuously since 2004 as a nursing care performance measure by the National Quality Forum. The EOMII (Schmalenberg and Kramer 2008) was designed to (a) measure attributes of a work environment based on Donabedian's (1966, 1988) structure-process-outcome paradigm and (b) represent the Magnet Hospital Standards. Dimensions in the EOMII are support for education, nurse-physician relations, working with clinically competent peers, clinical autonomy, control over nursing practice, perceived adequacy of staffing, patient-centered values, nurse manager support, and professional job satisfaction. The Healthy Work Environment Assessment Tool (AACN n.d.) is based on the AACN Healthy Work Environments Standards (AACN 2016) and measures the dimensions of skilled communication, true collaboration, effective decision-making, appropriate staffing, meaningful recognition, and authentic leadership.

Measures of Joy in Work
Although there are currently no direct measures of joy in work, the IHI recommends a suite of proxy instruments for assessing joy in work (Perlo et al. 2017, Appendix C, pp. 33–37). Among these measures are leadership, safety attitudes, burnout, and job satisfaction.

Measures of Safety Culture

The two most commonly used measures of safety culture are the Safety Attitudes Questionnaire (SAQ) and the Agency for Healthcare Research and Quality Hospital Survey on Patient Safety Culture (AHRQ HSOPSC) (DiCuccio 2015). Both questionnaires are based on the safety culture definition of "the product of individual and group values, attitudes, perceptions, competencies, and patterns of behavior that determine the commitment to, and the style and proficiency of, an organization's health and safety management" (Sorra et al. 2016). The SAQ measures six dimensions of clinicians' attitudes: teamwork climate, job satisfaction, perceptions of management, safety climate, working conditions, and stress recognition (Sexton et al. 2006). It has been adapted for use in intensive care units, operating rooms, general inpatient settings, and ambulatory clinics. The HSOPSC asks all workers in an organization to rate 12 dimensions: communication openness, feedback and communication about error, frequency of events reported, handoffs and transitions, management support for patient safety, nonpunitive response to error, organizational learning-continuous improvement, overall perceptions of patient safety, staffing, supervisor/manager expectations and actions promoting patient safety, teamwork across units, and teamwork within units. The HSOPSC also contains two questions on an overall grade for patient safety (AHRQ n.d.; Sorra et al. 2016). It has been adapted for medical offices, nursing homes, community pharmacies, and ambulatory surgical centers.

Measures of Incivility, Bullying, and Violence

Two commonly used workplace bullying measures are the Negative Acts Questionnaire-Revised (NAQ-R) and the Bergen Bullying Indicator (BBI). The NAQ-R measures the domains of personal bullying, work-related bullying, and physically intimidating bullying (Einarsen et al. 2009). Items are worded behaviorally; that is, they avoid the use of terms such as bullying and harassment. The NAQ-R is useful in detecting bullying targets and differentiating groups of employees with different levels of exposure to bullying. The BBI is a one-item self-labeling measure that asks the worker how often they experience bullying behaviors (Notelaer et al. 2006). The BBI can classify workers into six categories, ranging from "not bullied" to "victim."

Other measures of incivility and bullying exist. For example, the Incivility in Nursing Education-Revised (INE-R) is a 48-item survey with four additional open-ended survey questions. The INE-R is a unique instrument because it employs both qualitative and quantitative methodologies to measure perceptions of uncivil behaviors (Clark et al. 2015). Another unique feature of the INE-R is that it simultaneously gathers input for potential solutions to the identified incivility.

Incidences of violence and injury are collected nationally. The Bureau of Labor Statistics (BLS) monitors the incidence and prevalence of workplace violence and injuries in the USA. It serves as the primary source for reporting and analysis via the Survey of Occupational Injuries and Illness (SOII) (BLS 2017, 2018) and through mandatory Occupational Safety and Health Administration (OSHA) reporting. Guided by the Occupational Safety and Health Act of 1970 (OHSA 1970), the intention was that employers were required to track and record injury data. In 2016, a significant change in reporting requirements was implemented by OSHA, requiring employers to report this same data electronically directly to OSHA. Although work is still in progress to assure data integrity and full reporting, there is a promise of improved data accuracy through combined reporting between the BLS and OSHA (Pierce 2017).

Measures of Staffing

No one measure exists that effectively represents nurse staffing. A challenge with staffing measures is that many have yet to be standardized with universally accepted definitions and formulas. Only two unit-level nurse staffing measures are endorsed by the National Quality Forum (NQF): nursing hours per patient day (NQF 2019a) and skill mix (NQF 2019b). As detailed by NQF, both measures are intended for use in the hospital/inpatient setting only and are applicable to nursing units such as medical-surgical, pediatric, and critical care. The National Database of Nursing Quality Indicators® has expanded these nurse staffing measures to other unit types such as emergency department, perioperative units, labor and delivery, and ambulatory care.

Considerations for Selecting NWE Measures

When selecting NWE measures to use within the QHOM, one needs to be mindful of the measurement level—micro, meso, or macro. The QHOM allows for measurement at one level or more than one level. For example, nurse job satisfaction can be measured at the individual or micro-level. At the meso-level, nursing is practiced as a group on units in many work settings such as acute and long-term care (Kendall-Gallagher and Blegen 2009). Therefore, a patient will likely be cared for by multiple group members. Thus, some measures may need to be at the unit level. Examples are staffing (nursing hours per patient day and skill mix) and nursing specialty certification (percent of nurses on the unit with a nursing specialty certification, which captures nurse workgroup competence). Alternately, measures can be at more than one level. For example, in a typical organizational structure, individual nurses and other clinicians are nested in units or workgroups, units and workgroups are nested in organizations, organizations are often nested in corporate systems, and so forth. As individual nurses and clinicians in workgroups and organizations are exposed to common features, events, and processes over time, they develop consensual views of the workgroup and work environment through interacting and sharing (Kozlowski and Klein 2000). Consensual views of safety culture and morale at the meso-level are examples. These measures are taken at the individual level but are aggregated to the group level for analysis.

System Interventions

In keeping with the QHOM, interventions to enhance NWEs are targeted at the system and client. Further, interventions are generally at the meso-level (unit and organization). They include improving professional relationships, professional autonomy, safety culture, structural empowerment and engagement, appropriate staffing and resources, balanced work schedule, professional advancement opportunities, transformational leadership, and joy in work/clinician well-being. Two intervention programs with demonstrated outcomes (e.g., improved nurse satisfaction, better retention of nursing staff and nursing leaders, higher quality interprofessional teamwork and nursing practice, better fiscal outcomes) are the Magnet Recognition Program® (ANCC n.d.-a) and the Pathway to Excellence (PTE) Recognition Program (ANCC n.d.-b). Both programs are performance-driven organizational (system) level accreditations for nursing excellence from the American Nurses Credentialing Center. Magnet Recognition also includes excellence in patient outcomes. Magnet- and Pathway-designated institutions can display the respective ANCC logo on advertisements, publications, and presentations—offering a significant marketing, recruitment, and reputational advantage. To achieve Magnet or PTE designation, healthcare organizations undergo a lengthy rigorous journey in which they conduct self-assessments, create opportunities for organizational advancement, and transform the organizational culture. For example, on average, it takes an institution 4.25 years to attain Magnet designation (Jayawardhana et al. 2014). Accreditation lasts 4 years. Currently (October 2020), there are 540 Magnet and 192 PWE facilities worldwide, with only a few outside the USA.

Magnet® Recognition

Magnet Recognition has been in place for 30 years. It is based on the Magnet Model of 14 Forces of Magnetism that include nursing leadership, management style, organizational structure, personnel polies and programs, community and healthcare organization, image of nursing, professional development, professional models of care, consultations and resources, autonomy, nurses as teachers, interdisciplinary relationships, quality improvement, and quality of care (ANCC n.d.-a). The Forces are categorized into five Magnet Model components of transformation leadership, structural empowerment, exemplary professional practice, empirical quality results, and new knowledge, innovation, and improvement (ANCC n.d.-a). For instance, the Forces of Magnetism "nurse leadership" and "management style" are categorized under the model component of transformational leadership. The Magnet Model provides the overarching constructs for nursing practice and research. Nursing excellence drives measurable improvements in organizational outcomes related to safety, quality patient care, and financial savings. As part of the program, Magnet organizations are required to measure and report nurse job satisfaction, nurse-sensitive clinical measures, and patient satisfaction (ANCC n.d.-a). Because Magnet Recognition is resource intensive, both personnel and financial, mostly larger hospitals have pursued it.

Pathway to Excellence® Recognition

The newer ANCC recognition program is the Pathway to Excellence Program (PTE). In 2003, the State of Texas developed the "Nurse-Friendly" program mainly for smaller hospitals that do not have the organizational resources to become Magnet accredited (Merviglia et al. 2008). In 2007, the ANCC acquired the program, renamed it the Pathway to Excellence program, and offered it to hospitals nationwide and internationally. PTE differs from Magnet Recognition in several ways, but the most significant difference is that the performance standards exclusively address the work environment and nursing engagement. Patient and quality outcomes are not directly measured as a part of the criteria for recognition. PTE Recognition entails demonstrated achievement of six standards—shared decision-making, leadership, safety, quality, well-being, and professional development—and evidence to support 181 performance elements.

Implications and Future Directions

As depicted in the QHOM, the system characteristic of a healthy NWE is linked with improved outcomes—nurse, patient, and organizational. Over 40 years of nursing leadership and research have provided growing knowledge and improvement of NWEs. Current and future challenges include how to improve joy in work and clinician well-being, ways to support clinician resilience and organizational agility, methods for building stronger cultures to promote safety, and ways to eliminate systemic racism in health care.

Improving Joy in Work, Clinician Well-Being, and Resilience

The aforementioned NAM Conceptual Model of Factors Affecting Clinician Well-Being and Resilience provides a framework for future research in nursing practice and education to increase understanding of the phenomena of joy in work, clinician well-being, and resilience. These phenomena are affected by patient well-being, clinician-patient relationships, and other individual and external factors. More importantly, effective strategies for enhancing joy in work, clinician well-being, and resilience are needed (Brigham et al. 2018). The model's application should be embraced by nurses, educators, researchers, and scholars. Further examination of the linkages among joy, well-being, and resilience will likely be solidified, and additional improvement strategies developed.

Building a Stronger Safety Culture

Within the IHI Framework for Safe, Reliable, and Effective Care (Frankel et al. 2017), the concept of leadership needs further development. Senior leaders hold the keys to safety performance through culture change (Maccoby et al. 2013). Safety-specific transformational leadership (SSTFL) is one area that could assist with this change. However, it is an under-researched concept in health care, especially when contrasted with other high-risk industries (Fischer 2016). Transportation,

manufacturing, aviation, and nuclear power have monitored and studied safety performance and outcomes much longer than health care and, subsequently, have much
better safety track records than health care (Barling et al. 2002; Conchie and Donald
2009; Conchie et al. 2012; Curcuruto et al. 2016; de Vries et al. 2016; Kelloway
et al. 2006). In contrast with health care, these other industries have fully embraced
the concept of SSTFL (Fischer 2016). SSTFLs promote individual and collective
safety efforts and drive a healthy safety climate, thereby potentially influencing
patients' and workers' health and well-being. Both research and development of
consistent language to describe the complexity of safety phenomena provide current
and future leaders at all levels with knowledge and tools that help decrease harm to
patients and workers from preventable error, as well as generate new ways of thinking about safety (Fischer 2016).

Addressing the Quintuple Aim of Systemic Racism

Given the recent introduction of the Quintuple Aim (Matheny et al. 2019)—which
adds equity and inclusion to the Quadruple Aim—considerations for equity and
inclusion in health care and the NWE require sharper focus. Paradigms previously
accepted in health care are now being challenged and changed. Health and healthcare disparities based on ethnicity, race, gender identity, and sexual orientation are
no longer considered acceptable or unchangeable (Bonvicini 2017; Wheeler and
Bryant 2017). Public awareness of systemic racism and momentum for change is
growing. Chapter 3 contains a discussion of nursing workforce diversity issues.
Further discussion and consideration of the timely and appropriate Quintuple Aim
and its effect on the NWE and, subsequently, patient, nurse, and organizational
outcomes are needed.

References

Agency for Healthcare Research and Quality (AHRQ) (n.d.) Surveys on patient safety culture.
    https://www.ahrq.gov/sops/index.html
American Association of Colleges of Nursing (2003) Hallmarks of the professional practice envi-
    ronment. https://www.aacnnursing.org/News-Information/Position-Statements-White-Papers/
    Hallmarks-Practice
American Association of Critical-Care Nurses (2016) AACN standards for establishing and sus-
    taining healthy work environments: a journey to excellence, 2nd edn. American Association of
    Critical-Care Nurses, Aliso Viejo, CA
American Association of Critical-Care Nurses (n.d.) AACN healthy work environment assess-
    ment tool. https://www.aacn.org/nursing-excellence/healthy-work-environments/aacn-healthy-
    work-environment-assessment-tool
American Nurses Association (2015) Incivility, bullying, and workplace violence. https://www.
    nursingworld.org/practice-policy/nursing-excellence/official-position-statements/id/incivility-
    bullying-and-workplace-violence/
American Nurses Association (2019) Nurse staffing advocacy. https://www.nursingworld.org/
    practice-policy/nurse-staffing/nurse-staffing-advocacy/

American Nurses Association (2020) ANA's principles for nurse staffing, 3rd edn. American Nurses Association, Silver Spring, MD

American Nurses Association (n.d.) The nurses bill of rights. https://www.nursingworld.org/practice-policy/work-environment/

American Nurses Credentialing Center (n.d.-a) ANCC magnet recognition program. https://www.nursingworld.org/organizational-programs/magnet/

American Nurses Credentialing Center (n.d.-b) ANCC pathway to excellence program. https://www.nursingworld.org/organizational-programs/pathway/

American Organization for Nursing Leadership (2019) Elements of a healthy practice environment. https://www.aonl.org/elements-healthy-practice-environment

Anusiewicz CV, Shirey MR, Patrician PA (2019) Workplace bullying and newly licensed registered nurses. Workplace Health Saf 67:250–261. https://doi.org/10.1177/2165079919827046

Barling J, Loughlin C, Kelloway EK (2002) Development and test of a model linking safety-specific transformational leadership and occupational safety. J Appl Psychol 87(3):488–496. https://doi.org/10.1037/0021-9010.87.3.488

Bodenheimer T, Sinsky C (2014) From triple to quadruple aim: care of the patient requires care of the provider. Ann Fam Med 12(6):573–576. https://doi.org/10.1370/afm.1713

Bonvicini KA (2017) LGBT healthcare disparities: what progress have we made? Patient Educ Couns 100(12):2357–2361. https://doi.org/10.1016/j.pec.2017.06.003

Boyle DK, Baernholdt M, Adams J, McBride S, Harper E, Poghosyan L, Manges K (2019) Improve nurses' well-being and joy in work: implement true interprofessional teams and address electronic documentation systems usability issues. Nurs Outlook 67:783–789. https://doi.org/10.1016/j.outlook.2019.10.002

Brigham T, Barden C, Dopp AL, Hengerer A, Kaplan J, Malone B, Martin C, McHugh M, Nora LM (2018) A journey to construct an all-encompassing conceptual model of factors affecting clinician well-being and resilience. NAM Perspectives. Discussion Paper. National Academy of Medicine, Washington, DC. https://doi.org/10.31478/201801b. https://nam.edu/journey-construct-encompassing-conceptual-model-factors-affecting-clinician-well-resilience/

Bureau of Labor Statistics (2017) Survey of occupational injuries and illnesses. https://www.bls.gov/opub/hom/soii/pdf/soii.pdf

Bureau of Labor Statistics (2018) Occupational injuries and illnesses among registered nurses. https://www.bls.gov/opub/mlr/2018/article/occupational-injuries-and-illnesses-among-registered-nurses.htm

Cimiotti JP, Aiken LH, Sloane DM, Wu ES (2012) Nurse staffing, burnout, and health care-associated infection. Am J Infect Control 40(6):486–490. https://doi.org/10.1016/j.ajic.2012.02.029

Clark CM, Barbosa-Leiker C, Gill LM, Nguyen D (2015) Revision and psychometric testing of the Incivility in Nurse Education (INE) Survey: introducing the INE-R. J Nurs Educ 54:306–315. https://doi.org/10.3928/01484834-20150515-01

Conchie SM, Donald IJ (2009) The moderating role of safety-specific trust on the relation between safety-specific leadership and safety citizenship behaviors. J Occup Health Psychol 14(2):137–147. https://doi.org/10.1037/a0014247

Conchie SM, Taylor PJ, Donald IJ (2012) Promoting safety voice with safety-specific transformational leadership: the mediating role of two dimensions of trust. J Occup Health Psychol 17(1):105–115. https://doi.org/10.1037/a0025101

Copanitsanou P, Fotos N, Brokalaki H (2017) Effects of work environment on patient and nurse outcomes. Br J Nurs 26(3):172–176. https://doi.org/10.12968/bjon.2017.26.3.172

Curcuruto M, Mearns KJ, Mariani MG (2016) Proactive role-orientation toward workplace safety: psychological dimensions, nomological network and external validity. Saf Sci 87:144–155. https://doi.org/10.1016/j.ssci.2016.03.007

de Vries J, de Koster R, Stam D (2016) Safety does not happen by accident: antecedents to a safer warehouse. Prod Oper Manag 25(8):1377–1390. https://doi.org/10.1111/poms.12546

DiCuccio MH (2015) The relationship between patient safety culture and patient outcomes: a systematic review. J Pat Saf 11(3):135–142. https://doi.org/10.1097/PTS.0000000000000058

Donabedian A (1966) Evaluating the quality of medical care. Milbank Mem Fund Quart 44(part 2):166–206

Donabedian A (1988) The quality of care: how can it be assessed? JAMA 260:1743–1748. https:// doi.org/10.1001/jama.1988.03410120089033

Dyrbye LN, Shanafelt TD, Sinsky CA, Cipriano PF, Bhatt J, Ommaya A, West CP, Meyers D (2017) Burnout among health care professionals: a call to explore and address this under- recognized threat to safe, high quality care. Discussion Paper. NAM Perspectives. National Academy of Medicine, Washington, DC. https://doi.org/10.31478/201707b. https://nam.edu/ wp-content/uploads/2017/07/Burnout-Among-Health-Care-Professionals-A-Call-to-Explore- and-Address-This-Underrecognized-Threat.pdf

Edward K, Ousey K, Warelow P, Lui S (2014) Nursing and aggression in the workplace: a system- atic review. Br J Nurs 23:653–659. https://doi.org/10.12968/bjon.2014.23.12.653

Einarsen S, Hoel H, Notelaers G (2009) Measuring exposure to bullying and harassment at work: validity, factor structure and psychometric properties of the Negative Acts Questionnaire- Revised. Work Stress 23(1):24–44. https://doi.org/10.1080/02678370902815673

Einarsen S, Hoel H, Zapf D, Cooper CL (2011) The concept of bullying and harassment at work: the European tradition. In: Einarsen S, Hoel H, Zapf D, Cooper CL (eds) Bullying and harass- ment in the workplace. Developments in theory, research, and practice, 2nd edn. CRC Press, Taylor and Francis Group, New York, pp 3–39

Fischer SA (2016) Transformational leadership in nursing: a concept analysis. J Adv Nurs 72(11):2644–2653. https://doi.org/10.1111/jan.13049

Frankel A, Haraden C, Federico F, Lenoci-Edwards J (2017) A Framework for safe, reliable, and effective care. White paper. Institute for Healthcare Improvement and Safe and Reliable Health- care, Cambridge, MA. http://www.ihi.org/resources/Pages/IHIWhitePapers/Framework-Safe- Reliable-Effective-Care.aspx.

Grant S, Davidson J, Manges K, Dermenchyan A, Wilson E, Dowdell E (2020) Creating healthful work environments to deliver on the quadruple aim. J Nurs Administr 50:314–321. https://doi. org/10.1097/NNA.0000000000000891

Halm M (2019) The influence of appropriate staffing and healthy work environments on patient and nurse outcomes. Am J Crit Care 28:152–156. https://doi.org/10.4037/ajcc2019938

Institute of Medicine (2000) To err is human: building a safer health system. The National Acad- emies Press, Washington, DC

Institute of Medicine (2004) Keeping patients safe: transforming the work environments of nurses. The National Academies Press, Washington, DC

International Council of Nurses (2017) Position statement: prevention and management of work- place violence. https://www.icn.ch/sites/default/files/inline-files/PS_C_Prevention_mgmt_ workplace_violence_0.pdf

Jayawardhana J, Welton JM, Lindrooth RC (2014) Is there a business case for magnet hospitals? Estimates of the cost and revenue implications of becoming a magnet. Med Care 52:400–406. https://doi.org/10.1097/MLR.0000000000000092

Johnson Foundation's Wingspread Center (2017) A gold bond to restore joy in nursing: a col- laborative exchange of ideas to address burnout [White paper]. https://ajnoffthecharts.com/ wp-content/uploads/2017/04/NursesReport_Burnout_Final.pdf

Kelloway EK, Mullen J, Francis L (2006) Divergent effects of transformational and passive leader- ship on employee safety. J Occup Health Psychol 11(1):76–86. https://doi.org/10.1037/1076- 8998.11.1.76

Kendall-Gallagher D, Blegen MA (2009) Competence and certification of registered nurses and safety of patients in intensive care units. Am J Crit Care 18(2):106–113. https://doi.org/10.4037/ ajcc2009487

Kramer M, Schmalenberg C, Maguire P (2010) Nine structures and leadership practices essential for a magnetic (healthy) work environment. Nurs Adm Q 34(1):4–17. https://doi.org/10.1097/ NAQ.0b013e3181c95ef4

Kozlowski SWJ, Klein KJ (2000) A multilevel approach to theory and research in organizations: contextual, temporal, and emergent processes. Jossey-Bass, San Francisco

Lake ET (2002) Development of the practice environment scale of the nursing work index. Res Nurs Health 25:172–177. https://doi.org/10.1002/nur.10032

Lake ET, Sanders J, Duan R, Riman KA, Schoenauer KM, Chen Y (2019) A meta-analysis of the associations between the nurse work environment in hospitals and 4 sets of outcomes. Med Care 57:353–361. https://doi.org/10.1097/MLR.0000000000001109

Larrabee JH, Wu Y, Persily CA, Simoni PS, Johnston PA, Marcischak TL, Mott CL, Gladden SD (2010) Influence of stress resiliency on RN job satisfaction and intent to stay. West J Nurs Res 32(1):81–102. https://doi.org/10.1177/0193945909343293

Lee SE, Scott LD (2018) Hospital nurses' work environment characteristics and patient safety outcomes: a literature review. West J Nurs Res 40:121–145. https://doi.org/10.1177/0193945916666071

Lulat Z, Blain-McLeod J, Grinspun D, Penney T, Harripaul-Yhap A, Rey M (2018) Seventy years of RN effectiveness: a database development project to inform best practice. Worldviews Evid-Based Nurs 15(4):281–289. https://doi.org/10.1111/wvn.12283

Maccoby M, Norman C, Norman C, Margolies R (2013) Transforming health care leadership: a guide to improve patient care, decrease costs, and improve population health. Jossey-Bass, San Francisco

Manomenidis G, Panagopoulou E, Montgomery A (2019) Resilience in nursing: the role of internal and external factors. J Nurs Manag 27(1):172–178. https://doi.org/10.1111/jonm.12662

Marshall ES, Broome ME (2017) Transformational leadership in nursing: from expert clinician to influential leader, 2nd edn. Springer, New York

Matheny M, Thadaney Israni S, Ahmed M, Whicher D (eds) (2019) Artificial intelligence in health care: the hope, the hype, the promise, the peril. NAM Special Publication. National Academy of Medicine, Washington, DC. https://nam.edu/artificial-intelligence-special-publication/?gclid=Cj0KCQiAh4j-BRCsARIsAGeV12DBAk8QqNdnJmMXvt6j9f7ciXkBP6sSXjwy-BIfMIZQzvu3ZnxLqbEaAomhEALw_wcB

McAllister M (2013) Resilience: a personal attribute, social process and key professional resource for the enhancement of the nursing role. Profess Infermieris 66(1):55–62. https://doi.org/10.7429/pi.2013.661055

McBride S, Tietze M, Robichaux C, Stokes L, Weber E (2018) Identifying and addressing ethical issues with use of electronic health records. Online J Issues Nurs 23:1. https://doi.org/10.3912/OJIN.Vol23No01Man05

McClure ML, Poulin MA, Sovie MD, Wandelt MA (2002) Magnet hospitals: attraction and retention of professional nurses (The original study). In: McClure ML, Hinshaw AS (eds) Magnet hospitals revisited: attraction and retention of professional nurses. American Nurses Publishing, Silver Spring

Mealer M, Hodapp R, Conrad D, Dimidjian S, Rothbaum B et al (2017) Designing a resilience program for critical care nurses. AACN Adv Crit Care 28:359–365. https://doi.org/10.4037/aacnacc2017252

Medicare.gov (n.d.) Linking quality to payment. https://www.medicare.gov/hospitalcompare/linking-quality-to-payment.html

Merviglia M, Grobe SJ, Tabone S, Wainwright M, Shelton S, Yu L, Jordan C (2008) Nurse-friendly hospital project: enhancing nurse retention and quality of care. J Nurs Care Qual 23:305–313. https://doi.org/10.1097/01.NCQ.0000314728.65721.7c

Mitchell PH, Ferketich S, Jennings BM (1998) Quality health outcomes model. Image J Nurs Sch 30(1):43–46. https://doi.org/10.1111/j.1547-5069.1998.tb01234.x

Nascimento A, Jesus E (2020) Nursing work environment and patient outcomes in a hospital context: a scoping review. JONA 50:261–266. https://doi.org/10.1097/NNA.0000000000000881

National Quality Forum (2019a) Nursing hours per patient day. https://www.qualityforum.org/QPS/0205

National Quality Forum (2019b) Skill mix. https://www.qualityforum.org/QPS/0204

National Steering Committee for Patient Safety (2020) Safer together: a national action plan to advance patient safety. Institute for Healthcare Improvement, Boston, MA. www.ihi.org/SafetyActionPlan

Notelaer G, Einarsen S, De Witte H, Vermunt JK (2006) Measuring exposure to bullying at work: the validity and advantages of the latent class cluster approach. Work Stress 20(4):289–302. https://doi.org/10.1080/02678370601071594

Occupational Safety and Health Act of 1970 (1970) Public Law 91-596, 84 STAT. 1590. https://www.osha.gov/laws-regs/oshact/completeoshact

Padesky CA, Mooney KA (2012) Strengths-based cognitive-behavioural therapy: a four-step model to build resilience. Clin Psychol Psychother 19(4):283–290. https://doi.org/10.1002/cpp.1795

Perlo J, Balik B, Swensen S, Kabcenell A, Landsman J, Feeley D (2017) IHI framework for improving joy in work [White paper]. http://www.ihi.org/resources/Pages/IHIWhitePapers/Framework-Improving-Joy-in-Work.aspx

Petit Dit Dariel O, Regnaux JP (2015) Do Magnet®-accredited hospitals show improvements in nurse and patient outcomes compared to non-Magnet hospitals: a systematic review. JBI Database System Rev Implement Rep 13(6):168–219. https://doi.org/10.11124/jbisrir-2015-2262

Pierce B (2017) Prospects for combining survey and non-survey data sources to improve estimated counts of certain work-related injuries. https://www.bls.gov/iif/jsm2017-soii-osha.pdf

Pipe TB, Buchda VL, Launder S et al (2012) Building personal and professional resources of resilience and agility in the healthcare workplace. Stress Health 28(1):11–22. https://doi.org/10.1002/smi.1396

Plsek P (2001) Redesigning health care with insights from the science of complex adaptive systems. In: Institute of medicine committee on quality of health care in America. Crossing the Quality Chasm. National Academy Press, Washington, DC, pp 309–322

Schmalenberg C, Kramer M (2008) Essentials of a productive nurse work environment. Nurs Res 57:2–13. https://doi.org/10.1097/01.NNR.0000280657.04008.2a

Serpa S, Ferreira CM (2019) Micro, meso, and macro levels of social analysis. Int J Soc Stud 7(3). https://doi.org/10.11114/ijsss.v7i3.4223

Sexton JB, Helmreich RL, Neilands TB et al (2006) The safety attitudes questionnaire: psychometric properties, benchmarking data, and emerging research. BMC Health Serv Res 6:44. https://doi.org/10.1186/1472-6963-6-44; https://psnet.ahrq.gov/issue/safety-attitudes-questionnaire-psychometric-properties-benchmarking-data-and-emerging#

Sikka R, Morath JM, Leape L (2015) The quadruple aim: care, health, cost and meaning in work. BMJ Qual Saf 24:608–610. https://doi.org/10.1136/bmjqs-2015-004160

Sorra J, Gray L, Streagle S, Famolaro T, Yount N, Behm J (2016) AHRQ Hospital Survey on Patient Safety Culture: User's Guide. AHRQ Publication No. 15-0049-EF (Replaces 04-0041). Agency for Healthcare Research and Quality, Rockville, MD. http://www.ahrq.gov/professionals/quality-patient-safety/patientsafetyculture/hospital/index.html

Stagman-Tyrer D (2014) Resiliency and the nurse leader: the importance of equanimity, optimism, and perseverance. Nurs Manag 45(6):46–50. https://doi.org/10.1097/01.NUMA.0000449763.99370.7f

Stalpers D, de Brouwer BJM, Kaljouw MJ, Schuurmans MJ (2015) Associations between characteristics of the nurse work environment and five nurse-sensitive patient outcomes in hospitals: a systematic review of literature. Int J Nurs Stud 52:817–835. https://doi.org/10.1016/j.ijnurstu.2015.01.005

The Joint Commission (2001) Health care at the crossroads: strategies for addressing the evolving nursing crisis. https://www.jointcommission.org/-/media/deprecated-unorganized/imported-assets/tjc/system-folders/topics-library/health_care_at_the_crossroadspdf.pdf?db=web&hash=262C8CFD6F7CAFE1B083A6E77CB52D6B

Ulrich B, Barden C, Cassidy L, Varn-Davis N (2019) Critical care nurse work environments 2018: findings and implications. Crit Care Nurse 39(2):67–84. https://doi.org/10.4037/ccn2019605

Wei H, Sewell KA, Woody G, Rose MA (2018) The state of the science of nurse work environments in the United States: a systematic review. Int J Nurs Sci 5:287–300. https://doi.org/10.1016/j.ijnss.2018.04.010

Wheeler SM, Bryant AS (2017) Racial and ethnic disparities in health and health care. Obstet Gynecol Clin N Am 44(1):1–11. https://doi.org/10.1016/j.ogc.2016.10.001

Zhang YY, Han WL, Qin W et al (2018) Extent of compassion satisfaction, compassion fatigue and burnout in nursing: a meta-analysis. J Nurs Manag 26:810–819. https://doi.org/10.1111/jonm.12589

Workflow, Turbulence, and Cognitive Complexity

Bonnie Mowinski Jennings

Introduction

The concept of workflow is problematic when applied to nurses and clinical practice. Flow suggests smoothness and continuity. Rather than smooth, nurses' work is inherently turbulent; the flow is nonlinear (Phillips 2018), disorderly, unstable (Gleick 1987), and "irregular" (Cornell et al. 2011, p. 410). Turbulence is evident as nurses move among patients throughout the shift as well as to and from centralized work areas such as the nurses' station and medication rooms (Cornell et al. 2010; Jennings et al. 2011; Potter et al. 2004; Tucker and Spear 2006). Turbulence is the unifying characteristic in the patterns of work complexity identified by Ebright and colleagues (Ebright et al. 2003). The importance of scrutinizing turbulence was affirmed by Browne and Braden (2020), who noted, "managing turbulence rather than patient needs is becoming a priority for nurses" (p. 184). Turbulence is perpetuated by the highly unpredictable nature of nurses' work. For example, nurses know that patient admissions will occur, but it is difficult to anticipate when they will happen (Jennings et al. 2013). Although medication administration seems orderly and predictable, it is filled with turbulence (Jennings et al. 2011), thereby altering workflow. As the workflow turbulence increases, the cognitive work of nursing becomes increasingly complex. The focus of this chapter, therefore, relates to workflow, turbulence, and cognitive complexity.

B. M. Jennings (✉)
Nell Hodgson Woodruff School of Nursing, Emory University, Atlanta, GA, USA
e-mail: bonnie.m.jennings@emory.edu

© Springer Nature Switzerland AG 2021
M. Baernholdt, D. K. Boyle (eds.), *Nurses Contributions to Quality Health Outcomes*, https://doi.org/10.1007/978-3-030-69063-2_5

Workflow, Turbulence, and Cognitive Complexity: Specific Linkages with the QHOM

The primary construct from the QHOM (Mitchell et al. 1998) showcased in this chapter is the system (organization and microsystem). Workflow and turbulence are major concepts within the system construct. Features of turbulence with the most robust evidence for illustrating its effect on nurses' work include interruptions, handoffs, and patient turnover. By reframing the client construct within the QHOM as the nurse, the way is opened to address the cognitive (mental) workload and resulting cognitive complexity that often stem from a turbulent workflow. To date, interventions to improve nurses' work (e.g., smoothing workflow and mitigating turbulence) remain few. Those interventions that have been tried (i.e., not interrupting medication administration) have not had an enduring effect in making the system better and reducing nurses' cognitive complexity.

Consequently, the focus in this chapter is on describing the characteristics within the system (turbulence and workflow) and the client (nurses' cognitive workload and complexity) that affect nurse outcomes (work stress and cognitive failures) (Fig. 5.1). Interventions will receive only brief mention. Nursing has been known as a high-stress profession since the 1960s (Menzies 1960). The role of turbulence as a potential contributor to work stress is a new slant on nurses' work conditions. Therefore, the chapter aims to depict the nature of nurses' work in the twenty-first century by exploring workflow, turbulence, cognitive workload, and cognitive complexity in acute care settings.

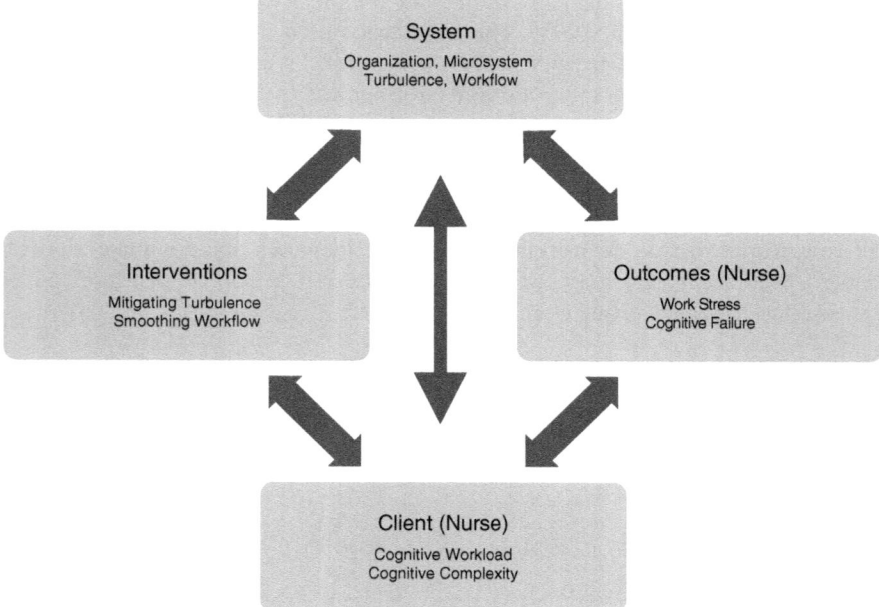

Fig. 5.1 Framework for workflow, turbulence, and cognitive complexity

System Characteristics

Workflow

The workflow concept originated in the early 1900s as factory managers sought to remove bottlenecks and improve efficiency in manufacturing plants (Derksen 2014). According to the dictionary, workflow is a "sequence of steps involved in moving from the beginning to the end of a work process" (https://www.meeriam-webster. com/dictionary/workflow). Cain and Hague (2008) proposed that workflow includes a set of tasks grouped chronologically into a process and the people and resources needed to complete the tasks. Thus, workflow suggests a pattern that is repeatable such as the work done on an assembly line. Some quality improvement initiatives are designed to enhance workflow. For instance, "lean" is a set of principles adapted from The Toyota Production System that focus on ways to eliminate waste, especially wasted time (i.e., waiting), by standardizing practices (Lawal et al. 2014). Despite the usefulness of importing principles from other industries (e.g., airlines, manufacturing), healthcare is less predictable than machines where parts and interconnections work linearly. Instead, healthcare is a human system with people as the parts, not bolts and screws. Variation is thus inherent in healthcare because of the human element.

Workflow in Healthcare

As a human system, healthcare is considered a complex adaptive system (CAS) where unpredictability, nonlinearity, and surprises prevail (McDaniel et al. 2003; Plsek 2001). In CASs, the unexpected is normative (Plsek 2001). Features of CASs are chaos (Plsek 2001), disorder, instability (Gleick 1987), and nonlinear flow, yielding similarities to turbulence (Phillips 2018). Although commonly used, turbulence is an unsolved problem in physics with tremendous practical importance; the most important flows are turbulent (Phillips 2018). Therefore, it is conceivable that turbulence reflects workflow in healthcare systems.

The lack of smooth workflow in healthcare often stems from poorly designed systems. System problems that impede workflow or facilitate turbulence were termed "operational failures" by Tucker (2004) and "performance obstacles" by Gurses et al. (2009). Such problems illustrate why Carayon and colleagues stated, "The entire [healthcare] work system needs to be well designed for optimal performance" (Carayon et al. 2007, p. i54), emphasizing that patient safety is about the system. Similarly, Karsh and colleagues advocated for system redesign to improve performance and reduce hazards, highlighting that systems need to support the healthcare professionals who are delivering care (Karsh et al. 2006). The need to support staff who work in healthcare systems is at the heart of a recent report from the National Academy of Medicine that focuses on clinician burnout and professional well-being (National Academies of Sciences, Engineering, and Medicine 2019).

Nevertheless, turbulent workflow prevails in healthcare settings. Altered workflow has been linked to surgical errors (Wiegmann et al. 2007). Moreover, even when systems are redesigned and the desired goals achieved, there may also be unintended, undesirable consequences. Such unintended consequences are illustrated by investigators who assessed hospital redesign focused on enhancing patient-centeredness (Mikesell and Bromley 2012). Along with making the hospital more patient centered, the changes also created many inconveniences for the staff, especially nurses: Walking and telephone interruptions increased; time at the bedside and face-to-face exchanges with both patients and coworkers decreased (Mikesell and Bromley 2012).

Regardless of system redesign, the idea of workflow for nurses is an oxymoron. "There is little 'flow' in nurse workflow" (Cornell et al. 2010, p. 366); "nurse workflow actually lacks flow" (Myny et al. 2012, p. 432). Instead, nurses' work is characterized by work complexity patterns (Ebright et al. 2003) and as noted earlier, the unifying characteristic in these patterns is turbulence. To understand nurses' work it, therefore, becomes vital to understand turbulence.

Turbulence

Turbulence is a term commonly used in meteorology, oceanography, mathematics, physics, and engineering. In these fields, turbulence characterizes irregularities in flow, such as the up and down currents that may be experienced in an airplane or the choppy seas sometimes experienced on a ship or sailboat. Organizations face turbulence too when changes occur that are "nontrivial, rapid, and discontinuous" (Cameron and Kim 1987, p. 225). Turbulence is further evident when change exceeds an organization's ability to adapt (McCann and Selsky 1984).

Turbulence in Healthcare

More than 35 years ago, Strauss and colleagues noted that hospital work was intrinsically complex and unpredictable (Strauss et al. 1997). Before the 1980s, acute care hospitals were regarded as placid settings, whereas in the 1980s, these same settings were considered turbulent (Beekun and Ginn 1993). The turbulence in the external healthcare environment (e.g., health policies, financing, and regulations) contributed to turbulence in the internal healthcare environment, those conditions within healthcare settings—both at the organizational and unit level (microsystem).

Turbulence in the External Environment

Acute care hospitals were confronted with turbulence in the 1980s when massive external changes were implemented to deal with the skyrocketing cost of healthcare (Bazzoli et al. 2004). The turbulence was primarily due to alterations in healthcare financing and restructuring. The financing changes (i.e., prospective vs. retrospective payment) imposed a business model onto the health systems; the restructuring efforts shifted patients from inpatient to outpatient settings (e.g., ambulatory surgery; Jennings 2008a).

The effects of hospital restructuring exerted a profound influence on the registered nurse's (RN) work role (e.g., less time for direct patient care), workload (a complex combination of higher patient acuity, scheduling, and fluctuating census), and control over work (bureaucratic hierarchy vs. professional, collegial control; Norrish and Rundall 2001). Turbulence has persisted: ongoing, "nontrivial, rapid" (Cameron and Kim 1987, p. 225) changes remain normative in twenty-first-century healthcare. In 2020, major upheaval was experienced in the external environment when the COVID-19 outbreak was deemed a pandemic by the World Health Organization (WHO 2020). The coronavirus pandemic exemplifies how external turbulence may yield turbulence within the internal healthcare environment. Although some external forms of turbulence may be inevitable, others can be reduced, potentially reducing their internal environment effects.

Turbulence in the Internal Environment

Although organizational turbulence is important, the focus here is on the unit level (microsystem) "where the work happens; it is where the 'quality' experienced by the patient is made or lost" (Berwick 2002, p. 84). Work at the unit level in acute care settings is described as occurring in a hyperdynamic, turbulent environment where nurses' workflow is "irregular" (Cornell et al. 2011, p. 410).

Tucker and Spear (2006) referred to the "staccato pace" (p. 650) of nurses' work, suggesting that workflow is choppy, not smooth: nurses switched among patients about every 11 min. They switched among locations about 13 times/hour (Tucker and Spear 2006). Choppy workflow suggests turbulence. In a decade-old characterization of turbulence in the acute care environment, Jennings (2008b) suggested that communication and workload were the major components comprising turbulence. Communication included interruptions, handoffs (where information might be lost), and noise. Workload included large patient assignments, patient turnover (admissions, discharges, transfers), and equipment/supply issues. In a later study, Cornell et al. (2011) connected turbulence to cognition by raising questions about how turbulence features affect critical thinking and the cognitive workload nurses must manage. In Jennings' characterization of turbulence, cognitive workload per se was not addressed (Jennings 2008b). Rather, ideas related to cognitive workload (i.e., decision-making, cognitive stacking, simultaneous demands, unfamiliar work, time pressure) were parsed into the communication and workload components, illustrating the interplay among these workplace characteristics.

Sources of Turbulence in Nurses' Work

Although little research has been done for the explicit purpose of examining turbulence in acute care settings, there is evidence that turbulence disrupts patient safety and quality care. In the 1990s, Salyer (1995) conducted the first known exploration of turbulence in acute care. Nurses on units with more turbulence—defined as higher patient turnover and fluctuating patient acuity—had poorer communication and interpersonal relationships (Salyer 1995). Poor communication is a factor in sentinel events (Comprehensive Accreditation Manual for Hospitals 2013) and preventable adverse events (Gosbee 1998). Poor interpersonal relationships impair teamwork (Chap. 10); together, good communication and teamwork can advance system safety (IHI Multimedia Team 2017). In this way, turbulence may diminish the quality of care.

In 2007, Bosco (2007) completed a secondary analysis using data from the Impact of Unit Characteristics on Patient Outcomes (IMPACT) study where turbulence serendipitously emerged as a latent variable (Verran et al. 2003). The investigators represented turbulence as a composite variable comprised of five constructs: (a) the number of patients per day on a unit, (b) accessibility of needed resources, (c) distance required to access resources, (d) responsiveness of support services, and (e) perceived environmental uncertainty. Bosco (2007) found that turbulence directly affected medication errors and patients' perception of being well cared for, further suggesting a link between turbulence, quality care, patient safety, and patient outcomes.

Jennings et al. (2011, 2013) sought to understand better how turbulence affected patients and staff by conducting an ethnographic study on inpatient medical and surgical units. Medication administration (Jennings et al. 2011) and patient turnover (Jennings et al. 2013) were related to, and at times the source of, turbulence; both were also strongly tied to patient safety and quality care.

Most recently, Browne and Braden (2020) initiated a study to develop a preliminary measure of nursing turbulence in critical care. Their work was prompted by a belief that workload, which does not have a standard definition, was inadequate to encompass all nursing activities. Although there are questions about how turbulence was operationalized, the initial findings illustrated that turbulence and workload are separate concepts, thereby contradicting the conceptual assertion that turbulence is a characteristic of nurses' workload (Swiger et al. 2016). Refinement of the relationship between turbulence and workload warrants further exploration as the turbulent healthcare environment (i.e., lack of smooth workflow) appears to elevate nurses' cognitive workload (Cornell et al. 2011; Myny et al. 2012). Greater cognitive workload contributes to the cognitive complexity of nurses' work. Primary sources of turbulence for which the evidence is most robust include interruptions, handoffs, and patient turnover. Also, nurses may use workarounds to overcome system impediments created by turbulence to get the work done.

Interruptions

Interruptions are characteristic of nurses' work (Jennings et al. 2011) and a significant source of turbulent workflow. More than 20 years ago, it was noted that "being 'interrupted' is an unremarkable and normative experience of nursing practice and one that is taken for granted" (Waterworth et al. 1999, p. 165). More recent explorations illuminating the inseparability of the tasks comprising nurses' work underscore that nursing remains inherently and highly interruptive (Hopkinson and Weigand 2017; Jennings et al. 2011).

Most interruptions (similar although not synonymous terms are distractions and disruptions) are communication and relationship driven (Reed et al. 2018). They are a product of healthcare workers' preference to communicate synchronously, face to face or via the telephone (Coiera and Tombs 1998; Edwards et al. 2009; Fairbanks et al. 2007; Parker and Coiera 2000). They also are a product of verbal interactions with patients (Rivera-Rodriguez and Karsh 2010; Weigl et al. 2017) and patients' families (Rivera-Rodriguez and Karsh 2010).

Technology represents a communication modality that serves as a significant source of interruptions (Chap. 6). Some technologies facilitate human communication (e.g., mobile work phones, patient intercoms). Other technologies communicate with nurses by alarming (e.g., physiological monitors, bar code medication administration [BCMA], intravenous infusion pumps; Powell-Cope et al. 2008; Zuzelo et al. 2008). These technologies exert "a profound impact on workflow" (Aarts et al. 2007, p. S4). When alarms are continually sounding, nurses may experience sensory and cognitive overload, referred to as alarm or alert fatigue (Sendelbach and Funk 2013), which may increase cognitive workload (Woods and Patterson 2001).

Although concerns with patient safety have yielded an emphasis on the potentially harmful effects of interruptions, it is essential to remember that there are benefits as well (Grundgeiger and Sanderson 2009; Hopkinson and Jennings 2013; Li et al. 2012; Rivera-Rodriguez and Karsh 2010). For instance, interruptions may direct attention to avoiding a medication error or creating a pause that might otherwise have yielded an error. Thus, reducing or stopping interruptions is unrealistic and perhaps even unwise. For the most part, however, interruptions are viewed as undesirable.

The Anatomy of an Interruption
Interruptions are highly complicated phenomena due, in part, to the many components comprising an interruption. Components include the complexity of the primary task, the duration of the interruption (longer interruptions have a bigger impact), the type of interruption, when the interruption occurs in the task sequence (interruptions that occur at the beginning of a task are the least disruptive; Couffe and Michael 2017; Magrabi et al. 2011), and whether memory prompts are used to facilitate recovery after an interruption (Coiera 2012). Additional considerations surrounding interruptions include the complexity of both the primary and interrupting tasks, the similarity of the primary and interrupting tasks, and the interruption's modality (e.g., face to face or a device alarm; Magrabi et al. 2011).

Regardless of the components comprising an interruption, all interruptions share three attributes: (a) intrusion of a secondary, unplanned, unscheduled task; (b) a break in continuity when the primary task currently in progress is suspended unexpectedly before its completion; and (c) the resumption of the primary task after the interruption (Brixey et al. 2007). An often overlooked feature of interruptions is that they occur internally; people can choose to acknowledge or ignore an interruption regardless of the interruption source (e.g., people, telephones, alarms; Brixey et al. 2007; Jett and George 2003; Rivera-Rodriguez and Karsh 2010). Such choices often come easier for more experienced nurses (Patterson et al. 2011).

An important feature of interruptions involves the temporal context of nurses' work. When time is fixed, such as with shift lengths, interruptions compete for time, potentially contributing to a sense of feeling hurried and fostering the use of workarounds (Brown 2019; Coiera 2012). Over 20 years ago, Perlow (1999) referred to time pressure at work, the sense of having too much to do and not enough time to do it, as "time famine" (p. 57). More recently, Krichbaum et al. (2011) addressed how unexpected occurrences during a nurse's shift create a sense of time scarcity.

Nevertheless, managing time in the context of an interruption-filled environment is accomplished by task-switching and multitasking, both of which affect cognition. Task-switching involves shifting from one task to another (Rubinstein et al. 2001; Walter et al. 2014). For instance, a nurse might stop medication administration to answer a question from a family member. By contrast, multitasking involves doing more than one task at a time (Mark 2015; Morgan et al. 2013; Walter et al. 2014). For instance, a nurse might continue with medication administration while answering a mobile work telephone call.

Multitasking is more common than task-switching. Findings from a US study showed that nurses on inpatient units used multitasking 34% of the time (Kalisch and Aebersold 2010). Findings from an Australian study showed that of 28,809 tasks observed among nurses on inpatient units, 800 involved task-switching and 4482 involved multitasking (Walter et al. 2014). This amount of multitasking equates to dealing with 14.1 multitasking events/hour (Walter et al. 2014), close to twice the number of task-switching events. Multitasking has many additional considerations. These include whether the multitasking is voluntary (internally motivated; the individual chooses) or forced (externally prompted) and the task modalities involved (e.g., button pressing, visual, auditory; Douglas et al. 2017). Issues surrounding task-switching and multitasking further reveal the turbulent nature of nurses' workflow.

Interruptions, including task-switching and multitasking, may create a perception of higher workload (Grundgeiger and Sanderson 2009; Myny et al. 2012), including higher cognitive workload (Rivera-Rodriguez and Karsh 2010). The causal chain, however, remains unclear. For instance, is it that more interruptions leave workers with perceptions of higher workloads, or is it that higher workloads yield more chances for being interrupted (Coiera 2012; Weigl et al. 2012)?

Handoffs

Numerous terms are used for care transition events (e.g., handoff, handover; Cohen and Hilligoss 2010). From their critical literature review, Cohen and Hilligoss (2010) proposed handoff as the prevailing term defining it as "the exchange between health professionals of information about a patient accompanying either a transfer of control over, or of responsibility for that patient" (p. 494). The care transition itself alters workflow and, if ineffective, these communication events create patient safety risks (Dracup and Morris 2008; Gandhi 2005; Kohn et al. 2001; Ong and Coiera 2011; Wachter and Shojania 2005). The information exchange inherent to handoffs raised concerns with The Joint Commission in 2006 (Friesen et al. 2008). Because of the potential safety risks associated with inadequate communication during handoffs and the complexity involved in handoff communication, patient handoffs were earmarked as a potential sentinel event (The Joint Commission 2017).

Adequate communication, however, is complex and involves more than passing along information. The information must be correct, complete, and understood by the receiver (Hilligoss and Cohen 2011). Thus, a handoff is not a one-way communication event but rather a conversation in which there is "active co-construction of an understanding of the patient" (Cohen et al. 2012, p. 4). Also affecting communication is whether the exchange occurs between individuals from the same profession or between individuals with different professional backgrounds (Chap. 10). Nurses, for instance, tend to focus on the "big picture" using "broad and narrative" descriptions (Leonard et al. 2004, p. i86); physicians tend to focus on bullet points of critical information (Leonard et al. 2004). This chapter focuses on handoffs between nurses, both within-unit handoffs, typically referred to as shift reports, and between-unit handoffs, or intrahospital transfers.

Shift report is a frequently studied, routinely occurring within-unit handoff where nurses ending their shift handoff responsibilities and patient information to nurses starting their shift. Report at shift change creates an anticipatable pause in the usual workflow. The flow of report information, however, is altered by interruptions during the reporting process and high noise levels, such as when a report occurs in a central place like the nurses' station (Staggers and Jennings 2009). Turbulent workflow is also typical during shift reports because oncoming nurses rarely receive reports from a single nurse due to how patient assignments are made. The flow of shift reports becomes choppy or turbulent as nurses go "through a process of 'finding' each other" to give and receive a report (Staggers and Jennings 2009, p. 395). Shift length (e.g., 12 h, 8 h) also adds to the turbulent workflow of shift report. In one of the few investigations in which varied shift schedules were addressed (i.e., a mixture of 8- and 12-h shifts), the schedules were viewed as "disjointed and confused" (Kalisch et al. 2008, p. 134) and an impediment to handoffs.

Templates for standardizing handoffs pertain primarily to shift report handoffs. Yet, these must be viewed with caution because of differing informational needs and expectations among nurses giving reports, nurses receiving the report, and the nurse's level of experience (Carroll et al. 2012; Welsh et al. 2010). Standardized communication protocols are exemplified by the well-known SBAR (Situation, Background, Assessment, Recommendation; Cornell et al. 2013) and the more recently developed I-PASS (Illness severity, Patient summary, Action list, Situation awareness and contingency plans, and Synthesis by the receiver; Starmer et al. 2014, 2017). Although various regulatory agencies recommend standardizing handoffs, the need for a two-way conversation and co-construction with the patient argues against rigid standardization (Hilligoss and Cohen 2011).

Handoffs related to intrahospital transfers involve nurses from different units; a nurse from the sending unit reports to a nurse on the receiving unit. Between-unit handoffs vary based on where the patient is coming from and going to (e.g., from intensive care to acute care; Ong and Coiera 2011). Between-unit handoffs are highly unpredictable because, unlike shift reports, they do not occur at a designated time (Hilligoss and Cohen 2013). Between-unit transfers and their associated handoffs, therefore, create disruptions in care and workflow (Blay et al. 2017; Jennings et al. 2013). Although between-unit handoffs have more layers of complexity than shift report handoffs, between-unit handoffs have received less attention in the literature.

Communication is especially prone to compromise during between-unit hand-offs because patients are moving across unit (Hilligoss and Cohen 2013) and departmental (Ong and Coiera 2011) boundaries, "from one entire clinical microsystem to another" (Beach et al. 2017, p. 1190). Staff from different clinical microsystems do not know each other very well, or at all. The staff from each unit is unaware of what is occurring on the other unit. Also, the nurses involved in the handoff are not co-located, often communicating via telephone, and unable to observe body language.

Regardless of whether nurses are on the sending or receiving units (Ong and Coiera 2011), the turbulent workflow exhibits common properties that alter nurses' work. For instance, delays occur when a nurse on the receiving unit is not available to take the sending unit report. Delays may prolong a patient's stay on the sending unit, disrupting the workflow on that unit, as well as possibly hurrying through the hand-off when it finally occurs, potentially yielding a less complete and accurate report (Abraham and Reddy 2010). Microsystem culture also comes into play. Emergency department (ED) nurses, for example, strive to move patients quickly to be ready for the arrival of more acute patients (Rosenberg et al. 2018). Also, the rapid movement of patients from the ED to inpatient beds is regarded as a quality indicator (www.ihi.org/resources/Pages/Measures/TimefromEDtoInpatientBEdmedian.aspx). Thus, the goals of the ED microsystem may contribute to turbulence on the admitting unit.

The layers of complexity associated with between-unit transfers also involve whether an intermediary is a part of the information exchange. Charge nurses or clinical leaders, for example, may give or take a report, passing the information from or to the bedside nurse (Whittaker and Ball 2000). In these instances, important information often is lost, yielding inadequate handoffs (Lin et al. 2013).

Patient Turnover

Patient arrivals and departures also create disruptions and contribute to turbulent workflow (Blay et al. 2017, 2014). However, patient turnover—admissions, discharges, and transfers—is a major component of nurses' work. When patient turnover is high, workload increases (Myny et al. 2012; Park et al. 2016), and nursing care may become fragmented (Lin et al. 2013).

Much of the interest in patient turnover relates to staffing (Chap. 4). Although the midnight census is commonly used to reflect staffing needs, in a review article, Park et al. (2016) concluded that the midnight census was inadequate because it could lead to understaffing. There also is not a standard way to measure patient turnover rates. Moreover, turnovers vary by day of the week, time of day, and unit type (Park et al. 2016). For instance, Jennings and colleagues found that patient turnover rates were 1.6 times higher on a surgical unit than a medical unit (Jennings et al. 2013). In practical terms, there were times when surgical nurses cared for twice as many patients as suggested by the number of patients at the beginning and end of their shifts because their entire set of patients had turned over—all five or six patients were discharged, and five or six new patients were admitted (Jennings et al. 2013). These findings illustrate that different nursing specialties may be exposed to different turbulence sources from patient turnover. For instance, despite the high turnover in the surgical unit, they could better predict when most patients would arrive based on the operating room schedule. On the medical unit, by contrast, the number of ED and direct admissions was "predictably unpredictable" (Jennings et al. 2013, p. 558).

Misconceptions and nuances involving patient turnover include that the events are not equivalent: they vary by type, whether they can be anticipated, the intensity of the work involved, and the turnover event's timing (Jennings et al. 2013). Evaluating turnover *type* showed that admissions were more turbulent than discharges. There were subtypes within admissions that varied based on how the patient entered an inpatient unit—direct admissions, ED, postanesthesia care, or a transfer from another floor. Direct admissions created the greatest turbulence; they were likened to "a code" because of workflow disruption. *Anticipating* patient turnover was possible with discharges; they were known in advance, offering nurses some ability to plan their shift. The turnover event's *intensity* was related to what tasks were done before the patient reached the unit and how many were left for the admitting nurse to complete. The *timing* of turnover events made a difference in the degree of the turbulent workflow. Turnovers that occurred proximate to shift report created tremendous turbulence—these events were usually admissions with patients moving from one microsystem to another (e.g., ED to acute care). Admissions that were clustered in quick succession, rather than staggered, also were more disruptive. Moreover, regardless of when it occurred, each turnover event was associated with a handoff, creating the potential for a communication failure.

Workarounds as a Sign of Turbulence

Articulation work refers to organizing tasks and workers' efforts "in the service of workflow" to overcome bottlenecks (Strauss 1988, p. 164). Articulation work is used to manage time (Star 1991; Star and Strauss 1999; Strauss 1985, 1988). As time contracts (i.e., more to do in a finite period), the importance of articulation work expands (Hampson and Junor 2005). In more recent years, the idea of workarounds has replaced the concept of articulation work as a way to consider system impediments that obstruct workflow (Koopman and Hoffman 2003). Workarounds are ways to "circumvent or temporarily 'fix' an evident or perceived workflow block" (Debono et al. 2013, p. 4). Thus, workarounds are a form of articulation work (Jennings et al. 2011).

Workarounds, however, tend to be viewed more negatively than positively (Debono et al. 2013). The negative view of workarounds is illustrated in a comment about bar code medication administration (BCMA), where deviations from prescribed protocols were referred to as "violations or workarounds" (Koppel et al. 2008, p. 409). In an extensive analysis of BCMA, however, these same authors concluded that shortcomings of the technology and workflow disruptions "encourage workarounds" (Koppel et al. 2008, p. 408). In general, automated technologies contribute to workarounds (Koopman and Hoffman 2003) and workarounds accompany the introduction of technology into healthcare (Ash et al. 2004; Novak and Lorenzi 2008; Patterson et al. 2002; Pingenot et al. 2009).

At the crux of workarounds is the need for nurses to save time, avoid waiting, and overcome system inefficiencies to care for patients (Brown 2019). Thus, workarounds are not about bad actors, but clumsy system designs and turbulent workflow. Workarounds are best viewed as a sign of turbulence in the environment.

"Understanding nurses' practice and their perception of workaround behaviours is at the heart of … improve[ing] healthcare at the bedside, where care is delivered" (Debono et al. 2013, p. 14).

Client Characteristics

Cognitive Complexity

Whereas workflow and turbulence are system characteristics, cognitive issues relate to the mental demands required of nurses to manage the turbulent workflow (Baethge and Rigotti 2013; Cornell et al. 2011; Grundgeiger and Sanderson 2009; Laxmisan et al. 2007; Myny et al. 2012; Patterson et al. 2011; Rivera-Rodriguez and Karsh 2010; Woods and Patterson 2001). More than the tasks per se, turbulence heightens the cognitive workload that contributes to the cognitive complexity of nurses' work. Nurses "weave together the many facets of the [healthcare] service and create order in a fast flowing and turbulent work environment" (Allen 2004, p. 279). As such, the "nature of nursing practice … involves covert cognitive behaviors as well as overt physical activities …" (Potter et al. 2004, p. 102). The covert behaviors equate to nurses' invisible work (Star and Strauss 1999). Invisible cognitive behaviors like "… attention switching … decisions … play the most critical role" in errors (Zhang et al. 2004, p. 194).

The literature addressing cognition is voluminous. This section is limited to considering the role of turbulence and altered workflow in creating cognitive complexity. The invisible work of nursing—cognitive workload (mental effort) and cognitive stacking—are cognitive challenges that illustrate the cognitive complexity of nurses' work.

Visible and Invisible Work

Nursing is often depicted as a set of visible tasks, many of which are portrayed as straightforward and routine, although few are. The visible tasks overshadow much of nurses' work, the work that is "hidden" (Star 1991, p. 270), reflecting a "tension between formal task descriptions and overt … 'behind the scenes' work" (Star and Strauss 1999, p. 9). Nurses from neonatal, pediatric, and adult intensive care units included invisible work, such as mental and temporal demands, as part of their subjective workload (Tubbs-Cooley et al. 2018). In a synthesis of 54 publications, Allen (2004) identified nurses' overarching role as an intermediary. This role was less visible than the tasks nurses accomplished in caring for individual patients. Intermediary functions included managing the multiple agendas within healthcare systems, managing interprofessional relationships, and serving as "information broker[s]" (Allen 2004, p. 276).

Also, the simplistic view of nurses' work as tasks disguises the cognitive complexity often involved in completing each task. Medication administration exemplifies this complexity; more is involved than following the five rights (right patient, drug, dose, route, time; Grissinger 2010). Moreover, medication work is not a discrete task with identifiable beginnings and endings (Jennings et al. 2011). Instead, medication administration is inseparable from other nursing work because care activities are woven together as nurses strive to manage time well (Jennings et al. 2011), thus increasing the cognitive complexity. Medication administration has mistakenly been referred to as a procedural task executed automatically (Li et al. 2012). The idea of automatic execution is refuted by findings from several studies in which nurses' thought processes and clinical reasoning during medication administration were identified (Dickson and Flynn 2012; Eisenhauer et al. 2007; Jennings et al. 2011; Pingenot et al. 2009). Nurses must also manage interruptions during medication administration (Biron et al. 2009; Dickson and Flynn 2012; Jennings et al. 2011), including those arising from technology and physical space limitations (Jennings et al. 2011). Strategies to "administer as many medications 'on time' as possible" (Jennings et al. 2011, p. 1448) further illustrate that medication administration exemplifies the invisible, highly complex cognitive work that is embedded in a visible task.

Cognitive Workload

Cognition and cognitive abilities are features of cognitive workload. Cognition involves intellectual activities like thinking, reasoning, or remembering (https://www.merriam-webster.com/dictionary/cognitive) and thus relates to information processing. Cognitive abilities involve three interdependent concepts: (a) attention or deciding which stimuli to process and act upon (e.g., working memory; Couffe and Michael 2017; Parker and Coiera 2000); (b) storing information for later retrieval (Grundgeiger and Sanderson 2009; Li et al. 2012; Rivera-Rodriguez and Karsh 2010); and (c) executive processes or goal-directed behavior (e.g., planning, reasoning, problem-solving; Patterson et al. 2011; Sitterding and Ebright 2015).

Cognitive workload refers to short-term or working memory (i.e., attention), where information is actively processed (Parker and Coiera 2000). The limits of working memory were noted in Miller's (1956) classic paper, where he suggested that we can remember seven digits—plus or minus two. Along with its limited capacity, working memory is limited in duration, with accuracy persisting for 20 s or less (Parker and Coiera 2000). When working memory is taxed, in other words when cognitive workload is high, errors are more likely (Reason 1990). Nursing workload measures, however, typically focus on the number of patients assigned to each nurse (Carayon and Gurses 2008; Holden et al. 2011; Swiger et al. 2016), a metric that fails to consider cognitive workload.

Communication, time pressure, and cognitive shifts all contribute to nurses' cognitive workload. Communication events are defined as "any action taken in order to relay information to another clinician" (Edwards et al. 2009, p. 630). Communication may also occur as a part of multitasking, such as completing documentation while talking (Edwards et al. 2009). As noted previously, communication is a major contributor to interruptions. Both high communication load and interruptions create demands on working memory (Parker and Coiera 2000).

Time pressure is also associated with increased cognitive workload and possibly cognitive failure (Elfering et al. 2013). Woods and Patterson (2001) noted that as operational tempo increases and situations become more critical, information processing must also increase to keep pace with the activities, thereby increasing the cognitive workload and yielding greater cognitive complexity. For instance, Grayson et al. (2005) found that nursing personnel, 84% of whom were RNs, reported more errors when they perceived their work conditions as more hectic; errors were often related to missing patient information.

Potter et al. (2004, 2005) added to the understanding of nurses' cognitive workload by illustrating the repetitive pathways nurses traveled, the interruptions nurses experienced, and the cognitive shifts that nurses had to make. For instance, while observing one nurse caring for six patients over 10 h, investigators documented 128 links (physical movement between locations such as a patient's room and the nurse's station), 43 interruptions, and 71 cognitive shifts. These observations illustrate the challenge to short-term memory due to the cognitive shifts involved in task-switching (Potter et al. 2004).

Cognitive Stacking

Ebright et al. (2003) identified three patterns in RN work performance: work complexity, cognitive factors, and care management strategies. One care management strategy was labeled "stacking" and defined as the nurses' ability to "[move] on to other activities to prevent downtime when not able to complete something because of waiting … or the inability to access resources" (Ebright et al. 2003, p. 636). Stacking involves managing time and changing priorities. Nurses constantly shift among tasks as they reorganize their work to avoid waiting (Biron et al. 2009; Ebright et al. 2003; Hall et al. 2010; Jennings et al. 2011; Tucker and Spear 2006) and to alter priorities based on patients' clinical conditions (Ebright et al. 2003; Patterson et al. 2011).

Potter et al. (2005) built on Ebright's idea of stacking (Ebright et al. 2003) and developed a way to calculate cognitive stacking to reflect the cognitive demands nurses handle. Based on observations of seven RNs, Potter et al. (2005) determined that nurses managed an average cognitive stack of 11 tasks and a maximum cognitive stack of 16. Both the average and the maximum stack exceed Miller's (1956) magic number of working memory being able to handle seven plus or minus two, illustrating that working memory is stressed if not exceeded because of the increased cognitive workload. Although similar to a mental "to-do" list, a nurse's cognitive stack has more potential patient safety consequences (Patterson et al. 2011).

To advance the concept of cognitive stacking, Patterson et al. (2011) sought to understand how RNs prioritize activities. They developed a 7-level hierarchy of priorities among nursing tasks. Threatening clinical concerns were at the top of the hierarchy, as were activities with high uncertainty (Patterson et al. 2011). Experienced nurses prioritized differently than those with less experience. For instance, they understood trade-offs better, such as how delaying some tasks could increase the workload at the end of the shift (Patterson et al. 2011). More recently, task juggling, which resembles stacking, is another term to help nurses stay on track (Renolen et al. 2018). Juggling and stacking contribute to nurses' cognitive complexity and thus influence the outcomes of work stress and cognitive failure.

Client (Nurse) Outcomes

Work Stress

Nursing has long been regarded as a stressful profession, largely due to the nature of the work and the working conditions (Jennings 2008c). Stress is a complicated phenomenon because it may be a stimulus, a response, or an interaction (Jennings 2008c). Consequently, various perspectives seek to explain stress, all of which note that stress involves perception and interpretation of incidents in the work setting. Lazarus and Folkman (1984), for instance, adopted a psychological stance stating that stress is "a particular relationship between the person and the environment that is appraised by the person as taxing or exceeding his or her resources and endangering his or her well-being" (p. 19).

Work stress is at the crux of concerns about nurses' work environment and patient safety. Findings from two studies conducted in Switzerland showed that conditions such as time pressure, cognitive demands, and workflow interruptions contributed to high job stress (Elfering et al. 2006) and low job satisfaction (Baethge and Rigotti 2013). Although turbulence per se was not mentioned in the Swiss studies, the findings reflect that workflow issues and cognitive demands contribute to work stress. One might surmise that reducing environmental turbulence or diminishing nursing workflow irregularities could reduce some of nurses' work-related stress.

Cognitive Failure

Cognitive failure refers to lapses in memory, perception, and action (Broadbent et al. 1982), yielding "mistakes on everyday tasks that a person normally is capable of completing without error" (Elfering et al. 2011, p. 194). Carrigan and Barkus (2016) conducted a systematic review of 45 articles focused on healthy people (e.g., US military personnel, undergraduate students) who experienced cognitive failures or "brain farts" (p. 30). From their review, Carrigan and Barkus noted a variety of factors that contributed to cognitive failures—some were stable characteristics, such as neuroticism and trait anxiety, and some were variable characteristics, such as times of high stress and chaotic environmental conditions. High work stress and turbulent workflow may predispose healthcare workers to cognitive failures.

Elfering et al. (2011) illustrated an association between job characteristics and work-related cognitive failures among 96 nurses in 11 Swiss hospitals. As expected, cognitive workload increased when task stressors (e.g., interruptions, time pressure) increased, enhancing the likelihood of cognitive failure. In a second study involving 165 nurses in 7 Swiss hospitals, the investigators confirmed that workflow interruptions (i.e., turbulence) were likely triggers of errors (Elfering et al. 2015). Elfering et al. (2015) recommended work redesign to reduce cognitive failure and improve patient safety.

Implications and Future Directions

As showcased in this chapter, turbulent workflow is a significant characteristic of the system within which nurses work. Turbulence adds to the cognitive complexity of nurses' work with the potential to contribute to work stress and cognitive failure. The implications are clear. First, attention is needed to focus on how systems might be redesigned to improve nurses' workflow and reduce turbulence. Second, and perhaps more immediately achievable, interventions are needed to improve nurses' work (e.g., smoothing workflow and mitigating turbulence). Third, and very achievable, is to increase simulation training in nursing education to better prepare student nurses for the practice setting's reality. Perhaps less time on learning bed baths and more time learning to manage interruptions would alleviate some work stress and cognitive failures.

Leaders at the organizational and unit levels need to be educated to recognize workarounds and turbulence as warning signs and examine other data reflective of turbulence. Patient turnover and handoffs are two such data points. Examining patient flow resulting from turnover can pinpoint hours of the day when turnover is least disruptive for all units involved, affording opportunities for optimizing workflow. Because handoffs are a companion to patient turnover, examining patient turnover might also improve information exchange during the handoff. As part of patient turnover, early identification of patients for discharge and arranging for discharges early in the day might be used as incentives.

New hospital construction needs to involve a cadre of individuals such as architects, human factors engineers, and practicing nurses to ensure that clunky features within existing work systems are not replicated in new facilities. Healthcare leaders and administrators need to participate in this work too, helping to design hospitals of the future that are built to maximize efficiency and minimize turbulence. Any additional costs associated with designing and constructing turbulence-reducing hospitals must be weighed against the cost of continually recruiting nurses to replace those who leave the workplace due to stress and burnout, as well as the cost associated with unsafe patient care.

It might also be helpful to develop measures of turbulent workflow; human factors engineers would be important allies in such endeavors. It seems there is sufficient evidence, however, that the nurses' work environment is turbulent. Thus, rather than measure what seems like a given, it would be more beneficial to invest time and resources into improving practice environments. Diminishing turbulence was an explicit suggestion from Myny et al. (2012). More generally, Carayon and Gurses (2008) recommended redesigning work systems to reduce nurses' workload. Even modest investments might yield substantial returns. For instance, mobile work telephones were implemented to minimize nurses need to walk to a central nurses' station to get or return telephone calls. What was not anticipated, however, was the highly interruptive nature of mobile work telephones. These interruptions are one of many examples of practices that need to be thought through more fully to minimize unwanted consequences of work system redesign. Similarly, it is essential to determine whether care quality is affected by implementing interventions to improve the practice environment (Swiger et al. 2017).

Finally, a word of caution for the future of existing measures of nurses' work environments (Chaps. 4 and 13); workflow and turbulence are not reflected in these measures. Moreover, a family of measures was developed using data from the 1980s. Nursing practice has changed immensely since those measures were developed. The trio of measures are the Nursing Work Index (NWI; Kramer and Hafner 1989), the Nursing Work Index-Revised (NWI-R; Aiken and Patrician 2000), and the Practice Environment Scale of the Nursing Work Index (PES-NWI; Lake 2002, 2007) (Chap. 4). The PES-NWI is especially prominent because of its wide use (Swiger et al. 2017; Warshawsky and Havens 2011). Therefore, leaders must consider what work environment measures reflect about contemporary environments, realizing that turbulence sources are not represented.

Workflow for nurses is an oxymoron—nurses' work in a flow that is turbulent. Although workflow is a significant issue within the nursing profession, there is little evidence of remediating the turbulent working conditions. Practicing nurses deal with turbulence from many sources. They use ingenious strategies to function as best they are able for patients and themselves despite the turbulent workflow. To keep nurses interested in acute care and bedside practice, it is imperative that we reduce the turbulent flow that prevails in acute care settings, making them safer for patients and better for the nurses who practice in them.

References

Aarts J, Ash J, Berg M (2007) Extending the understanding of computerized physician order entry: implications for professional collaboration, workflow and quality of care. Int J Med Inform 76S:S4–S13

Abraham J, Reddy MC (2010) Challenges to inter-departmental coordination of patient transfers: a workflow perspective. Int J Med Inform 79:112–122

Aiken LJ, Patrician PA (2000) Measuring organizational traits of hospitals: the revised nursing work index. Nurs Res 49:146–153

Allen D (2004) Re-reading nursing and re-writing practice: towards an empirically based reformulation of the nursing mandate. Nurs Inq 11:271–283

Ash JS, Berg M, Coiera E (2004) Some unintended consequences of information technology in health care: the nature of patient care information system-related errors. J Am Med Inform Assoc 11:104–112

Baethge A, Rigotti T (2013) Interruptions to workflow: their relationship with irritation and satisfaction with performance, and the mediating roles of time pressure and mental demands. Work Stress 27:43–63

Bazzoli GJ, Dynan L, Burns LR, Yap (2004) Two decades of organizational change in health care: what have we learned. Med Care Res Rev 613:247–331

Beach C, Cheung DS, Apker J, Horwitz LI, Howell EE, O'Leary KJ, Patterson ES et al (2017) Improving interunit transitions of care between emergency physicians and hospital medicine physicians: a conceptual approach. Acad Emerg Med 19:1188–1195

Beekun RI, Ginn GO (1993) Business strategy and interorganizational linkages within the acute care hospital industry: an expansion of the Miles and Snow typology. Hum Relat 46:1291–1318

Berwick DM (2002) A user's manual for the IOM's 'Quality Chasm' report. Health Aff 21:80–90

Biron AD, Lavoie-Tremblay M, Loiselle CG (2009) Characteristics of work interruptions during medication administration. J Nurs Scholarsh 41(4):330–336

Blay N, Duffield CM, Gallagher R, Roche M (2014) A systematic review of time studies to assess the impact of patient transfers on nurse workload. Int J Nurs Pract 20:662–673

Blay N, Roche MA, Duffield C, Gallagher R (2017) Intrahospital transfers and the impact on nursing workload. J Clin Nurs 26:4822–4829

Bosco CL (2007) The relationship between environmental turbulence, workforce ability and patient outcomes. University of Arizona, Tucson, AZ

Brixey JJ, Robinson DJ, Johnson CW, Johnson TR, Turley JP, Zhang JJ (2007) A concept analysis of the phenomenon interruption. Adv Nurs Sci 30(1):E26–E42

Broadbent DE, Cooper PF, FitzGerald P, Parkes KR (1982) The cognitive failures questionnaire (CFQ) and its correlates. Br J Clin Psychol 21:1–16

Brown T (2019) The American medical system is one giant workaround. The New York Times, Section A, Sept 6. p. 23.

Browne J, Braden CJ (2020) Nursing turbulence in critical care: relationships with nursing workload and patient safety. Am J Crit Care 29:182–191

Cain C, Hague S (2008) Organizational workflow and its impact on work quality. In: Hughes R (ed) Patient safety and quality: an evidence-based handbook for nurses, AHRQ Publication No. 08-0043. Agency for Healthcare Research and Quality, Rockville, MD, pp 2-217–2-244

Cameron KS, Kim MU (1987) Organizational effects of decline and turbulence. Adm Sci Q 32(2):222–240

Carayon P, Gurses AP (2008) Nursing workload and patient safety—A human factors engineering perspective. In: Hughes R (ed) Patient safety and quality: an evidence-based handbook for nurses, AHRQ Publication No. 08-0043. Agency for Healthcare Research and Quality, Rockville, MD, pp 2-203–2-216

Carayon P, Hundt AS, Karsh B-T, Gurses AP, Slvarado CJ, Smith M, Brennan PF (2007) Work system design for patient safety: the SEIPS model. Qual Saf Health Care 15(Suppl 1):i50–i58

Carrigan N, Barkus E (2016) A systematic review of cognitive failures in daily life: healthy populations. Neurosci Biobehav Rev 63:29–42

Carroll JS, Williams M, Gallivan TM (2012) The ins and outs of change of shift handoffs between nurses: a communication challenge. BMJ Qual Saf 21:586–593

Cohen MD, Hilligoss PB (2010) The published literature on handoffs in hospitals: deficiencies identified in an extensive review. BMJ Qual Saf Health Care 19:493–497

Cohen MD, Hilligoss B, Amaral ACK-B (2012) A handoff is not a telegram: an understanding of the patient is co-constructed. Crit Care 16:303

Coiera E (2012) The science of interruption. [Editorial]. BMJ Qual Saf Health Care 21:357–360

Coiera E, Tombs V (1998) Communication behaviours in a hospital setting: an observational study. Br Med J 316:673–676

Comprehensive Accreditation Manual for Hospitals (2013) Sentinel events (SE). https://www.jointcommission.org/-/media/deprecated-unorganized/imported-assets/tjc/system-folders/topics-library/camh_2012_update2_24_sepdf.pdf?db=web&hash=FD320B7BAF3E08EC28B44AA51CB21ABE

Cornell P, Herrin-Griffith D, Keim C, Petschonek S, Sanders AM, D'Mello S et al (2010) Transforming nursing workflow, Part 1. The chaotic nature of nurse activities. J Nurs Adm 40:366–373

Cornell P, Riordan M, Townsend-Gervis M, Mobley R (2011) Barriers to critical thinking. Workflow interruptions and task switching among nurses. J Nurs Adm 41:407–414

Cornell P, Gervis MT, Yates L, Vardaman JM (2013) Improving shift report focus and consistency with the Situation, Background, Assessment, Recommendation protocol. J Nurs Adm 43:422–428

Couffe C, Michael GA (2017) Failures due to interruptions or distractions: a review and a new framework. Am J Psychol 130(2):163–181

Debono DS, Greenfield D, Travaglia JF, Long JF, Black D, Johnson J, Braithwaite J (2013) Nurses' workarounds in acute healthcare settings: a scoping review. BMC Health Serv Res 13:175

Derksen M (2014) Turning men into machines? Scientific management, industrial psychology, and the "human factor". J Hist Behav Sci 50(2):148–165

Dickson GL, Flynn L (2012) Nurses' clinical reasoning: processes and practices of medication safety. Qual Health Res 22:3–16

Douglas HE, Raban MZ, Walter SR, Westbrook JI (2017) Improving our understanding of multitasking in healthcare: drawing together the cognitive psychology and healthcare literature. Appl Ergon 59:45–55

Dracup K, Morris PE (2008) Passing the torch: the challenge of handoffs. [Editorial]. Am J Crit Care 17:95–97

Ebright PR, Patterson ES, Chalko BA, Render M (2003) Understanding the complexity of registered nurse work in acute care settings. J Nurs Adm 33:630–638

Edwards A, Fitzpatrick L-A, Augustine S, Trzebucki A, Cheng SL, Presseau C et al (2009) Synchronous communication facilitates interruptive workflow for attending physicians and nurses in clinical settings. Int J Med Inform 78:629–637

Eisenhauer LA, Hurley AC, Dolan N (2007) Nurses' reported thinking during medication administration. J Nurs Scholarsh 39(1):82–87

Elfering A, Semmer NK, Grebner S (2006) Work stress and patient safety: observer-rated work stressors as predictors of characteristics of safety-related events reported by young nurses. Ergonomics 49:457–469

Elfering A, Grebner S, Dudan A (2011) Job characteristics in nursing and cognitive failure at work. Saf Health Work 2:194–200

Elfering A, Grebner S, de Tribolet-Hardy F (2013) The long arm of time pressure at work: cognitive failure and commuting near accidents. Eur J Work Organ Psychol 22:737–749

Elfering A, Grebner S, Ebener C (2015) Workflow interruptions, cognitive failure and near-accidents in health care. Psychol Health Med 20:139–147

Fairbanks RJ, Bisantz AM, Sunm M (2007) Emergency department communication links and patterns. Ann Emerg Med 50:396–406

Friesen MA, White SV, Byers JF (2008) Handoffs: implications for nurses. In: Hughes R (ed) Patient safety and quality: an evidence-based handbook for nurses, AHRQ Publication No. 08-0043. Agency for Healthcare Research and Quality, Rockville, MD, pp 2-285–2-332

Gandhi TK (2005) Fumbled handoffs: one dropped ball after another. Ann Intern Med 142:352–358

Gleick J (1987) Chaos. Making a new science. Penguin Books, New York, NY, pp 121–123

Gosbee J (1998) Communication among health professionals: human factors engineering can help make sense of the chaos. Br Med J 316(7132):642

Grayson D, Boxerman S, Potter P, Wolf L, Dunagan C, Sorock G, Evanoff B (2005) Do transient working conditions trigger medical errors? In: Henriksen K, Battles JB, Marks ES, Lewin DI (eds) Advances in patient safety: from research to implementation. Vol. 1, Research findings, AHRQ Publication No. 05-0021-1. Agency for Healthcare Research and Quality, Rockville, MD, pp 53–64

Grissinger M (2010) The five rights. A destination without a map. PT 35:542

Grundgeiger T, Sanderson P (2009) Interruptions in healthcare: theoretical views. Int J Med Inform 78:293–307

Gurses AP, Carayon P, Wall M (2009) Impact of performance obstacles on intensive care nurses' workload, perceived quality and safety of care, and quality of working life. HSR: Health Service Res 44(part 1):422–443

Hall LM, Pedersen C, Fairley L (2010) Losing the moment. Understanding interruptions to nurses' work. J Nurs Adm 40:169–176

Hampson I, Junor A (2005) Invisible work, invisible skills: interactive customer service as articulation work. New Technology. Work Employm 20:166–181

Hilligoss B, Cohen MD (2011) Hospital handoffs as multi-functional situated routines: implications for researchers and administrators. Adv Health Care Manag 11:91–132

Hilligoss B, Cohen MD (2013) The unappreciated challenges of between-unit handoffs: negotiating and coordinating across boundaries. Ann Emerg Med 61:155–160

Holden RJ, Scanlon MC, Patel NR, Kaushal R, Escoto KH, Brown RL et al (2011) A human factors framework and study of the effect of nursing workload on patient safety and employee quality of working life. BMJ Qual Saf 20:15–24

Hopkinson SG, Jennings BM (2013) Interruptions during nurses' work: a state-of-the-science review. Res Nurs Health 36:38–53

Hopkinson SG, Weigand DL (2017) The culture contributing to interruptions in the nursing work environment: an ethnography. J Clin Nurs 26:5093–5102

Institute for Healthcare Improvement [IHI] Multimedia Team (2017) Teamwork and communication: the keys to building a strong patient safety culture. IHI_%20Teamwork%20and%20 Communication_%20Multimedia%202017.html

Jennings BM (2008a) Restructuring and mergers. In: Hughes R (ed) Patient safety and quality: an evidence-based handbook for nurses, AHRQ Publication No. 08-0043. Agency for Healthcare Research and Quality, Rockville, MD, pp 2-93–2-109

Jennings BM (2008b) Turbulence. In: Hughes R (ed) Patient safety and quality: an evidence-based handbook for nurses, AHRQ Publication No. 08-0043. Agency for Healthcare Research and Quality, Rockville, MD, pp 2-193–2-202

Jennings BM (2008c) Work stress and burnout among nurses: role of the work environment and working conditions. In: Hughes R (ed) Patient safety and quality: an evidence-based handbook for nurses, AHRQ Publication No. 08-0043. Agency for Healthcare Research and Quality, Rockville, MD, pp 2-137–2-158

Jennings BM, Sandelowski M, Mark B (2011) The nurse's medication day. Qual Health Res 21:1441–1451

Jennings BM, Sandelowski M, Higgins MK (2013) Turning over patient turnover: an ethnographic study of admissions, discharges, and transfers. Res Nurs Health 36:554–566

Jett QR, George JM (2003) Work interrupted: a closer look at the role of interruptions in organizational life. Acad Manag Rev 28:494–507

Kalisch BJ, Aebersold M (2010) Interruptions and multi-tasking in nursing care. Jt Comm J Qual Patient Saf 36:126–132

Kalisch BJ, Begeny S, Anderson C (2008) The effect of consistent nursing shifts on teamwork and continuity of care. J Nurs Adm 38:132–137

Karsh B-T, Holden RJ, Alper SJ, Or CKL (2006) A human factors engineering paradigm for patient safety: designing to support the performance of the healthcare professional. BMJ Qual Saf Health Care 15:i59–i65

Kohn LT, Corrigan JM, Donaldson MS (eds) (2001) To err is human. Building a safer health system. National Academy Press, Washington, DC

Koopman P, Hoffman RR (2003) Work-arounds, make-work, and kludges. IEEE Intell Syst 18(6):70–75

Koppel R, Wetterneck T, Telles JL, Karsh B-T (2008) Workarounds to barcode medication administration systems: their occurrences, causes, and threats to patient safety. J Am Med Inform Assoc 15:408–423

Kramer M, Hafner LP (1989) Shared values: impact on staff nurse satisfaction and perceived productivity. Nurs Res 38:172–177

Krichbaum KE, Peden-McAlpine C, Diemert C, Koenig P, Mueller C, Savik K (2011) Designing a measure of complexity compression in registered nurses. West J Nurs Res 33(1):7–25

Lake ET (2002) Development of the practice environment scale of the nursing work index. Res Nurs Health 25:176–188

Lake ET (2007) The nursing practice environment: measurement and evidence. Med Care Res Rev 64:104S–122S

Lawal AK, Rotter T, Kinsman L, Sari N, Harrison L, Jeffery C et al (2014) Lean management in health care: definition, concepts, methodology and effects reported (systematic review protocol). Syst Rev 3:103

Laxmisan A, Hakimzada F, Sayan OR, Green RA, Zhang J, Patel VL (2007) The multi-tasking clinician: decision-making and cognitive demand during and after team handoffs in emergency care. Int J Med Inform 76:801–811

Lazarus RS, Folkman S (1984) Stress, appraisal, and coping. Springer, New York, NY

Leonard M, Graham S, Bonacum D (2004) The human factor: the critical importance of effective teamwork and communication in providing safe care. Qual Saf Health Care 13(Suppl 1):i85–i90

Li SYW, Magrabi F, Coiera E (2012) A systematic review of the psychological literature on interruption and its patient safety implications. J Am Med Inform Assoc 19:6–12

Lin F, Chaboyer W, Wallis M, Miller A (2013) Factors contributing to the process of intensive care patient discharge: an ethnographic study informed by activity theory. Int J Nurs Stud 50:1054–1066

Magrabi F, Li SYW, Dunne AG, Coiera E (2011) Challenges in measuring the impact of interruption on patient safety and workflow outcomes. Methods Inf Med 50:447–453

Mark G (2015) Multi-tasking in the digital age. Morgan & Claypool, San Rafael, CA

McCann JE, Selsky J (1984) Hyperturbulence and the emergence of type 5 environments. Acad Manag 9:460–470

McDaniel RR, Jordan ME, Fleeman BF (2003) Surprise, surprise, surprise! A complexity science view of the unexpected. Health Care Manag Rev 28:266–278

Menzies IEP (1960) Nurses under stress. Int Nurs Rev 7:9–16

Mikesell L, Bromley E (2012) Patient centered, nurse averse? Nurses' care experiences in a 21st-century hospital. Qual Health Res 22:1659–1671

Miller GA (1956) The magical number seven, plus or minus two: some limits on our capacity for processing information. Psychol Rev 63:81–97

Mitchell PH, Ferketich S, Jennings B (1998) Quality health outcomes model. Image J Nurs Sch 30(1):43–46

Morgan B, D'Mello S, Abbott R, Radvansky G, Haass M, Tamplin A (2013) Individual differences in multi-tasking ability and adaptability. Human Fact J Human Fact Ergon Soc 55:776–788

Myny D, Van Hecke A, De Bacquer D, Verhaeghe S, Gobert M, Defloor T, Van Goubergen D (2012) Determining a set of measurable and relevant factors affecting nursing workload in the acute care hospital setting: a cross-sectional study. Int J Nurs Stud 49:427–436

National Academies of Sciences, Engineering, and Medicine (2019) Taking action against clinician burnout: a systems approach to professional well-being. The National Academies Press, Washington, DC

Norrish BR, Rundall TG (2001) Hospital restructuring and the work of registered nurses. Milbank Quart 79(1):55–79

Novak LL, Lorenzi NM (2008) Barcode medication administration: supporting transitions in articulation work. AMIA Symp Proc 2008:515–519

Ong M-S, Coiera E (2011) A systematic review of failures in handoff communication during intrahospital transfers. Jt Comm J Qual Patient Saf 37:274–284, AP1–AP6

Park SH, Weaver L, Mejia-Johnson L, Vukas R, Zimmerman J (2016) An integrative literature review of patient turnover in inpatient hospital settings. West J Nurs Res 38:629–655

Parker J, Coiera E (2000) Improving clinical communication: a view from psychology. J Am Med Inform Assoc 7:453–461

Patterson ES, Cook RI, Render ML (2002) Improving patient safety by identifying side effects from introducing bar coding in medication administration. J Am Med Inform Assoc 9: 540–553

Patterson ES, Ebright PR, Saleem JJ (2011) Investigating stacking: how do registered nurses prioritize their activities in real-time? Int J Ind Ergon 41:389–393

Perlow LA (1999) The time famine: toward a sociology of work time. Adm Sci Q 44:57–81

Phillips L (2018) Turbulence, the oldest unsolved problem in physics. arstechnica.com/science/2018/10/turbulence-the-oldest-unsolved-problem-in-physics

Pingenot A, Shanteau J, Sengstacke DN (2009) Description of inpatient medication management using cognitive work analysis. CIN: Comput Informat Nurs 27:379–392

Plsek P (2001) Redesigning health care with insights from the science of complex adaptive systems. In: Institute of Medicine Committee on Quality of Health Care in America (Ed.), Crossing the Quality Chasm. National Academy Press, Washington, DC, pp 309–322

Potter P, Boxerman S, Wolf L, Marshall J, Grayson D, Sledge J, Evanoff B (2004) Mapping the nursing process. A new approach for understanding the work of nursing. J Nurs Adm 34:101–109

Potter P, Wolf L, Boxerman S, Grayson D, Sledge J, Dunagan C, Evnaoff B (2005) Understanding the cognitive work of nursing in the acute care environment. J Nurs Adm 35:327–335

Powell-Cope G, Nelson AL, Patterson ES (2008) Patient care technology and safety. In: Hughes R (ed) Patient safety and quality: an evidence-based handbook for nurses, AHRQ Publication No. 08-0043. Agency for Healthcare Research and Quality, Rockville, MD, pp 3-207–3-220

Reason J (1990) Human error. Cambridge. Cambridge University Press, England

Reed C, Minnick AF, Dietrich MS (2018) Nurses' responses to interruptions during medication tasks: a time and motion study. Int J Nurs Stud 82:113–120

Renolen A, Hoye S, Hjalmhult E, Danbolt LJ, Kirkevold M (2018) "Keeping on track"—Hospital nurses' struggles with maintaining workflow while seeking to integrate evidence-based practice into their daily work: a grounded theory study. Int J Nurs Stud 77:179–188

Rivera-Rodriguez AJ, Karsh B-T (2010) Interruptions and distractions in healthcare: review and reappraisal. Qual Saf Health Care 19:304–312

Rosenberg A, Britton MC, Feder S, Minges K, Hodshon B, Chaudhry SI et al (2018) A taxonomy and cultural analysis of intra-hospital patient transfers. Res Nurs Health 41:378–388

Rubinstein JS, Meyer DE, Evans JE (2001) Executive control of cognitive processes in task switching. J Exp Psychol 27:753–797

Salyer J (1995) Environmental turbulence. Impact on nurse performance. J Nurs Adm 25(4):12–20

Sendelbach S, Funk M (2013) Alarm fatigue. A patient safety concern. AACN Adv Crit Care 24:378–386

Sitterding MC, Ebright P (2015) Information overload: a framework for explaining the issues and creating solutions. In: Sitterding MC, Broome ME (eds) Information overload. American Nurses Association, Silver Spring, MD, pp 11–33

Staggers N, Jennings BM (2009) The content and context of change of shift report on medical and surgical units. J Nurs Adm 39:393–398

Star SL (1991) The sociology of the invisible: the primacy of work in the writings of Anselm Strauss. In: Maines DR (ed) Social organization and social process. Essays in honor of Anselm Strauss. Aldine de Gruyter, Hawthorne, NY, pp 265–283

Star SL, Strauss AL (1999) Layers of silence, arenas of voice: the ecology of visible and invisible work. Comput Support Cooperat Work (CSCW) 8:9–30

Starmer AJ, Spector ND, Srivastava R, West DC, Rosenbluth G, Allen AD, et al for the I-PASS Study Group (2014) Changes in medical errors after implementation of a handoff programs. N Engl J Med 371:1803–1812

Starmer AJ, Schnock KO, Lyons A, Hehn RS, Graham DA, Keohane C, Landrigan CP (2017) Effects of the I-PASS nursing handoff bundle on communication quality and workflow. BMJ Qual Saf 26:949–957

Strauss A (1985) Work and the division of labor. Sociol Q 26:1–19

Strauss A (1988) The articulation of project work: an organizational process. Sociol Q 29:163–178

Strauss A, Fagerhaugh S, Suczek B, Wiener C (1997) Social organization of medical work. Transaction, New Brunswick, NJ

Swiger PA, Vance DE, Patrician PA (2016) Nursing workload in the acute-care setting: a concept analysis of nursing workload. Nurs Outlook 64:244–254

Swiger PA, Patrician PA, Miltner RS, Raju D, Breckenridge-Sproat S, Loan LA (2017) The practice environment scale of the nursing work index: an updated review and recommendations for use. Int J Nurs Stud 74:76–84

The Joint Commission (September 12, 2017) Sentinel event alert 58: inadequate handoff communication. https://www.jointcommission.org/-/media/tjc/documents/resources/patient-safety-topics/sentinel-event/sea_58_hand_off_comms_9_6_17_final_(1).pdf

Tubbs-Cooley HL, Mara CA, Carle AC, Gurses AP (2018) The NASA Task Load Index as a measure of overall workload among neonatal, paediatric and adult intensive care nurses. Intens Crit Care Nurs 46:64–69

Tucker AL (2004) The impact of operational failures on hospital nurses and their patients. J Oper Manag 22:151–169

Tucker AL, Spear SJ (2006) Operational failures and interruptions in hospital nursing. HSR: Health Service Res 41(3, Part 1):643–662

Verran JA, Effken J, Lamb G (2003) Impact of nursing unit characteristics on outcomes. RO1HS11973. Agency for Healthcare Research & Quality

Wachter RM, Shojania KG (2005) Handoffs and fumbles. In: Internal bleeding. Rugged Land, New York, NY, pp 159–179

Walter SR, Li L, Dunsmuir WTM, Westbrook JI (2014) Managing competing demands through task-switching and multi-tasking: a multi-setting observational study of 200 clinicians over 1000 hours. BMJ Qual Saf 23:231–241

Warshawsky NE, Havens DS (2011) Global use of the practice environment scale of the nursing work index. Nurs Res 60:17–31

Waterworth S, May C, Luker K (1999) Clinical 'effectiveness' and 'interrupted' work. Clin Eff Nurs 3(4):163–169

Weigl M, Muller A, Vincent C, Angerer P, Sevdalis N (2012) The association of workflow interruptions and hospital doctors' workload: a prospective observational study. BMJ Qual Saf 21:399–407

Weigl M, Beck J, Wehler M, Schneider A (2017) Workflow interruptions and stress at work: a mixed-methods study among physicians and nurses of a multidisciplinary emergency department. BMJ Open:7

Welsh CA, Flanagan ME, Ebright P (2010) Barriers and facilitators to nursing handoffs: recommendations for redesign. Nurs Outlook 58:148–154

Whittaker J, Ball C (2000) Discharge from intensive care: a view from the ward. Intens Crit Care Nurs 16:135–143

Wiegmann DA, ElBardissi AW, Dearani JA, Daly RC, Sundt TM (2007) Disruptions in surgical flow and their relationship to surgical errors: an exploratory investigation. Surgery 142:658–665

Woods DD, Patterson ES (2001) How unexpected events produce an escalation of cognitive and coordinative demands. In: Hancock PA, Desmond PA (eds) Stress, workload, and fatigue. Lawrence Erlbaum, Mahwah, NJ, pp 290–301

World Health Organization (2020) WHO Director-General's opening remarks at the media briefing on COVID-19—11 March 2020. https://www.who.int/dg/speeches/detail/who-director-general-s-opening-remarks-at-the-media-briefing-on-covid-19%2D%2D-11-march-2020

Zhang J, Patel VL, Johnson TR, Shortliffe EH (2004) A cognitive taxonomy of medical errors. J Biomed Inform 37:193–204

Zuzelo PR, Gettis C, Hansell AW, Thomas L (2008) Describing the influence of technologies on registered nurses' work. Clin Nurse Spec 22:132–140

Health Information Technology and Electronic Health Records

Susan McBride and Mari Tietze

Introduction

The QHOM (Mitchell et al. 1998) considers the system as an organized agency that includes hospitals and provider networks. The model further identifies system structural elements that interact with treatment processes to impact outcomes. Structural elements identified include the size of the organization, ownership, client demographics, and technology. Specifically noted is that technology can positively impact outcomes. Health information technology (Health IT) in the context of the QHOM should be considered a significant intervention or tool imposed by the federal legislative agenda to promote and encourage the adoption and implementation of electronic health records (EHRs) and other types of Health IT. This chapter ties the QHOM to the optimization of Health IT. It concludes with a call to address usability, unintended consequences, burden of documentation, and importance of Health IT competencies to improve health outcomes.

Health IT: Linkages to the QHOM

The QHOM is an excellent framework for addressing technology optimization for nursing and the interprofessional team because the model captures essential factors that influence the overall outcomes for individuals, groups, and

S. McBride (✉)
Nursing Informatics, School of Nursing, Texas Tech University Health Sciences Center, Lubbock, TX, USA
e-mail: susan.mcbride@ttuhsc.edu

M. Tietze
Texas Woman's University, T. Boone Pickens Institute of Health Sciences-Dallas Center, Dallas, TX, USA
e-mail: mtietze@twu.edu

© Springer Nature Switzerland AG 2021
M. Baernholdt, D. K. Boyle (eds.), *Nurses Contributions to Quality Health Outcomes*, https://doi.org/10.1007/978-3-030-69063-2_6

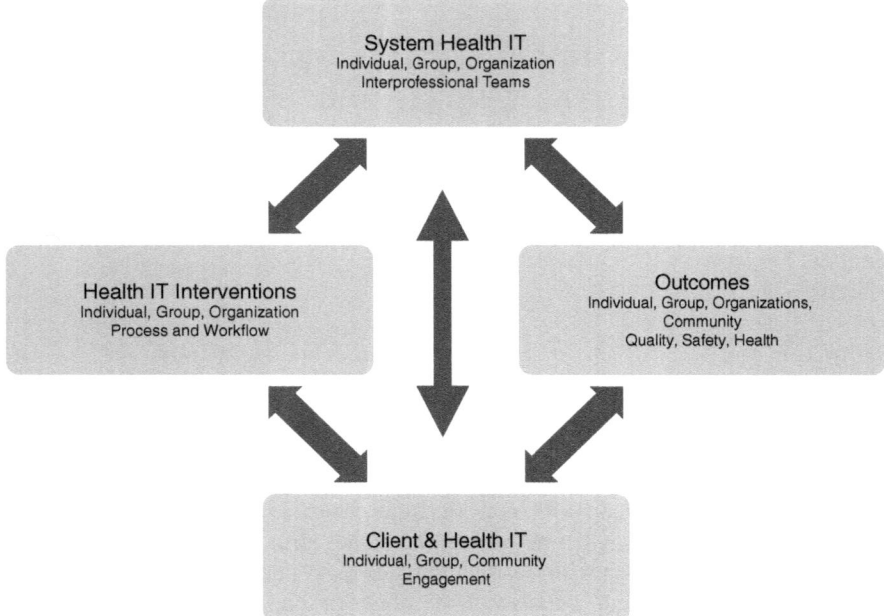

Fig. 6.1 Framework for Health IT

communities. The capacity to reach ideal patient outcomes depends on *system* Health IT expansions and improvements to the EHR that promote interoperability across care settings and foster healthcare consumer engagement and activation.

The QHOM components of system characteristics, interventions, client, and outcomes will be described in terms of Health IT optimization. The individuals, groups, and organizations within each of the QHOM components will be addressed with clinical examples to emphasize the impact on the three levels with respect to Health IT optimization to improve outcomes. Mitchell and colleagues discuss the QHOM as follows: "Interventions affect and are affected by both system and client characteristics in producing desired outcomes … and no single intervention acts directly through either system or client alone" (Mitchell et al. 1998, p. 44). This statement can be directly related to the optimization of technology, mainly seen as an intervention focused on process improvement to use technology as a tool to enhance outcomes. Health IT is impacted by system characteristics and influences individual, group, and community health outcomes. Figure 6.1 reflects these relationships. These relationships are dynamic reciprocal relationships that exist and act upon each other (Mitchell et al. 1998).

Environmental Context of Healthcare Regulation in the USA

With the massive expansion of Health IT throughout the USA, new approaches are needed to wholly realize the vision of a fully interoperable national Health IT infrastructure established by the Office of the National Coordinator (ONC) for Health IT. The ONC was initially established by executive order in 2004 by the Bush Administration. The ONC has federal oversight under Health and Human Services for Health IT regulation. The ONC defines IT as "The application of information processing involving both computer hardware and software that deals with the storage, retrieval, sharing, and use of healthcare information, data, and knowledge for communication and decision making" (ONC 2020a). The ONC's mission is to promote the wellness and health of individuals and communities through the use of Health IT (ONC 2019).

Baernholdt et al. (2018) conducted a study under the American Academy of Nursing Quality Expert Panel, expanding on the QHOM to include important environmental contextual influences. The authors examined Health IT and the development of electronic measures including the collection, storage, and use of data, all of which were impacted by interventions and changes within the healthcare context. An important contextual factor for Health IT is policy and regulation that significantly expanded the US Health IT infrastructure and the capacity to collect and use data. See Chap. 2 for other policy interventions that have affected US healthcare.

Important Health IT Regulatory Milestones

In 2009, the Health Information Technology for Economic Clinical Health (HITECH) Act was enacted as a component of the American Recovery and Reinvestment Act (ARRA).

The HITECH Act had several key goals:

- Improve quality and efficiency.
- Improve the exchange of information to promote better care coordination between hospitals, providers, labs, and other healthcare organizations.
- Maintain privacy and security of personal health information.
- Establish mechanisms to detect, prevent, and manage chronic illnesses (US Congress 2009).

The HITECH Act was an important legislation for health information technology that propelled the adoption and implementation of Health IT forward exponentially. Based on this legislation, the Centers for Medicare & Medicaid Services (CMS) established the Electronic Health Record (EHR) Incentive Program in 2011 (CMS 2019). In the next several years, the national EHR penetration rate improved substantially. By 2016, 78% of providers and 96% of hospitals had adopted a federally certified EHR system that meets federal requirements for meaningful use of EHRs (see Table 6.1 for stages of meaningful use). Although impressive, the improvement

Table 6.1 Stages of meaningful use and respective years (ONC 2020b)

Years	Stage	Goals
2011–2012	1	Data capture and sharing
2014	2	Advanced clinical processes
2016	3	Improved outcomes

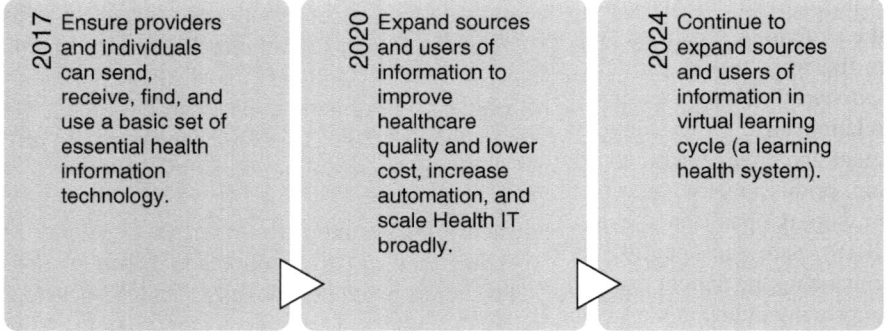

Fig. 6.2 Milestones for promoting interoperability and a learning healthcare system focused on quality

in EHR adoption presents challenges with optimizing certified technology within institutions and across regions, states, and the nation.

The adoption of EHR technology is only one step toward the effective use of Health IT. The decision by organizations to adopt, implement, and reach the meaningful use measures was largely impacted by CMS's financial incentives to implement EHRs, followed by penalties for organizations that did not reach certain levels of adoption and use of EHRs. The CMS EHR incentive program became the framework for promoting EHR adoption. Meaningful use established the specific objectives that providers and hospitals needed to meet to be eligible for financial incentives under the CMS Incentive Program. Meaningful use was defined within the federal regulations specifying a certified EHR's functions and capabilities under the Incentive Program. Three stages were defined and are noted in Table 6.1. These stages of meaningful use pushed to achieve higher levels of adoption and implementation, advancing many of the capabilities of certified EHRs for better interoperability.

Additional important milestones that followed the HITECH Act was the 21st Century Cures Act, which was enacted in 2016 to accelerate the design, development, and use of new technologies needed to support care delivery and outcomes. Finally, in 2014, the ONC released a 10-year road map with a vision established for a fully interoperable learning healthcare system nationwide. This interoperability vision includes hospitals, providers, labs, and other healthcare organizations using Heath IT to exchange important healthcare information to promote health and better care for populations. Figure 6.2 notes several essential milestones for interoperability.

Structural Components of Health IT Established Under Meaningful Use

Certified EHRs under "meaningful use" include electronic prescribing, computer provider order entry (CPOE), clinical decision support systems (CDSS), patient portals, personal health records, and an ability to capture data for electronic clinical quality measures. These components rely on a standardized approach to capturing data to create interoperability within and across institutions and communities. Through the use of all of these structural components, the ultimate national vision for certified technology is a digital highway that connects providers and hospitals and supports healthcare consumers in accessing their personal health information worldwide. This national goal has the potential to impact individuals, groups, and communities as a profound intervention to impact overall outcomes.

The Health IT structural components, coupled with quality improvement methods, constitute Health IT interventions defined in Table 6.2. Within the QHOM framework, the interventions are delivered to individuals, families, or communities to improve outcomes.

The electronic clinical quality measures (eCQMs) within healthcare reform address both process and outcome measures, and the eCQMs are tied to the Triple Aim outlined within the national quality strategy (NQS) (McBride et al. 2019). The Triple Aim is better care, improved population health, and affordable costs (Berwick et al. 2008). Further, the eCQMs are guided by CMS' measurement strategy and the six NQS priorities: care coordination, safety, clinical quality of care, person and caregiver experience and outcomes, population/community health, and efficiency and cost reduction. The CMS measurement strategy includes measurements at multiple levels such as community, practice setting, and individual clinician/provider levels (Agency for Healthcare Research and Quality 2014a).

System Characteristics that Influence Health IT Adoption

Characteristics of the healthcare system within the QHOM model constitute structural components. The QHOM proposes relationships among components such that interventions act upon and through characteristics of the system and the client, and vice versa. Health IT and all its components can be viewed as a significant intervention deployed by "the system" to influence outcomes, particularly when coupled with quality improvement strategies. In other words, the effect of the Health IT intervention is mediated by or interacts with client and system characteristics and it has no independent direct effect on the outcome.

For example, environmental contextual factors, such as federal policy enacted to encourage and regulate Health IT for hospitals and providers, can be viewed within the QHOM framework as influencing the system to adopt certified EHRs. However, organizations elect which EHR to adopt and how quickly to implement it. For instance, many organizations elected "the big bang" approach to certified EHR adoption. Big bang implementation means the system is elected to move over from

Table 6.2 Health IT terminology with definitions (ONC 2020a)

Component	Definition
Electronic prescribing (ePrescribing)	Computer-based electronic generation, transmission, and filling of a medical prescription, taking the place of paper and faxed prescriptions
Computer provider order entry (CPOE)	Computerized provider order entry (CPOE) refers to the process of providers entering and sending treatment instructions—including medication, laboratory, and radiology orders—via a computer application rather than paper, fax, or telephone
Clinical decision support systems (CDSS)	Clinical decision support (CDS) provides clinicians, staff, patients, or other individuals with knowledge and person-specific information, intelligently filtered or presented at appropriate times, to enhance health and healthcare. CDS encompasses a variety of tools to enhance decision-making in the clinical workflow
Patient portals	A patient portal is a secure online website that gives patients convenient, 24-hour access to personal health information from anywhere with an Internet connection. Using a secure username and password, patients can view health information such as recent doctor visits, discharge summaries, and medications
Personal health records	A personal health record, or PHR, is an electronic application through which patients can maintain and manage their health information (and that of others for whom they have authorized) in a private, secure, and confidential environment
Health information exchange	Electronic health information exchange (HIE) allows doctors, nurses, pharmacists, other healthcare providers, and patients to appropriately access and securely share a patient's vital medical information electronically—improving the speed, quality, safety, and cost of patient care
Interoperability	The ability of computer systems or software to exchange and make use of information, "interoperability between devices made by different manufacturers"
Data standards	In the context of healthcare, the term data standards encompasses methods, protocols, terminologies, and specifications for the collection, exchange, storage, and retrieval of information associated with healthcare applications, including medical records, medications, radiological images, payment, and reimbursement
Electronic clinical quality measures (eCQMs)	Electronic clinical quality measures (eCQMs) use data electronically extracted from electronic health records (EHRs) and/or health information technology systems to measure the quality of healthcare provided

the old way of documenting (paper or an older legacy electronic record) overnight. One day, clinicians are on one system. The next day, the entire system moves over to a new way of doing things. System characteristics influence many organizations' decisions of how, when, and what type of technology to implement. Further, the environmental context (federal regulations) influences organizations (systems) to reach meaningful use of EHRs through financial incentives. System structural components influence the rapid adoption of clinical processes and workflows, which significantly influences how care processes are delivered.

In many institutions, EHRs were deployed as a technology implementation project and were not coupled with quality improvement strategies. System characteristics of an organization's culture led by an IT department rather than quality improvement likely influenced this approach. Unfortunately, this approach resulted in clinician dissatisfaction primarily due to the negative impact on clinicians' workflow and unnecessary documentation burden (Bodenheimer and Sinsky 2014; McBride et al. 2017).

Staff resources and competencies also influenced how hospitals and providers adopted the new EHR, implemented it, and trained their clinicians to use the new system. The characteristics of an organization would also influence the long-term maintenance of an EHR. Holmgren et al. (2018) reported that several hospital characteristics influenced EHR selection. These include ownership (private nonprofit, private for-profit, or public nonfederal); size (number of beds); participation in payment reform models; rural or urban location; teaching status; critical access hospital status; and participation in a health information exchange program. As a result of the rapid decisions and deployment of Health IT across the nation in the past decade and a half, EHRs and other Health IT components negatively influence the care delivered. Using the QHOM model, these challenges can be examined as opportunities to improve the use of technology and deploy quality improvement strategies discussed under the next section.

Health IT Interventions

The EHR and other point-of-care technologies that support and connect to the EHR, including device integration, are important considerations that impact patient safety and care quality in both positive and negative ways. Point-of-care technologies that supplement the EHR are devices that connect through interoperable connectivity standards to add additional patient care functionality. Examples of this type of technology include but are not limited to intravenous (IV) pumps, smart beds, and barcode administration mobile devices. Certified EHRs created many challenges that impact clinical workflow and, when coupled with additional point-of-care devices, result in better functionality, but at the same time added complexity with additional challenges and often unintended consequences of the technology. This section ties the QHOM to the optimization of technology and emphasizes the use of quality improvement science as a solution to better use Health IT.

The science of quality improvement (QI) is defined by the Institute for Healthcare Improvement (IHI) as follows: "… a unique approach to working with health systems, countries, and other organizations on improving quality, safety, and value in healthcare. This approach is called the science of improvement. The science of improvement is an applied science that emphasizes innovation" (IHI.org 2019, p. 1). As such, QI can be considered as the backbone for improving Health IT. The healthcare industry continues to "innovate" with the use of technology. Yet, many of our fundamental QI tools and strategies have not been used to adopt and implement technology innovations. An examination of a few of these fundamental tools that can be coupled with structural Health IT components to improve clinical processes and outcomes is given next.

Quality Improvement Tools to Improve Structural Components of Health

The QHOM framework creates an excellent foundation for examining technology's effect as an intervention and its impact on process and outcome for individuals, groups, and communities. In this context, the Health IT intervention is implemented using QI tools. As noted, the QHOM (Mitchell et al. 1998) proposes relationships among bidirectional components, with interventions or processes acting through characteristics of the system and of the client, and vice versa. An example of how this occurs is IV pump integration with the EHR. The intended outcome is at least twofold, with improved outcomes for individuals within the system that might be measured by an overall reduction in medication errors or pump infusion errors. The second outcome is improved processes. The process might involve pump integration to increase efficiency in the process of administering and monitoring IV medications on a hospital medical-surgical unit. With this integration, suggested process outcomes might be the total time to administer medications from computer provider order entry (CPOE) to IV pump start and the rate of pump integration errors. The medical-surgical unit's characteristics, such as nurse-to-patient ratio, influence the relationship between the process of administering medications and the outcome of medication errors. Other unit characteristics include the complexity of patients on the unit, day shift compared to evening and night shift, and day of the week. To address unintended consequences, monitoring of the improvement might include measuring patient, physician and nurse satisfaction (the client). In this example, QI tools can improve the process that impacts the outcomes by developing strategies to optimize Health IT's structural components. Useful QI tools include project charter, Plan-Do-Study-Act (PDSA) cycles, control charts, and workflow redesign.

The Project Charter
The project charter establishes "the game plan" for QI by outlining fundamental process improvement components, establishing the overall aim, scope of the project, and plan of action. A well-designed project charter also includes the process, outcome measures, and balancing parameters. When applied to technology optimization or to addressing a flaw or unintended consequence of technology, these measures align with the QHOM by establishing improvement strategies and tools to optimize technology for improved care processes and outcomes. For the example of the IV pump integration, the project charter's aim might be stated as follows: IV smart pump integration within 3 months to improve outcomes for a reduction in IV pump medication errors by 20%.

Plan-Do-Study-Act (PDSA) Cycles

The PDSA cycles originally proposed by Deming (1986) frame an *approach* to QI, upon which the entire QI activity is conceptualized as a more extensive process that is preplanned, executed, and evaluated in a logical, stepwise fashion. Inherent in the PDSA cycle is the assumption that to improve outcomes, processes must also improve. The PDSA model has been used on many occasions as a useful way to map the processes and outcomes of an implementation (Harrison and Lyerla 2012; Murphy 2013). The PDSA cycles can be utilized to plan a project for improving or optimizing Health IT. This approach is very effective when examining technology and its impact on clinician workflow and overall quality of patient care. For example, the PDSA cycles can be used to frame an improvement strategy for the IV pump integration to improve medication errors (outcome), mitigate pump integration errors (structure/process), and improve patient and clinician satisfaction (client). The PDSA approach to the IV pump integration might start with small tests of change in one area following the PDSA cycles and then adding another change depending on the outcome.

However, before starting a PDSA cycle, the QI team should first consider process mapping of the current workflow to lay out the entire process of administering IV medications. Second, the team should consider using a failure mode effect analysis (FMEA) to examine steps in the process and score the steps according to the risk of failure, with the highest risk receiving the highest score. Many system characteristics and client characteristics, including staff and patient, influence the process and risk within the process. A well-executed FMEA helps clarify where the process might fail, how often that failure might occur and how to optimize the technology integration to prevent medication error (Subramanyam et al. 2016). Once the areas of failure are identified, the workflow redesign's focus is determined, and a new process can be mapped using PDSA cycles to optimize the Health IT (structure) for better outcomes. Measuring the process pre- and post-improvement with control charts is a critical step to evaluate if a process is in control and if the improvement has positively impacted the process and outcomes.

Control Charts

A control chart, designed originally by Shewhart, is a chart that displays data over time or units of measure with upper and lower control limits (Best and Neuhauser 2006; McNeese 2016). Control charts are an effective way to differentiate between common cause (chance) and special cause variation (assignable) (Best and Neuhauser 2006). These methods can determine if a process is in control before implementing improvement strategies. Once implemented, detect special cause variation that reflects the impact of the improvement.

Control charts can be applied to Health IT improvement strategies to examine if a process is in control and whether special cause variation is present that should be fully understood before improvement occurs, and to measure the impact of pre- and post-improvement. For example, in the earlier IV pump integration example, integration can result in unintended consequences. These might include significant patient safety incidents or even a sentinel event that might require a root-cause

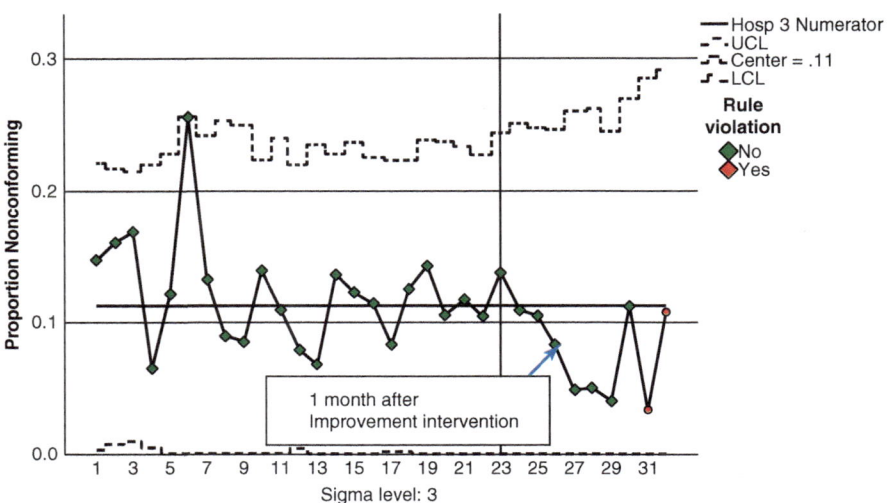

Fig. 6.3 Control chart for proportion of pump integration errors per month

analysis to fully understand the etiology or "root" of the issue. Also, control charts can be deployed to map relevant process measures. Figure 6.3 is a control chart displaying a successful intervention to optimize IV pump technology integration over time. The chart shows the proportion of errors in pre- and post-implementation. In this example, nonconforming is the proportion of errors on the *y*-axis, and time is noted on the *x*-axis. Time can vary by month, day, or quarter depending on the time-line for the improvement. The vertical line denotes 1 month after improvement. Month 23 reflects the onset of the improvement strategy to mitigate errors.

Workflow Redesign to Optimize EHRs and Other Point-of-Care Technologies

Research indicates that EHRs and other point-of-care devices have negatively impacted providers' clinical workflow (McBride et al. 2017). As such, workflow redesign methods are a critical QI tool to deploy for optimizing and rethinking technology within clinicians' workflow. The Health IT structural components can be redesigned to improve both process and outcomes by utilizing this QI tool. Workflow is defined by the Agency for Healthcare Research and Quality as "the sequence of physical and mental tasks performed by various people within and between work environments" (Agency for Healthcare Research and Quality 2014b). Workflow redesign is a method to map "as is" or current-state workflows. It examines opportunities to improve upon the workflow with a designed "to be" or future state based on the evidence and best practices. For example, the workflow of IV pump integration has several considerations related to clinical process and workflow. The following are key questions to consider, as noted by the American Society of Health-System Pharmacists (AHSP) (2020):

- How will automation of IV preparation change current processes?
- What is the new workflow?
- Does the new workflow make the process lean or add extra steps?
- How does the new technology impact the time to perform the task?
- Will there be a need to adjust other preparation or distribution workflows to enable incorporation of the new technology into daily, weekly, or off-shift use?
- Does the new workflow require an increase or decrease in the number of technicians and/or pharmacist staff during automation operations?
- Will the pharmacy department be able to repurpose staff assignments due to the implementation of the new technology (AHSP, p. 4)?

When considering these questions, the device integration implementation presents an excellent tie to how Health IT impacts clinical process and outcomes within the context of the healthcare environment influenced by system characteristics such as staffing and resources.

Health IT Competencies

Along with the introduction of Health IT into the healthcare delivery system came the need to educate clinicians, specifically nurses for whom Health IT education was of most importance. Educating nurses was crucial because of their pivotal role in coordinating patient care delivery. The advancement of technology in patient care delivery has been an ongoing evolution since the late 1990s. However, one can argue that the needed accompanying education in Heath IT has been slow to develop. Current examples are the needed competencies available through online course content such as the HITComp.org program (HITCOMP 2020) and the EU-US Initiative (EU*US eHealth Work 2018).

Along with the needed competencies, various nursing competency-based frameworks or models have evolved. The Nursing Education for Health Informatics (NEHI) is one example where competencies in teaching health informatics are emphasized (McBride et al. 2013). The framework organizes the informatics focus in three main domains: point-of-care technology, data management and analytics, and patient safety and quality for population health (see Fig. 6.4). The development of competencies for teaching in these three domains then yields the central aim of improved healthcare based on the union of each domain with the "nursing role." The next step is integrating the nursing role in an interprofessional approach with other healthcare team members. The ultimate goal of the framework and the competencies from each domain is creating an organizational culture where the healthcare team can collectively address today's care delivery challenges.

Nursing Informatics Content

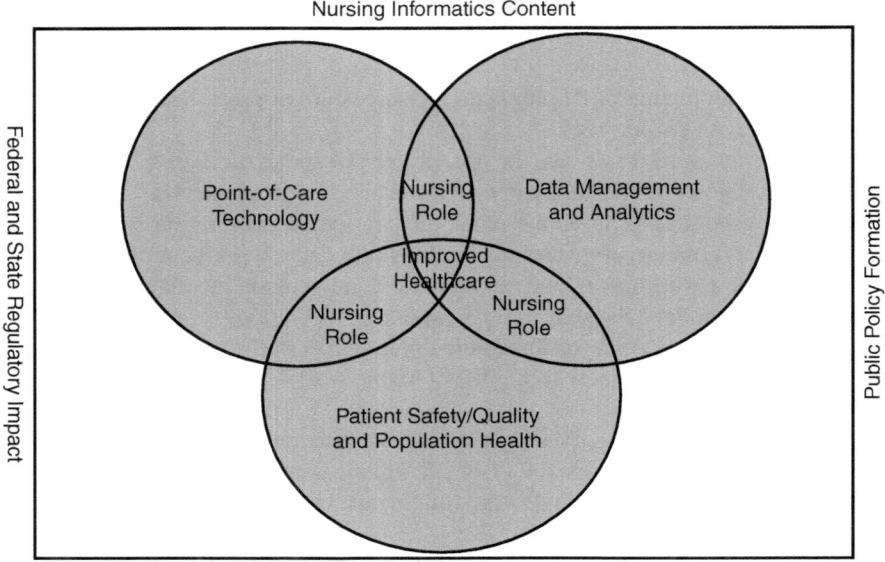

Fig. 6.4 The NEHI model. Framework for the development of curriculum to align with key information technology IOM recommendations (IOM Future of Nursing report) and the American Association of Colleges of Nursing DNP Essentials (with permission from McBride, S. G., Tietze, M., & Fenton, M. V. (2013). Developing an applied informatics course for a Doctor of Nursing Practice program. *Nurse Educator, 38*(1), 37–42. doi: https://doi.org/10.1097/NNE.0b01 3e318276df5d)

Technology Informatics Guiding Education Reform (TIGER)

One area where technology-based competencies have been consistently and significantly embraced over time is the Technology Informatics Guiding Education Reform (TIGER) initiative (TIGER Initiative 2014). TIGER initiated with a focus on nursing care delivery using technology, but it quickly morphed to an interdisciplinary focus, often the nature of technology in healthcare delivery. Beginning in the early 1990s, TIGER is now a global organization with more than 30 member countries. Besides, research and development of Health IT competencies, a virtual learning environment (VLE), houses the educational programs for teaching these competencies (HIMSS.org 2018b). The TIGER Competency Synthesis Project was comprised of international deployment of a survey questionnaire composed of 24 areas of core competencies in clinical informatics within five domains: (1) clinical nursing, (2) nursing management, (3) quality management, (4) IT management in nursing, and (5) coordination of interprofessional care (Hübner et al. 2016). The questionnaire was sent to 21 countries yielding participation from 43 experts to capture a global perspective.

These TIGER competencies have shed light on the role of executive leaders and what it takes for an organization to be truly technically safe and of high quality (HIMSS.org 2018a; Hübner et al. 2019). For the *Coordination of Interprofessional Care* with a focus on leadership competencies, specific sub-competencies emerge such as those listed here along with the proportion of respondents for each category:

- Data protection and security (85.9%)
- Information knowledge management (85.4%)
- Nursing documentation (83.4%)
- Process management (83.2%)
- Information communication systems (81.5%)
- Ethics and IT (78.8%) (Hübner et al. 2016)

These interprofessional, leadership-focused competencies are being further developed to improve their understanding and application.

Client

This section focuses on the client or healthcare consumer using technology to engage in healthcare delivery management. Patient, or consumer, engagement in their healthcare is a recent purposeful focus of healthcare delivery to achieve optimal patient outcomes. Several researchers have developed consumer engagement scales. One is the Stanford Self-Efficacy Scale (SES) (Ritter and Lorig 2014). The SES has 6 items where the patients report their degree of confidence on a 10-point scale in key aspects of chronic condition management such as fatigue, physical discomfort, and medications. Another scale measuring consumer engagement is the Patient Activation Measure (PAM) (Hibbard and Greene 2013; Hibbard et al. 2005). The PAM is much like the SES except that it contains 13 items, and the responses are on a 4-point Likert scale from strongly disagree to strongly agree (Hibbard et al. 2005). Both the SES and the PAM are extremely useful in quantifying the various levels of consumer engagement, which then guides the clinicians in efforts to support consumers and their family members in becoming optimally engaged in their healthcare, including while using Health IT. Studies have indicated that consumer engagement is associated with an improvement in healthcare outcomes (Centers for Medicare and Medicaid Services 2014; Coulter 2012; Graffigna et al. 2015) and with some decrease in the cost of healthcare delivery (Hibbard and Greene 2013).

Technology tools such as mobile health, telehealth services, and patient portals are commonly used to increase consumer engagement in healthcare delivery and manage their conditions (Tietze and Brown 2019). For example, with their secure online websites, portals give patients convenient, 24-hour access to personal health information from anywhere with an Internet connection. Portals can be accessed using a computer, laptop, iPad, or mobile phone. Portals are an example of a tool that can facilitate self-management in patients with complex chronic conditions (Powell and Myers 2018). Unfortunately, many patients are not taking advantage of this resource. In addition to patient portals, remote patient monitoring (RPM) in the home via technology is another way to engage consumers. The use of RPM is associated with a significant reduction in readmissions (Blum and Gottlieb 2014) and a decrease in emergency department use (Courtney et al. 2009). However, while convenient for patients, nurses, and other clinicians to use, measurements of the associated outcomes from these technology tools are difficult to capture and therefore are a much-needed focus for healthcare practice and research (Schulte and Fry 2019).

Outcomes

This section focuses on the impact of Health IT on positive and negative outcomes. In 2011, post-HITECH Act, Buntin et al. (2011) conducted a literature review to determine Health IT's positive and negative outcomes. They found that 92% of the articles reflected positive overall outcomes as defined by quality, efficiency, and satisfaction measures. More recently, Kruse and Beane (2018), following methods used by Buntin et al., also conducted a systematic review of the literature examining the impact of Health IT adoption on medical outcomes. Their findings also found a positive impact on medical outcomes defined as measures of efficiency and effectiveness. Although both reviews found a positive impact on outcomes, others have indicated that technology also results in unintended consequences with the potential for negative outcomes.

It has been said that Health IT positive outcomes for care delivery are directly related to the leadership's competencies in detecting and managing the unintended consequences of Health IT implementation. Sittig and Ash (2011) found nine unique ways clinicians are subjected to unintended consequences of Health IT. Their study used a retrospective review of over 10,000 patient charts. Numerous unintended consequences of technology-based patient care delivery were noted and grouped into nine major types. The types, along with proportion in each category, are

- More/new work for clinicians (19.8%)
- Workflow issues (17.6%)
- Never-ending system demands (14.8%)
- Paper persistence (10.8%)
- Changes in communication patterns and practices (10.1%)
- Emotions (7.7%)
- New kinds of errors (7.1%)
- Changes in power structure (6.8%)
- Overdependence on technology (5.2%) (Sittig and Ash 2011)

This description's critical aspect is that sometimes the use of Health IT results in patient harm and even contributes to death, without clinicians knowing that they have done so (Sittig and Ash 2011). Rigorous leadership training and education on preventing the issues listed can yield positive patient care outcomes.

As healthcare providers and hospitals continue to be encouraged by regulatory requirements to expand upon technology and to report quality measures for pay-for-performance models, the impact of technology on the client or patient, the clinicians, the organization, and the society is critical to consider.

Summary

In summary, this chapter has examined Health IT in the form of EHRs and other point-of-care technologies. The explosion of technology in the past 10 years has created a new digital healthcare age that creates both positive and negative challenges to processes and outcomes of patient care. As such, the QHOM emphasized throughout the chapter sets up an excellent approach to using QI methods to optimize technology. Several effective QI tools and methods to support Health IT optimization are presented. Both system and client components influence the optimization of Health IT. As per the QHOM model, outcomes must be reflected in both the client and clinician, and characteristics of the system or organization influence both. For example, a safety culture will emphasize competencies to prepare an organization to address outcomes.

Further, the commitment to measurement to positively impact the organization is fundamental. According to Baernholdt et al. (2018), for quality measures to be useful, they must be clearly defined, valid, reliable, and readily available to all stakeholders, i.e., the client, clinicians, organizational leaders, and policymakers. Finally, organizations' Health IT infrastructure ability to capture and report data for measuring process, outcome, and structural measures for all stakeholders is essential. This ability requires that Health IT staff, clinical informatics professionals and leadership maintain competencies in measurement, QI science and an interprofessional team approach to optimize technology for improved processes and health outcomes.

References

21st Century Cures Act, Pub. L. No. 114-255 (2016)
Agency for Healthcare Research and Quality (2014a) CMS framework for measurement maps to the six national quality strategy priorities [slide 15]. https://www.ahrq.gov/workingforquality/events/webinar-using-measurement-for-quality-improvement.html
Agency for Healthcare Research and Quality (2014b) What is workflow? https://healthit.ahrq.gov/health-it-tools-and-resources/evaluation-resources/workflow-assessment-health-it-toolkit/workflow
American Recovery and Reinvestment Act of 2009, Pub. L. No. 111-5, 123 Stat. 115 (2009)
American Society of Health-System Pharmacists (2020) Current state of IV workflow systems and IV robotics. https://www.ashp.org/-/media/assets/pharmacy-informaticist/docs/sopit-current-state-of-iv-workflow-systems-and-iv-robotics.pdf
Baernholdt M, Dunton N, Hughes RG, Stone PW, White KM (2018) Quality measures: a stakeholder analysis. J Nurs Care Qual 33(2):149–156. https://doi.org/10.1097/NCQ.0000000000000292
Berwick DM, Nolan TW, Whittington J (2008) The Triple Aim: care, health, and cost. Health Aff 27(3):759–769. https://doi.org/10.1377/hlthaff.27.3.759

Best M, Neuhauser D (2006) Walter A Shewhart, 1924, and the Hawthorne factory. Qual Saf Health Care 15(2):142–143. https://doi.org/10.1136/qshc.2006.018093

Blum K, Gottlieb SS (2014) The effect of a randomized trial of home telemonitoring on medical costs, 30-day readmissions, mortality, and health-related quality of life in a cohort of community-dwelling heart failure patients. J Card Fail 20(7):513–521. https://doi.org/10.1016/j.cardfail.2014.04.016

Bodenheimer T, Sinsky C (2014) From Triple to Quadruple Aim: care of the patient requires care of the provider. Ann Fam Med 12(6):573–576. https://doi.org/10.1370/afm.1713

Buntin MB, Burke MF, Hoaglin MC, Blumenthal D (2011) The benefits of health information technology: a review of the recent literature shows predominantly positive results. Health Affairs (Project Hope) 30(3):464–471. https://doi.org/10.1377/hlthaff.2011.0178

Centers for Medicare and Medicaid Services (2014) Partnership for patients: patient and family engagement. http://partnershipforpatients.cms.gov/about-the-partnership/patient-and-family-engagement/the-patient-and-family-engagement.html

Centers for Medicare and Medicaid Services (2019) Promoting interoperability programs. https://www.cms.gov/Regulations-and-Guidance/Legislation/EHRIncentivePrograms/index.html?redirect=/ehrincentiveprograms/

Coulter A (2012) Patient engagement—what works? J Ambulat Care Manag 35(2):80. http://www.ncbi.nlm.nih.gov/pubmed/22415281

Courtney M, Edwards H, Chang A, Parker A, Finlayson K, Hamilton K (2009) Fewer emergency readmissions and better quality of life for older adults at risk of hospital readmission: a randomized controlled trial to determine the effectiveness of a 24-week exercise and telephone follow-up program. J Am Geriatr Soc 57(3):395–402

Deming WE (1986) Out of the crisis. Massachusetts Institute of Technology, Cambridge, MA

EU*US eHealth Work (2018) Welcome to EU*US eHealth work. https://ehealthwork.org/

Graffigna G, Barello S, Bonanomi A, Lozza E (2015) Measuring patient engagement: development and psychometric properties of the patient health engagement (PHE) scale. Front Psychol 6:274. https://doi.org/10.3389/fpsyg.2015.00274

Harrison RL, Lyerla F (2012) Using nursing clinical decision support systems to achieve meaningful use. CIN: Comput Informat Nurs 30(7):380–385. https://doi.org/10.1097/NCN.0b013e31823eb813

Health Information Technology for Economic and Clinical Health (HITECH) Act, Title XIII of Division A and Title IV of Division B of the American Recovery and Reinvestment Act of 2009 (ARRA), Pub. L. No. 111-5, 123 Stat. 226 (February 17, 2009), codified at 42 USC. §§300jj et seq.; §§17901 et seq.

Hibbard JH, Greene J (2013) What the evidence shows about patient activation: better health outcomes and care experiences; fewer data on costs. Health Affairs (Project Hope) 32(2):207. https://www.insigniahealth.com/products/pam-survey

Hibbard JH, Mahoney ER, Stockard J, Tusler M (2005) Development and testing of a short form of the patient activation measure. Health Serv Res 40(6):1918–1930

HIMSS.org (2018a) TIGER international informatics competency synthesis project http://www.himss.org/professional-development/tiger-initiative/tiger-international-informatics-competency-synthesis-project

HIMSS.org (2018b) TIGER virtual learning environment: what is the virtual learning environment? http://www.himss.org/professional-development/tiger-initiative/virtual-learning-environment

HITCOMP (2020) Health information technology competencies: empowering a digitally skilled health workforce. http://hitcomp.org/

Holmgren J, Alder-Milstein J, McCullough J (2018) Are all certified EHRs created equal? Assessing the relationship between EHR vendor and hospital meaningful use performance. J Am Med Inform Assoc 25:654–660. https://doi.org/10.1093/jamia/ocx135

Hübner U, Shaw T, Thye J, Egbert N, Marin H, Ball M (2016) Towards an international framework for recommendations of core competencies in nursing and inter-professional informatics: the TIGER competency synthesis project. Stud Health Technol Informat 228:655. https://www.ncbi.nlm.nih.gov/pubmed/27577466

Hübner U, Thye J, Shaw T, Elias B, Egbert N, Saranto K et al (2019) Towards the TIGER international framework for recommendations of core competencies in health informatics 2.0: extending the scope and the roles. Stud Health Technol Informat 264:1218. https://www.ncbi.nlm.nih.gov/pubmed/31438119

IHI.org (2019) Institute for healthcare improvement (IHI): about us. http://www.ihi.org/about/Pages/ScienceofImprovement.aspx

Kruse CS, Beane A (2018) Health information technology continues to show positive effect on medical outcomes: systematic review. J Med Internet Res 20(2):e41. https://doi.org/10.2196/jmir.8793

McBride S, Tietze MF, Fenton M (2013) Developing an applied informatics course for a doctor of nursing practice program. Nurse Educ 38(1):37–42. https://doi.org/10.1097/NNE.0b013e318276df5d

McBride S, Tietze M, Hanley MA, Thomas L (2017) Statewide study to assess nurses' experiences with meaningful use-based electronic health records. CIN: Comput Informat Nurs 35(1):18–28. https://doi.org/10.1097/CIN.0000000000000290

McBride S, Bodine KM, Johnson L (2019) Chapter 23: Electronic clinical quality measures: building an infrastructure for success. In: McBride S, Tietze M (eds) Nursing informatics for the advanced practice nurse: patient safety, quality, outcomes, and interprofessionalism, 2nd edn. Springer Publishing Company, LLC, New York, NY, pp 557–588

McNeese B (2016) Control chart rules and interpretation. (Report No. 2016). 2016 BPI Consulting, LLC, Katy, TX. https://www.spcforexcel.com/knowledge/control-chart-basics/control-chart-rules-interpretation

Mitchell PH, Ferketich S, Jennings BM (1998) Quality health outcomes model. Image J Nurs Sch 30(1):43

Murphy JI (2013) Using plan do study act to transform a simulation center. Clin Simulat Nurs 9(7):e264. https://doi.org/10.1016/j.ecns.2012.03.002

Office of the National Coordinator for Health Information Technology (2014) Connecting health and care for the nation: a shared nationwide interoperability roadmap. https://www.healthit.gov/sites/default/files/hie-interoperability/nationwide-interoperability-roadmap-final-version-1.0.pdf

Office of the National Coordinator for Health Information Technology (2019) About ONC: what we do. https://www.healthit.gov/topic/about-onc

Office of the National Coordinator for Health Information Technology (2020a) Glossary: Health IT terms. https://www.healthit.gov/topic/health-it-basics/glossary

Office of the National Coordinator for Health Information Technology (2020b) What is meaningful use? https://www.healthit.gov/faq/what-meaningful-use

Powell KR, Myers CR (2018) Electronic patient portals: patient and provider perceptions. On-Line J Nurs Informat 22(1):1–1. https://search.proquest.com/docview/2033726655

Ritter PL, Lorig K (2014) The English and Spanish self-efficacy to manage chronic disease scale measures were validated using multiple studies. J Clin Epidemiol 67(11):1265–1273. https://doi.org/10.1016/j.jclinepi.2014.06.009

Schulte F, Fry E (2019) Death by 1,000 clicks: where electronic health records went wrong. https://khn.org/news/death-by-a-thousand-clicks/

Sittig DF, Ash JS (2011) Clinical information systems: overcoming adverse consequences. Jones and Bartlett Publishers, Sudbury, MA

Subramanyam R, Mahmoud M, Buck D, Varughese A (2016) Infusion medication error reduction by two-person verification: a quality improvement initiative. Pediatrics 138(6):e20154413. https://doi.org/10.1542/peds.2015-4413

Tietze M, Brown G (2019) Chapter 16: Telehealth and mobile Health. In: McBride S, Tietze M (eds) Nursing informatics for the advanced practice nurse: patient safety, quality, outcomes, and interprofessionalism, 1st edn. Springer Pub Co, New York, NY, pp 377–397

TIGER Initiative (2014) Technology informatics guiding education reform (TIGER initiative). http://www.thetigerinitiative.org/

Part IV

Client

Health Literacy and Social Determinants of Health

Terri Ann Parnell

Introduction

Health literacy is an essential component of each construct in the QHOM (Mitchell et al. 1998). However, in the QHOM, achieving optimal health outcomes depends on meeting clients where they are, providing individualized client interventions, and utilizing system resources. Improving social determinants of health, including health literacy, is vital to involving clients—individuals, groups, and communities—in their healthcare, and in turn improving client health outcomes. Social determinants of health (SDOH) refer to nonmedical factors that typically are considered outside the traditional healthcare setting. They include socioeconomic status, housing and physical environment, education, transportation, social and community support, access to food, and access to technology (Mogford et al. 2010). SDOH collectively are the conditions in which people are born, grow, live, work, and age, and the forces and systems shaping the conditions of daily life (US Department of Health and Human Services (USDHHS), Healthy People 2010, 2014). SDOH have an essential impact on the health status of individuals, families, and communities. The impact of SDOH, such as poverty, educational status, living environment (Sorenson et al. 2012), homelessness, and racism (Olshansky 2017), upon health outcomes has been reported widely. The World Health Organization (WHO) Commission on the Social Determinants of Health (CSDH) has proposed evidence that SDOH interventions can significantly reduce unacceptable inequity in health outcomes. The Commission shared specific action steps that included an enhanced

T. A. Parnell (✉)
Health Literacy Partners, LLC, Garden City, NY, USA
e-mail: Tparnell@healthliteracypartners.com

© Springer Nature Switzerland AG 2021
M. Baernholdt, D. K. Boyle (eds.), *Nurses Contributions to Quality Health Outcomes*, https://doi.org/10.1007/978-3-030-69063-2_7

understanding of the SDOH by the general public as an additional expansion of health literacy (CSDH 2008).

Historically, the term health literacy has had many definitions, analyses, and applications originating with an individual's skills or abilities, such as reading and comprehending health-related materials (Parnell et al. 2019). A more recent understanding of health literacy includes the multidimensional approach necessary to conceptualize the complex, dynamic nature of health literacy and the collaborative responsibility of patients, providers, and systems. Therefore, health literacy currently is defined as "a dynamic, collaborative, and mutually beneficial proficiency, incorporating prior health knowledge and experience, individual characteristics, health status, cultural and linguistic preferences, and cognitive abilities, influencing the ability of organizations, caregivers, and healthcare recipients to access, understand, and use health information and services to make informed, actionable decisions and enhance health outcomes" (Parnell et al. 2019, p. 8). A focus on health literacy is critical to addressing all social determinants of health and delivering equitable, safe healthcare. Many have considered health literacy a "new" SDOH due to its strong linkage to these factors (Rowlands et al. 2017) and its impact on health outcomes (Loan et al. 2018).

Like the SDOH, low health literacy skills also contribute to healthcare inequities and, ultimately, poor health outcomes. Although low health literacy can affect everyone at various times throughout their life, populations more likely to encounter low health literacy are older adults, individuals with less than high school education, racial and ethnic minorities, limited English proficient speakers, and those with low socioeconomic status (USDHHS, Office of Disease Prevention and Health Promotion 2010). These are many of the same population characteristics that align with the other SDOH and the current demographic transformation in the USA, which is projected to become a minority-majority population by 2044 when more than 50% of the population is nonwhite (US Census Bureau 2015). Other transformations include over 60 million people who speak a language other than English at home (US Census Bureau 2013) and the graying of America, with the nation's median age rising along with an increase in the 65 and older population from 35 million to approximately 49 million, between 2000 and 2016, respectively (US Census Bureau 2017). Research long ago demonstrated the significant health disparities between whites and nonwhite populations and documented the link between these disparities and SDOH (Heckler 1985).

Health Literacy: Specific Linkages to the QHOM

Health literacy is linked to all components of the QHOM (Mitchell et al. 1998) with multidirectional relationships whereby health literacy interventions act through client and system characteristics to improve health outcomes (Fig. 7.1). Further, client and system interactions affect health outcomes.

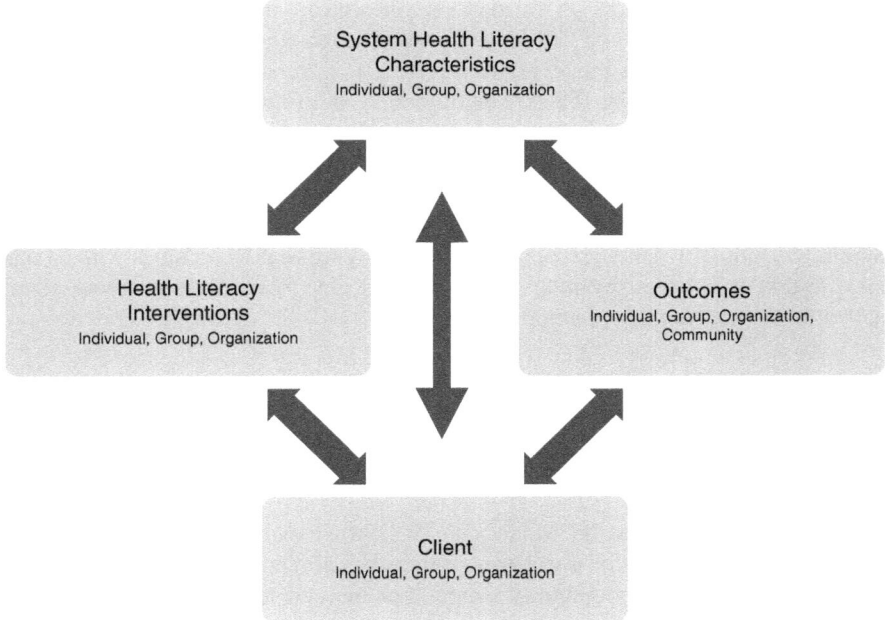

Fig. 7.1 Framework for health literacy

Client

In the QHOM, optimal outcomes are dependent upon interventions individualized to each client's characteristics and the resources available from the system. Because low health literacy is considered a limitation to accessing healthcare services, approaches for applying health literacy interventions focusing not only on specific clients but also on vulnerable groups and communities can improve health outcomes. Low health literacy implications include differences in health outcomes such as "poorer ability to demonstrate taking medications properly and interpret medication labels and health messages and, among elderly persons, poorer overall health status and higher mortality" (Berkman et al. 2011, p. 103). When linking health literacy to the QHOM, it is essential to recognize that clients or communities have varying characteristics and dynamic health literacy needs and will, therefore, require different interventions of engagement, education, and delivery of health services (Batterham et al. 2016).

Nurses play an essential role in ensuring that clients can access, understand, and use health information and services to make informed, actionable decisions that foster well-being and enhance health outcomes. Given the immense value of having enhanced health literacy skills for the client, healthcare professionals, and healthcare organizations, all nurses need to consider health literacy practices for every client and every client encounter (Barton et al. 2018). Nurses have a challenging but essential role in enhancing clients' health literacy skills and bridging the health literacy gap that so often exists between clients and providers (Parnell 2014). Nurses serve as client advocates and must have health literacy knowledge and agility needed to adapt to varying levels of health literacy by accessing various resources and implementing a variety of interventions. Nursing interventions that foster a collaborative, mutually beneficial approach to optimizing health outcomes with clients are presented, followed by interventions specifically focused on fostering client activation, engagement, and empowerment.

Interventions

Health Literacy Interventions Focused on the Client

The Health Literacy Tapestry Model (Fig. 7.2) provides a holistic nursing framework that incorporates six interwoven antecedent threads. These include demographics; the status of community support; media and marketplace; prior health

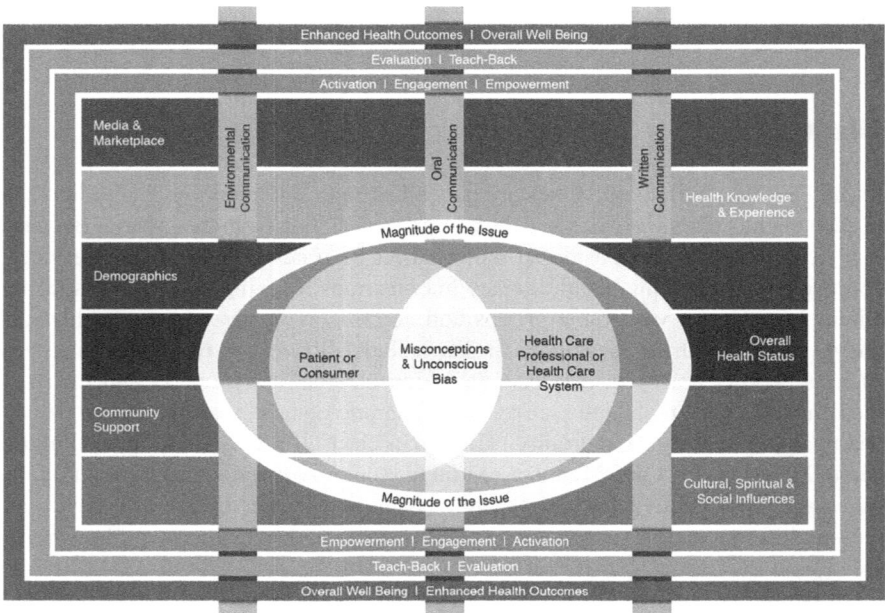

© 2014. *Health Literacy in Nursing: Providing Person-Centered Care.* Springer Publishing Company.

Fig. 7.2 The health literacy tapestry. Source: Parnell, T.A. (2015). Health literacy in nursing: Providing person-centered care. Springer Publishing Company LLC, NY, New York. ISBN: 9780826161727. (Reproduced with permission of Springer Publishing Company, LLC)

knowledge and experience; health status; and spiritual, cultural, or social factors (Parnell 2015). Collectively, the threads represent the dynamic, multidimensional conditions in which clients live, work, and age. The three basic fibers (domains) of the health literacy tapestry are oral communication, written communication, and environmental communication. The model was expanded recently to visually distinguish the essential role of empowerment, engagement, and activation, which are essential factors to foster well-being and enhanced health outcomes. Health literacy is vital for involving individuals in their healthcare, and therefore all engagement interventions also should integrate efforts to improve health literacy (Coulter 2012).

It is essential for nurses and all healthcare providers to have a foundational understanding of the depth and breadth of health literacy and the implications of low health literacy, and become competent in addressing interventions in clinical practice. Nurses can begin by creating a welcoming and respectful environment for all clients (Parnell 2015). Although many have expressed this as always being done, it is essential to understand that clients may feel uncomfortable sharing health-related concerns. This feeling of discomfort can be especially true when there are diverse cultural beliefs, linguistic differences, and a general lack of trust of healthcare clinicians. Building a foundation of trust and fostering dignity and respect start by recognizing each person's uniqueness, including taking time to assess their cultural and linguistic values, beliefs, and preferences (Parnell 2015). Whenever possible, ensure a private environment for communications. Other steps include asking how the client would like to be addressed and offering assistance in completing required forms. When providing education, nurses must assess the client's learning style, skills, and preferences to foster understanding (Parnell 2015). While communicating, nurses must also assess body language and make time to pause and listen. These techniques are used to accommodate teaching content to the client's preferences.

Health Literacy Universal Precautions

Nurses can advocate for always using a health literacy universal precautions approach (Brega et al. 2015). These precautions contain several principles, including speaking in plain, everyday language, confirming understanding, making the healthcare environment easier to access and navigate, and providing continuing support to clients (Brega et al. 2015).

Universal precautions include the use of an active voice when teaching clients (Dickens and Piano 2013; Parnell 2015), which helps to emphasize that the client is the one expected to perform the action being requested. Avoid lengthy discussions, pause periodically, and encourage questions by asking "what questions do you have for me?" It is common to provide too much information; therefore limit the content presented to "need-to-know" information rather than "nice-to-know" information (Dickens and Piano 2013; Parnell 2015). Avoid using medical jargon (Dickens and Piano 2013; Parnell 2015). For example, say "chest pain" rather than "angina" or "walk" rather than "ambulate."

Confirm understanding of teaching by incorporating the teach-back method (Dickens and Piano 2013; Parnell 2015). Ask the client to teach back the information discussed to ensure that provided information was clear. Clarify any misinformation right away. For example, the nurse may say, "We just reviewed some new medication instructions. I want to be sure I was clear when I explained these to you. Will you please tell me how you will describe these new instructions to your wife when you get home?" If information is not taught back correctly, then state, "I must not have been clear. Let's go over the instructions again." Then proceed with providing the information differently, using different terms, and repeat the teach-back until the client explains it sufficiently. When teach-back has been successfully completed encourage questions by asking "what questions do you have for me?" rather than "do you have any questions?" Asking clients to recall and restate what they have been told has been reported as a client safety practice during informed consent (Agency for Healthcare Research and Quality (AHRQ) 2013). Research on physicians' use of teach-back with diabetic clients to assess recall or comprehension resulted in better glycemic control (Schillinger et al. 2003). Finally, using written material to supplement teaching is an effective way to reinforce information and allow the client to refer back to the information and share with family members.

Other interventions, which can support a universal precautions approach, are designing the healthcare environment with the client burden lessened and making healthcare services easier to access and navigate (see System section below). All clients can thrive when nurses implement interventions to foster a health literacy universal precautions approach and support their efforts to manage their healthcare and improve their health safety.

Role of Health Literacy in Client Engagement, Empowerment, and Activation

Client engagement is a broad term, which incorporates empowerment and activation. Empowerment applies to providing information, education, and skills that help support the client when making decisions and taking action steps (Pelletier and Stichler 2013). Some have perceived health literacy as an educational means to empower individuals and inform and enlighten communities (CSDH 2008). The role of activation, or the client's skills and willingness to actively manage their health (Hibbard and Greene 2013), is critical to improving health outcomes. It has been reported that higher client activation levels are associated with better self-management and healthy behaviors, better use of screening services, and decreased costs for the healthcare system (Greene et al. 2015). "Health literacy is about the understanding of the social determinants of health and the knowledge of how to handle them and how to place the health of the individual, family and community in context" (Crondahl and Karlsson 2016, p. 2).

Nurses are well positioned to empower individuals and families with health information, client education, and skills necessary to manage their health. When planning interventions focusing on enhancing client engagement, nurses should also aspire to improve health literacy (Coulter and Ellins 2017). In a review of 67 studies of patient-focused interventions to improve health literacy, self-care, and patient safety, Coulter and Ellins (2017) identified best ways to support self-care in the management of chronic disease. Although the evidence regarding long-term outcomes and complex interventions remains limited, there were improved health outcomes for patients with depression, asthma, eating disorders, diabetes, and hypertension when self-help and educational programs were supported by clinicians (Coulter and Ellins 2017). Many of the previously mentioned health literacy interventions will foster empowerment and client's self-management. The teach-back method, previously described, encourages participation, promotes more informed clients, and facilitates shared decision-making. An additional intervention that can promote self-management is encouraging clients to participate in decisions about their goals for behavior change rather than assuming that they will comply with the clinician's plan (Coulter 2012).

Once client goals are determined, nurses can help clients draft action steps to help identify and break down tasks into manageable achievements. There is some evidence that e-learning programs and virtual support programs positively impact a patient's health behavior and enhanced clinical outcomes (Murray et al. 2005). When patient information is individualized and reviewed by clinicians, there is a more beneficial impact. In a literature review of patients with chronic heart failure, both structured telephone support and telemonitoring decreased heart failure-related hospitalizations (Ingis et al. 2010). Care planning and ongoing support offered after the clinical encounter via telehealth, or in-person health coaching, can support person-centered care and encourage activation and ongoing engagement.

The delivery of quality healthcare services relies on successful engagement, empowerment, and "actions individuals must take to obtain the greatest benefit from the healthcare services available to them" (Center for Advancing Health 2010, p. 2). Engaging clients in their healthcare foundationally relies on health literacy (Coulter 2012; Koh et al. 2013).

System

System characteristics consist of many structure and process factors and are differentiated based on client characteristics and healthcare organization type. Recognizing that health literacy is critical to delivering safe, effective, person-centered care, various organizations have prioritized the need to address system-level structure and processes that better align the healthcare demands and complexities with client skills and abilities (Brach et al. 2012). Health literacy is essential in providing culturally and linguistically safe, quality care for diverse populations. Healthcare organizations—including hospitals, inpatient facilities, ambulatory group practices and clinics, pharmacy practices, and large integrated health systems—are recognizing that operationalizing health literacy across structures and processes will benefit the majority of clients who experience difficulty accessing, understanding, and using health information and services (Brach et al. 2012).

Health Literacy Interventions Addressing the System

Investments in interventions that address SDOH, such as transportation, housing, health literacy, and environmental factors, can help both system and client characteristics achieve enhanced short- and long-term health outcomes. Health literacy is a dynamic, reciprocal proficiency that affects nurses, organizations, and clients' ability or inability to understand each other (Parnell et al. 2019). Therefore, health literacy should be a cross-cutting priority when proposing system-level interventions and evaluating quality improvement initiatives in a healthcare organization or system.

Fostering Health-Literate Healthcare Organizations

Communication is key to health literacy. Healthcare organizations often assume that they do a sufficient job communicating with clients and that the information provided was understood. Nurses have shared that they ask clients questions to ascertain how to teach, which is an inaccurate assessment of a client's health literacy ability. Examples of such questions are "what is your learning preference," "what was the last grade level completed," or "what are your learning barriers"? Instead, nurses should use the health literacy universal precautions described above. Despite client education and clear communication being core elements of a nurse's scope of practice, Macabasco-O'Connell and Fry-Bowers (2011) "surveyed 270 nurses; among 76 respondents, 80% reported that they never or rarely assessed health literacy using a validated tool and 60% responded that they used their gut feeling to estimate a client's health literacy level" (p. 62). Studies have also reported that most health information and education materials provided to clients are written well beyond most individuals' ability to comprehend them (Rudd 2010). Healthcare conversations about risk or benefit, explanation of benefits, insurance information, and cost of services are often delivered incomprehensibly (Institute of Medicine (IOM) 2004). A health-literate healthcare organization creates an environment that enables everyone to access and benefit from a range of healthcare services. Also, a health-literate healthcare organization strives to make it easy for all individuals to access, navigate, understand, and use information and services so they can take care of their health (Brach et al. 2012).

Nurse leaders can integrate health literacy in a variety of ways. They can begin by fostering a culture where clear, effective communication is a priority for all nurses. This culture can be enhanced by supporting values that center on the clients' perspectives and emphasize that communication is always a two-way interaction, with each person having equally essential roles (Brach et al. 2012). Nursing leadership can allocate roles and responsibilities to improve health literacy and establish accountability. A nursing culture that cultivates health literacy champions and prioritizes health literacy as a client safety concern will foster a health-literate organization (Loan et al. 2018). Annual education on health literacy should be incorporated into mandated topics and viewed as an equally important priority as handwashing. Health literacy is essential to client safety planning, and therefore health literacy should be incorporated into all quality improvement planning and process initiatives. Developing policies, procedures, metrics, or a dashboard and communicating trends will help identify successes and further improvement opportunities.

Several organizations support health professionals' training to enhance clear communication skills (Brach et al. 2012). Nursing leaders can foster a health-literate organization by preparing the workforce to be health literate. Health literacy education and training for the workforce can be incorporated during onboarding, annual mandated topics, and ad hoc throughout the year. Focusing on annual activities during Health Literacy Month in October will assist with raising awareness. Although a direct link between health literacy training and increased health outcomes has not been established (Coleman 2011), research shows that health professionals who attended health literacy training improved communication skills (Blake et al. 2010).

System Engagement of Community in Health Literacy

Another area where nursing interventions can encourage a health-literate organization is developing partnerships with the community. Consulting with community members when designing information or developing programs will result in products and services that more accurately meet the population's needs (Brach et al. 2012). Community members can also participate in advisory panels and committees. Some examples of partnering with community-based organizations are asking community members to participate in a "walk through" of the healthcare organization, provide guidance on new interventions, participate with material development, and share their own or the community members' experiences when accessing healthcare services (Brach et al. 2012).

Although health literacy and effective communication practices should be implemented for all clients, nurses can be instrumental in identifying high-risk areas or practices that may need additional attention. Areas that may require extra health literacy resources such as the emergency department, ambulatory clinics, care transitions, and palliative and end-of-life care present heightened opportunities to ensure safe communication and informed consent. Nurses have a vital role in leading interventions to support healthcare organizations when addressing the challenge of low health literacy. Clinician, system, and community interventions that enhance a person's health literacy improve healthcare outcomes for clients with low health literacy and benefit clients of all literacy levels (Sudore and Schillinger 2009).

Outcomes: Health Literacy Impact Upon Quality and Safety

Individual Outcomes

Health literacy and other SDOH are critical aspects of health promotion and disease prevention. Clients with less support, low health literacy, and lower activation levels tend not to participate in shared decision-making but instead go along with the clinician's decisions (Coulter 2012). Greene et al. (2015) examined the extent to which a single assessment of client engagement was associated with health outcomes and costs over time. They found an association between higher activation and improved health outcomes in addition to lower costs 2 years later. In another study of diabetic clients with low health literacy, the use of the teach-back method was shown to improve diabetes control (Schillinger et al. 2003). Although a wide range of stakeholders propose many health literacy interventions, not all interventions are appropriate for implementing in a clinical setting. Nurses should use a health literacy universal precautions approach, assess each situation, and select interventions and resources to provide safe person-centered care.

System/Organization Outcomes

Research findings suggest that the unequal quality of client-centered communication within a healthcare organization may contribute to poor health outcomes among people with low health literacy (IOM 2004). Therefore, organizational leaders must incorporate health literacy into the organization's vision, structure, and operations. The intervention should contain specific action steps; prioritize clear, effective communication; and assign responsibility and accountability for health literacy improvement across the workforce. Further, organizations need to build best practices to promote effective communication as a client safety imperative (National Quality Forum 2010) and foster an informed, activated client communicating with a proactive clinical team (Bodenheimer et al. 2002). Organizational health literacy is also an essential component for attaining increased client empowerment and engagement (Annarumma et al. 2016). Similar to suggestions for enhancing an individual's health literacy, a wide range of accreditation, quality, and professional organizations have recommended cross-cutting, system-level changes to address organizational health literacy (Brach et al. 2012). Leaders must create and prioritize an organizational culture of health literacy as part of continuous quality improvement.

Community/Group Outcomes

The National Prevention Strategy (2011) focuses on a community-centric approach for building healthy communities. This framework links education and health literacy to enhancing the quality of life. By eliminating educational and health literacy challenges to accessing healthcare, quality of life is improved. A focus on health-literate community partnerships will broaden community resources to address the SDOH (Koh et al. 2013). These partnerships can include community linkages to nonmedical support, wellness, and literacy resources. Nurses can assist by developing community referral relationships and providing assistance with, for example, referrals to adult basic education, discount prescriptions, financial assistance with medications, and food assistance programs.

The use of preventative services is mutually dependent upon the alignment of the healthcare system's ability to provide the appropriate services and the community members' understanding of the benefits of preventive care and their level of engagement and activation (National Prevention Strategy 2011). Quality of care will be improved if alignment and integration occur among clinical and community services. Providing community members with clear, accurate, culturally, and linguistically appropriate information that matches their health literacy skills will help them use health information and adopt healthy behaviors (Rudd et al. 2007). The evidence continues to grow in support of health literacy interventions in improving healthcare quality and outcomes (Berkman et al. 2011).

Implications and Future Directions

Health literacy is essential for improving clients, families, and communities' health and quality of life. The achievement of quality outcomes is dependent upon the interrelationship of client health literacy, system health literacy characteristics, and health literacy interventions focused on the individual, the organization, and the community. Nurses have limited knowledge of health literacy and the impact low health literacy has on client outcomes. Further, nurses tend to overestimate their clients' health literacy abilities (Macabasco-O'Connell and Fry-Bowers 2011). Therefore, organizations and schools of nursing must include health literacy education and skill development to adequately prepare nurses to deliver safe, quality healthcare services to an increasingly diverse client population.

Low health literacy is linked significantly to race, ethnicity, socioeconomic status, education level, and age (Kutner et al. 2003). Research suggests that health literacy is linked directly to key social determinants of health and health outcomes (Logan et al. 2015). Further, health literacy and all other SDOH elements need to be couched within a sociopolitical framework that includes racism and not just race (Boyd et al. 2020). As with health literacy, racism needs to be identified at different levels, such as implicit bias in individual clinicians and structural racism in organizations.

Future research addressing interventions targeting the organization (system) and the healthcare practitioners (e.g., nurses) is needed to evaluate what works to lessen the adverse client outcomes associated with low health literacy (Macabasco-O'Connell and Fry-Bowers 2011). Research and funding are also needed to integrate health literacy throughout all community interventions and advocate for policy development to advance health literacy as a priority area for client safety and quality improvement in nursing education, the healthcare system, and the community. Addressing health literacy is an essential component of mitigating healthcare inequities. The QHOM constructs incorporate various dynamic, contextual feedback opportunities between the client, healthcare system, and interventions to promote quality outcomes. Aligning system characteristics and individualized health literacy client interventions throughout the QHOM will foster client engagement, empowerment, and activation and ultimately achieve meaningful, quality health outcomes for all.

References

Agency for Healthcare Research and Quality (AHRQ) (2013) Making health care safer II: an updated critical analysis of the evidence for patient safety practices. Agency for Healthcare Research and Quality, Rockville, MD. http://www.ahrq.gov/research/findings/evidence-based-reports/ptsafetyuptp.html

Annarumma C, Palumbo R, Cavallone M (2016) Empowering patients by empowering health care organizations: a comparative study. In: Baccarani C, Martin J (eds) Proceedings of 19th toulon-verona international conference. University of Huelva, Spain, pp 1–14

Barton AJ, Allen PE, Boyle DK, Loan LA, Stichler JF, Parnell TA (2018) Health literacy: essential for a culture of health. J Contin Educ Nurs 49(2):73–78. https://doi.org/10.3928/00220124-20180116-06

Batterham RW, Hawkins M, Collins PA, Buchbinder R, Osborne RH (2016) Health literacy: applying current concepts to improve health services and reduce health inequalities. Public Health 132:3–12. https://doi.org/10.1016/j.puhe.2016.01.001

Berkman ND, Sheridan SL, Donahue KE, Halperin DJ, Crotty K (2011) Low health literacy and health outcomes: an updated systematic review. Ann Intern Med 155(2):97–107. https://doi.org/10.7326/0003-4819-155-2-201107190-00005

Blake SC, McMorris K, Jacobson KL, Gazmararian JA, Kripalani S (2010) A qualitative evaluation of a health literacy intervention to improve medication adherence for underserved pharmacy patients. J Health Care Poor Underserved 21(2):559–567

Bodenheimer T, Wagner EH, Grumbach K (2002) Improving primary care for patients with chronic Illness. J Am Med Assoc 288(14):1775–1779. https://doi.org/10.1001/jama.288.14.177

Boyd RW, Lindo EG, Weeks LD, McLemore MR (2020, July 2) On racism: a new standard for publishing on racial health inequities. Health Affairs Blog. https://www.healthaffairs.org/do/10.1377/hblog20200630.939347/full/?utm_medium=social&utm_source=twitter&utm_campaign=blog&utm_content=Boyd

Brach C, Keller D, Hernandez LM, Baur C, Parker R, Dreyer B, Schyve P, Schillinger D (2012) Ten attributes of health literate health care organizations. NAM Perspectives. Discussion Paper. National Academy of Medicine, Washington, DC. https://doi.org/10.31478/201206a

Brega AG, Barnard J, Mabachi NM, Weiss BD, DeWalt DA, Brach C, West DR (2015) AHRQ Health literacy universal precautions toolkit, Second Edition. Agency for Healthcare Research and Quality, Publication No. 15-0023-EF, Rockville, MD. https://www.ahrq.gov/professionals/quality-patient-safety/quality-resources/tools/literacy-toolkit/healthlittoolkit2.html

Center for Advancing Health (2010) A new definition of patient engagement: what is engagement and why is it important? http://www.cfah.org/pdfs/CFAH_Engagement_Behavior_Framework_current.pdf

Coleman C (2011) Teaching health care professionals about health literacy: a review of the literature. Nurs Outlook 59(2):70–78

Coulter A (2012) Patient Engagement-What Works? J Ambulat Care Manag 35(2):80–89. https://doi.org/10.1097/JAC.0b013e318249e0fd

Coulter A, Ellins J (2017) Effectiveness of strategies for informing, educating, and involving patients. Br Med J 335:24–27. https://doi.org/10.1136/bmj.39246.581169.80

Crondahl K, Karlsson LE (2016) The nexus between health literacy and empowerment: a scoping review. SAGE Open:1–7. https://doi.org/10.1177/2158244016646410

CSDH (2008) Closing the gap in a generation: health equity through action on the social determinants of health. In: Final Report of the Commission on Social Determinants of Health. World Health Organization, Geneva. https://www.who.int/social_determinants/thecommission/finalreport/en/index.html

Dickens C, Piano MR (2013) Health literacy and nursing: an update. Am J Nurs 113(6):52–57. https://doi.org/10.1097/01.NAJ.0000431271.83277.2f

Greene J, Hibbard JH, Sacks R, Overton V, Parrotta CD (2015) When patient activation levels change, health outcomes and costs change, too. Health Aff 34(3):431–437. https://doi.org/10.1377/hlthaff.2014.0452

Heckler M (1985) Report of the Secretary's task force on black and minority health. US Department of Health and Human Services, Washington, DC. https://minorityhealth.hhs.gov/assets/pdf/checked/1/ANDERSON.pdf

Hibbard JH, Greene J (2013) What the evidence shows about patient activation: better health outcomes and care experiences; fewer data on costs. Health Aff 32(2):207–214. https://doi.org/10.1377/hlthaff.2012.1061

Ingis SC, Clark RA, McAlister FA, Ball J, Lewinter C, Cullington D, Cleland JG (2010) Structured telephone support or telemonitoring of programmes for patients with chronic heart failure. Cochrane Database Syst Rev 8:CD007228. https://doi.org/10.1002/14651858.CD007228.pub2

Institute of Medicine (IOM) (2004) Health literacy: a prescription to end confusion. National Academies Press, Washington, DC

Koh KK, Brach C, Harris LM, Parchman ML (2013) A proposed health literate care model would constitute a systems approach to improving patients' engagement in care. Health Aff 3(2):357–367. https://doi.org/10.1377/hlthaff.2012.1205

Kutner M, Greenberg E, Jin Y, Paulsen C (2003) The health literacy of America's adults: results from the 2003 national assessment of adult literacy. NCES 2006-483. US Department of Education. National Center for Education Statistics, Washington, DC

Loan LA, Parnell TA, Stichler JF, Boyle DK, Allen P, VanFosson CA, Barton AJ (2018) Call for action: nurses must play a critical role to enhance health literacy. Nurs Outlook 66(1):97–100. https://doi.org/10.1016/j.outlook.2017.11.003

Logan RA, Wong WF, Villaire M, Daus G, Parnell TA, Willis E, Paasche-Orlow MK (2015) Health literacy: a necessary element for achieving health equity. Discussion Paper, Institute of Medicine. http://www.nam.edu/perspectives/2015/Health-literacy-anecessary-element-for-achieving-health-equity

Macabasco-O'Connell A, Fry-Bowers EK (2011) Knowledge and perceptions of health literacy among nursing professionals. J Health Commun 16(Suppl 3):295–307. https://doi.org/10.1080/10810730.2011.604389

Mitchell PM, Ferketich S, Jennings BM (1998) Quality health outcomes model. Image J Nurs Scholar 30(1):43–46

Mogford E, Gould L, Devoght A (2010) Teaching critical health literacy in the US as a means to action on the social determinants of health. Health Promot Int 26(1):4–13. https://doi.org/10.1093/heapro/daq049

Murray E, Burns J, See TS, Lai R, Nazareth I (2005) Interactive Health Communication Applications for people with chronic disease. Cochrane Database Syst Rev 4:CD004274. https://doi.org/10.1002/14651858.CD004274.pub4

National Prevention Council (2011) National prevention strategy. Department of Health and Human Services, Office of the Surgeon General. https://www.surgeongeneral.gov/priorities/prevention/strategy/report.pdf

National Quality Forum (2010) Safe practices for better healthcare—2010 update. National Quality Forum. https://www.qualityforum.org/Publications/2010/04/Safe_Practices_for_Better_Healthcare_-_2010_Update.aspx

Olshansky EF (2017) Social determinants of health: the role of nursing. Am J Nurs 117(12):11. https://doi.org/10.1097/01.NAJ.0000527463.16094.39

Parnell TA (2014) Nursing leadership strategies, health literacy, and patient outcomes. Nurse Leader 12(6):49–52

Parnell TA (2015) Health literacy in nursing: providing person-centered care. Springer Publishing Company LLC, NY, New York

Parnell TA, Stichler JF, Barton AJ, Loan LA, Boyle DK, Allen PA (2019) A concept analysis of health literacy. Nurs Forum 54(3):315–327. https://doi.org/10.1111/nuf.12331

Pelletier LR, Stichler JF (2013) Action brief: patient engagement and activation: a health reform imperative and improvement opportunity for nursing. Nurs Outlook 61:51–54

Rowlands G, Shaw A, Jaswal S, Smith S, Harpham T (2017) Health literacy and the social determinants of health: a qualitative model from adult learners. Health Promot Int 32:13–138. https://doi.org/10.1093/heapro/dav093

Rudd R (2010) Improving Americans' health literacy (perspective). N Engl J Med 363(24):2283–2285

Rudd RE, Anderson JE, Oppenheimer S, Nath C (2007) In: Comings JP, Garner B, Smith C (eds) Health literacy: an update of public health and medical literature. Lawrence Erlbaum Associates Review of Adult Learning and Literacy, Mahwah, pp 175–204

Schillinger D, Piette J, Grumbach K, Wang F, Wilson C, Daher C, Leong-Grotz K, Castro C, Bindman AB (2003) Closing the loop: physicians' application of interactive communication to assess recall or comprehension was associated with better glycemic control for diabetic patients. Arch Intern Med 163(1):83–90

Sorenson K, Broucke SV, Fullam J, Doyle G, Pelikan J, Slonska A, Brand H, HLS-EU Consortium Health Literacy Project European (2012) Health literacy and public health: a systemic review and integration of definitions and models. BMC Public Health 12:80. https://doi. org/10.1186/1471-2458/12/80

Sudore RL, Schillinger D (2009) Interventions to improve care for patients with limited health literacy. J Clin Outcomes Manag 21:867–873

US Census Bureau (2013, August) Language use in the United States: 2011. https://www.census. gov/library/publications/2013/acs/acs-22.html

US Census Bureau (2015) New census bureau report analyzes US populationprojections. https:// www.census.gov/newsroom/press-releases/2015/cb15-tps16.html

US Census Bureau (2017) The Nation's older population is still growing, Census Bureau Reports. https://www.census.gov/newsroom/press-releases/2017/cb17-100.html

US Department of Health and Human Services (2010) Office of disease prevention and health promotion. National action plan to improve health literacy. https://health.gov/communication/ initiatives/health-literacy-action-plan.asp

US Department of Health and Human Services (2014) Healthy People 2020. 2020 topics and objectives: social determinants of health. https://www.healthypeople.gov/2020/topics-objectives/ topic/social-determinants-of-health

Chronicity

Amy J. Barton

Introduction

The Centers for Disease Control and Prevention (2018a) indicate that six in ten adults in the United States have a chronic disease, with four in ten adults having two or more chronic diseases. Chronic diseases occur for a year or longer for which the client receives continual treatment and the disease(s) interfere with daily living activities. The most prevalent chronic diseases in the United States are heart disease, cancer, and diabetes (CDC 2018a). Further, of the $3.3 trillion spent on healthcare in the United States, 90% of that total is for people with chronic physical and mental health conditions (CDC 2018b). Merely the prevalence and cost of chronic conditions suggest the complexity associated with chronic care. Increasingly, across the globe, clients are experiencing more than one chronic disease, a phenomenon known as multimorbidity. Multimorbidity is "the coexistence of two or more chronic conditions, where each must be a noncommunicable disease (NCD), a mental health disorder, or an infectious disease of long duration" (The Lancet 2018, p. 391).

In contrast, chronicity is the experience of chronic disease over time. Martin and Sturmberg (2009) state:

> Chronicity is overtly conceptualized to encompass the phenomena of an individual journey, with simple and complicated, complex and chaotic phases, through long term *asymptomatic disease to bodily dysfunction and illness*, located in family and communities. Chronicity encompasses trajectories of *self-care and health care, as health, illness and disease co-exist and co-evolve in the setting of primary care, local care networks, and at times institutions* (p. 571).

A. J. Barton (✉)
Professor and Daniel and Janet Mordecai Endowed Chair in Rural Health Nursing,
College of Nursing, University of Colorado Anschutz Medical Campus, Aurora, CO, USA
e-mail: amy.barton@cuanschutz.edu

© Springer Nature Switzerland AG 2021
M. Baernholdt, D. K. Boyle (eds.), *Nurses Contributions to Quality Health Outcomes*, https://doi.org/10.1007/978-3-030-69063-2_8

Among the first to speak about illness trajectories were Glaser and Strauss (1968). A trajectory is the events throughout an illness shaped by the client's response to illness, interactions with others, and particular interventions (Reed and Corner 2015). Illness trajectories have been used as conceptual frameworks for research (Mackintosh and Sandall 2016), to identify study participants for research projects (Ruetsch et al. 2013), to redefine metastatic breast cancer as a chronic disease (Reed and Corner 2015), and to define functional decline (Huang et al. 2013). Trajectories have also been used at a policy level to inform service planning for end-of-life care (Canadian and Palliative Care Association 2013; Lynn and Adamson 2003; National Health Service Kidney Care End-of-Life Programme 2015). The key to trajectories in relation to the Quality Health Outcomes Model (QHOM) (Mitchell et al. 1998) is that they have been described as a phenomenon nested within "genetic, biological, behavioural, social, cultural, environmental, political, and economic contexts that change as a client develops" (Henly et al. 2011, p. S5). Trajectories have also been studied at the micro-, meso- (Mackintosh and Sandall 2016), and macro- (Canadian and Palliative Care Association 2013) levels. Managing trajectories from chronicity is critical to improving client outcomes—individuals, groups, and communities—and reducing healthcare costs. The QHOM provides a framework to discuss how these concepts interact with chronicity.

Chronicity: Linkages to the QHOM

Within the QHOM, it is clear that chronicity is experienced by the client as an individual with one or more chronic diseases (Fig. 8.1). Also, the impact on chronicity is experienced within the family and community aspects of the client concept. For the system, primary, acute, and public healthcare all have roles in managing chronicity to better outcomes. As such, interventions to facilitate improved outcomes can be through the care of the client experiencing chronicity at the individual and group (family) levels, or interventions can be directed at the system or organization within which care is delivered. Whether interventions target the client or the system, outcomes of care can be assessed at the individual, family, community, and organizational levels. Hence, chronicity is a fitting concept to explore within the QHOM.

Client

Client characteristics are essential to understanding the experience of chronicity. A potential framework for considering characteristics was created from a scoping review focused on client complexity attributable to multimorbidity. Five client characteristics and experiences noted from the literature are discussed further: health and social experiences, demographics, mental health, social determinants, and medical/physical health (Schaink et al. 2012).

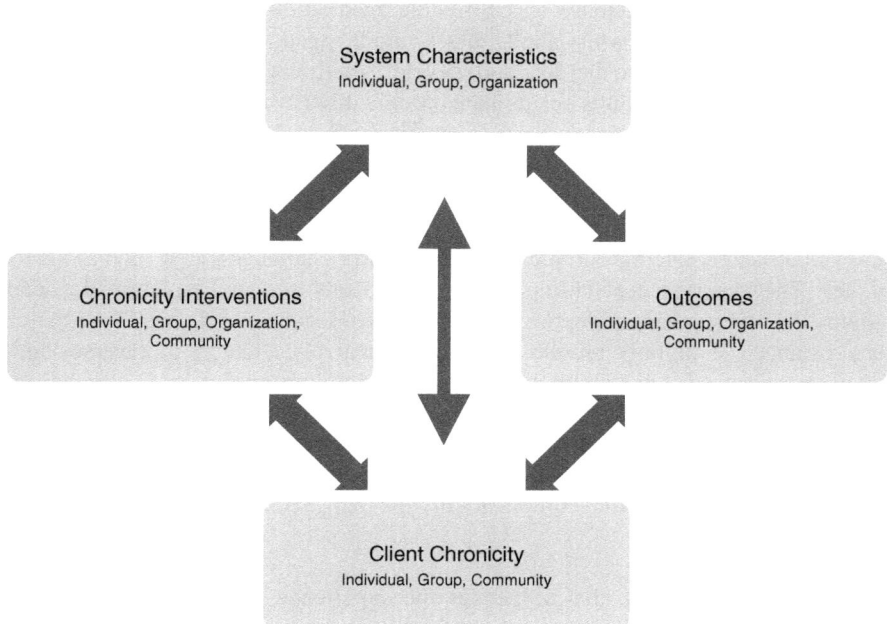

Fig. 8.1 Framework for chronicity

Client Characteristics

Health and Social Experiences

Health and social experiences encompass the utilization and cost of health services as well as challenges concerning self-care. For many clients with complex needs, the emergency department is an unavoidable point of care (Webster et al. 2015) that involves many resources and expenses. There are several dimensions within the healthcare system that require a better understanding to advance knowledge about chronicity and improve care. These include accessibility of care, continuity of care, client and caregiver access to information systems, and use of care teams (Bayliss et al. 2014).

Demographics

Within the United States, factors that influence complexity associated with multi-morbidity include older age, frailty, female gender, racial and ethnic disparities, and lower education (Schaink et al. 2012). Globally, factors such as urbanization, industrialization, and aging are associated with the rising rate of multimorbidity. A recent study from Sweden (Vermunt et al. 2018) indicated that older age, women, those with a lower level of education, a manual occupation, and poor social network accounted for increases in the number of chronic conditions. Racial and ethnic disparities are widely reported. For example, using the Health and Retirement Study

(HRS) representative database on US middle-aged adults, Quiñones et al. (2019) found that compared to white adults, black middle-aged adults start with a higher level of chronic disease burden and develop multimorbidities 4 years earlier. Hispanic middle-aged adults accumulate chronic disease at a faster rate than white adults. Thus, the client's demographic characteristics are essential in understanding the experience of chronicity and the trajectory pattern that unfolds.

Mental Health

Individuals experiencing chronicity often develop challenges with mental health issues. The experience of chronicity can lend itself to social isolation. In older adults, the development of depression is common (Hegeman et al. 2017). Addiction or substance use might be present, as well. Alternatively, a history of adverse childhood experiences is linked with the occurrence of multimorbidity, even after adjusting for related social, behavioral, and psychological factors (Sinnott et al. 2015b). When chronic psychiatric illness occurs with chronic medical illness, outcomes deteriorate as evidenced by poor self-care, increased symptom burden and functional impairment, increased complications, and higher cost (Chwastiak et al. 2014).

Social Determinants

The social environment also influences the experience of chronicity. Caregiver strain and burden, low socioeconomic status, and poor social support are concerns noted in the literature (Schaink et al. 2012). The client's health literacy level, which requires the ability to understand and use health information, strongly influences chronicity (van der Heide et al. 2018) (see Chap. 7). Another social determinant is structural racism, defined as "organized systems within societies that cause avoidable and unfair inequalities in power, resources, capacities and opportunities across racial or ethnic groups" (Paradies et al. 2015; p. 1). A meta-analysis of 293 studies on the effect of racism on clients found associations between racism and poor mental and physical health.

Medical/Physical Health

One of the primary challenges associated with physical health with multimorbidity is the limited applicability of clinical practice guidelines. The interplay of risk factors, disease complications, and shared pathophysiology and toxicities among chronic conditions must be considered (Oni et al. 2014). Following guidelines for specific diseases can result in polypharmacy and inappropriate prescribing. Physicians in primary care settings were found to use interventions such as relaxing targets, using hunches and best guesses, and negotiating a compromise in stabilizing the client's multimorbidity disease (and chronicity) trajectory (Sinnott et al. 2015a). Montori (2019) cautions providers that care guidelines are intended to manage a disease, not a person. In addition to the community in which a client lives, the client's personal and social contexts are important aspects of treating "this client," not a client with "this condition."

Interventions

Several evidence-based models have been developed to guide interventions that improve client outcomes of chronicity. Table 8.1 briefly defines four models: the Chronic Care Model (CCM) (Wagner et al. 1996), the Innovative Care for Chronic Conditions (ICCC) Framework (Nuno et al. 2012), the Chronic Disease Self-Management Program (CDSMP) (Bodenheimer et al. 2002), and the Transitional Care Model (TCM) (Naylor et al. 2004). Table 8.1 also provides a synopsis of the four models as they relate to client and system in the QHOM, with interventions targeted at the micro-, meso-, and macro-levels (Serpa and Ferreira 2019). For the client, the microlevel is the individual, and the meso-level is the community. For the system, the meso-level is within a clinical unit or the organization, whereas the macro-level is societal policies and regulations.

Chronicity Interventions Focused on the Client

Interventions directed toward the client include self-management, care coordination, and prevention. Each will be discussed within the evidence-based care model in which it was derived.

Self-Management Support

Facilitating self-management skills within clients is the primary intervention associated with chronicity. Self-management is the evidence-based intervention promoted by the Chronic Disease Self-Management Program, CDSMP. This model is based on self-efficacy theory, where self-efficacy is enhanced through skill mastery, modeling reinterpretation, and social persuasion (Lorig 2015). The fundamental tasks associated with self-management include solving problems, making decisions, utilizing resources, forming a patient-provider partnership, and making action plans for health behavior change and self-tailoring (Grover and Joshi 2014).

It is important to distinguish between the structured skill building associated with a self-management program and routine patient education. Traditional patient education involves relaying medical facts and providing direction for various treatments. Montori cautions that providers must be mindful of the burden created by the addition of "medical errands" (Montori 2019). These errands are the disease-related tasks that clients are expected to complete with the goal of better health or symptom relief. Examples of errands include taking medications, changing diet, monitoring and transmitting symptoms, and preparing questions for provider visits. Often clients experiencing chronicity are assigned an errand workload that may exceed their capacity or that of their caregivers. Montori advocates for "careful and kind care for all" (Montori 2019, p. 769), where providers are tuned into individual clients' needs and capabilities and work with them proactively to achieve care goals.

Table 8.1 Client and system interventions organized by evidence-based models of care

Model	Level	Client	System
The Chronic Care Model (CCM) organizes client-centered care through health system design, use of clinical information systems and decision support, self-management support, and community resources	Micro	Self-management support for an informed and activated client	
	Meso	Linking and using community resources	Delivery system design Decision support Clinical information systems Care coordination
	Macro		
The Innovative Care for Chronic Conditions model (ICCC) is an expansion of the CCM. It includes a focus on prevention, emphasis on quality of care, flexibility, adaptability, and integration. The model includes the importance of a favorable policy environment with interventions directed toward financing, legislation, and human resources	Micro	Informed, motivated, prepared client, family, community Emphasizes prevention	
	Meso	Raises awareness and reduces stigma Mobilizes and coordinates community resources	Uses healthcare personnel more effectively Builds integrated healthcare across settings, providers, time
	Macro		Coordinating financing across different phases of care Aligns sectoral policies to promote health Manages the political environment
The Chronic Disease Self-Management Program (CDSMP) is based on self-efficacy theory, includes peer teaching for specific conditions, and incorporates interventions concerning problem-solving, resource use, and action plans	Micro	Self-management support	
	Meso		
	Macro		

Table 8.1 (continued)

Model	Level	Client	System
The Transitional Care Model (TCM) is led by an advanced practice nurse and designed to facilitate coordination and continuity of healthcare as clients transfer between care levels within or across organizations	Micro	Identification of patient-specific concerns related to the transition process Medication adherence and persistence Assessing and supporting health literacy Utilization of remote patient monitoring Comprehensive plan of care	
	Meso		Advanced Practice Nurse Care Coordinator
	Macro		

Care Coordination

Care coordination is cited in several of the models as a client intervention for clients with chronicity. It is a care process based on a comprehensive plan of care that considers evidence and client preferences and values. An effective partnership with a care coordinator is characterized by the provider understanding and engaging with client preferences, improving client capacity, and decreasing client workload (Oni et al. 2014).

> Care coordination is the deliberate organization of patient care activities between two or more participants (including the patient) involved in a patient's care to facilitate the appropriate delivery of health care services. Organizing care involves the marshalling of personnel and other resources needed to carry out all required patient care activities, and is often managed by the exchange of information among participants responsible for different aspects of care (McDonald et al. 2007, p. 5).

Given that patients experiencing chronicity see several providers, the coordination of care among providers is essential to streamline interventions, monitor reactions to treatment, reduce redundancies, and enhance the quality of life. See Chap. 11 for specifics on care coordination.

Prevention

One of the most effective chronicity interventions is to prevent diseases from happening at all. The Innovative Care for Chronic Conditions (ICCC) Framework includes prevention as a strategy at both the micro- and macro-levels and emphasizes coordination and integration. Prevention strategies include early detection and behavioral lifestyle changes. Typical areas of emphasis include increasing physical activity, healthy eating, and reducing or eliminating tobacco use (Grover and Joshi 2014). The ICCC Framework is designed for clients to be "informed, motivated, and prepared" (Epping-Jordan et al. 2004, p. 301) across the health continuum. The focus on population health requires strategies to improve health behaviors to avoid the development of chronic conditions.

Chronicity Interventions Focused on the System

The current healthcare system is designed with a focus on acute care problems and needs. To appropriately care for clients with chronicity, systems must transform from an episodic model of care delivery to one that focuses on continuity, communication, coordination, and integration.

Delivery system design concerns assembling an interprofessional team of providers, each practicing to the full extent of their scope of practice to address the various nuances of chronicity. Departmental barriers within organizations need to be removed so clients can successfully and seamlessly navigate the system as they receive care. Finally, community resources are included to provide linkages to needed services outside of the healthcare arena. Providers and care coordinators must view the client within his/her community context and connect with the resources to facilitate optimal health.

Chronicity Interventions Within Healthcare Organizations

The CCM provides a distinct set of interventions targeting healthcare organizations (Wagner et al. 1996). Implementation of the model begins at the systems level, whether in an acute care facility or primary care clinic. It requires an organizational commitment to a model that effectively manages the complexity of chronic care. A robust clinical information system is necessary to track clients with specific diseases and promote information exchange between providers and clients. Given that clients experiencing chronicity tend to see multiple providers, information among providers must be shared, problem lists must be consistent, and medications must be streamlined. Decision support incorporates care guidelines that are consistent with the evidence as well as client preferences. As previously mentioned, care guidelines that are typically focused on one condition are not optimal for clients experiencing chronicity. It takes a deliberate assessment of the client, symptoms, and potential interactions between diseases and treatments to use the best evidence when multi-morbidity exists.

Chronicity Interventions Across Municipalities

The ICCC introduced interventions at the macro-level to address health policy issues concerning chronicity, especially in developing countries. The model's macroelements include the following: support a paradigm shift, manage the political environment, build integrated healthcare, and align sectoral policies for health (Grover and Joshi 2014). Managing the political environment is key to creating a system of care to support clients with chronicity. Even within the United States, the dialogue concerning whether insurance companies are required to provide coverage for preexisting conditions indicates that a "health for all" paradigm shift has not yet occurred. Further, systems are not aligned to support clients experiencing chronicity.

Recent emphasis on population health may contribute to looking beyond the walls of healthcare organizations, taking full advantage of community resources, and coordinating the care of clients experiencing chronicity within and outside of a traditional hospital or clinic. Although progress is occurring with the integration of behavioral health in primary care (Hunter et al. 2018), silos remain among specialty providers who treat disease-specific aspects of clients with chronicity. Once policies are aligned to support health across the life span, financing the healthcare system based on equity and effectiveness principles is essential (Epping-Jordan et al. 2004).

Implications and Future Directions

The prevalence of chronicity and the increasing occurrence of multimorbidity have prompted clinicians and researchers to explore complexity science as a more appropriate framework to inform work on chronicity. Complex adaptive care is client centered within a community context. It is an innovative and dynamic process that results in adaptability and empowerment (Martin and Sturmberg 2009). The complexity associated with multiple chronic conditions relates to the challenge that care protocols for individual diseases are not appropriate or effective for these clients. To meet their needs, clients must "(1) manage a high volume of information, visits, and self-care tasks, (2) coordinate, synthesize, and reconcile health information from multiple providers and about different conditions, and (3) serve as their own experts and advocates about health issues" (Zulman et al. 2015, p. 1065). A partnership between clients and their providers is essential to crafting practical, efficient, and reasonable solutions. The practice of complex adaptive care requires a provider to understand the client's capacity for a myriad of medical tasks and connect with community resources that will facilitate an improved state of health.

The Department of Human Services convened experts who made 11 recommendations concerning clinical guidelines for individuals experiencing multimorbidity across 3 categories: improving the stakeholder technical process, strengthening substance and content, and increasing the focus on client-centeredness (Goodman et al. 2014). Within the technical process, recommendations included harmonizing or coordinating guidelines across related disease groups and including experts in the process. Concerning substance and content, guidelines should prompt the clinician about the possibility of comorbidities, consider issues with adherence to self-management protocols, and integrate preventive measures and care coordination. Finally, guidelines should be client centered and highlight the importance of shared decision-making.

The challenges of research and care for those experiencing chronicity are shifting from a single disease focus to multimorbidity. A framework such as the QHOM provides a broad approach to identifying systems issues and interventions that may improve the client's outcomes. The study of chronicity as a health trajectory requires a measurement protocol that allows for the collection of variables over time, with the potential to note a pattern for clients, families, or populations (Henly et al. 2011).

Bayliss et al. (2014) call for the development of a partnership for collaborative action among healthcare providers, researchers, clients, caregivers, and community resources that are supported by payers and policy to advance understanding in the context of multiple chronic conditions. They recommend:

1. Establishing a measurement framework and prioritizing contextual factors at the individual, population, and system levels
2. Creating a national network of organizations to collect and disseminate best practices
3. Creating a public awareness campaign based on emerging research to empower further individuals experiencing multimorbidity
4. Activating an informed workforce to incorporate the vital contextual factors into practice and research
5. Fostering a supportive policy environment

The challenges of chronicity care and research will require interprofessional teams of dedicated clinicians and researchers to identify key factors and utilize qualitative and quantitative methodologies to advance the science.

References

Bayliss EA, Bonds DE, Boyd CM, Davis MM, Finke B, Fox MH et al (2014) Understanding the context of health for persons with multiple chronic conditions: moving from what is the matter to what matters. Ann Fam Med 12(3):260–269. https://doi.org/10.1370/afm.1643

Bodenheimer T, Lorig K, Holman H, Grumbach K (2002) Patient self-management of chronic disease in primary care. JAMA 288(19):2469–2475. https://doi.org/10.1001/jama.288.19.2469

Canadian and Palliative Care Association (2013) A model to guide hospice palliative care: based on national principles and norms. http://www.chpca.net/media/319547/norms-of-practice-eng-web.pdf

Centers for Disease Control and Prevention (2018a, November 19) About chronic diseases

Centers for Disease Control and Prevention (2018b) Health and economic costs of chronic diseases. https://www.cdc.gov/chronicdisease/about/costs/index.htm

Chwastiak L, Vanderlip E, Katon W (2014) Treating complexity: collaborative care for multiple chronic conditions. Int Rev Psychiat 26(6):638–647. https://doi.org/10.3109/0954026 1.2014.969689

Epping-Jordan JE, Pruitt SD, Bengoa R, Wagner EH (2004) Improving the quality of health care for chronic conditions. Qual Saf Health Care 13(4):299–305. https://doi.org/10.1136/qhc.13.4.299

Glaser B, Strauss A (1968) Time for dying. Aldine Press, Chicago, IL

Goodman RA, Boyd C, Tinetti ME, Von Kohorn I, Parekh AK, McGinnis JM (2014) IOM and DHHS meeting on making clinical practice guidelines appropriate for patients with multiple chronic conditions. Ann Fam Med 12(3):256–259. https://doi.org/10.1370/afm.1646

Grover A, Joshi A (2014) An overview of chronic disease models: a systematic literature review. Global J Health Sci 7(2):210–227. https://doi.org/10.5539/gjhs.v7n2p210

Hegeman JM, van Fenema EM, Comijs HC, Kok RM, van der Mast RC, de Waal MWM (2017) Effect of chronic somatic diseases on the course of late-life depression. Int J Geriatr Psychiat 32(7):779–787. https://doi.org/10.1002/gps.4523

Henly SJ, Wyman JF, Findorff MJ (2011) Health and illness over time: the trajectory perspective in nursing science. Nurs Res 60(3 Suppl):S5–S14. https://doi.org/10.1097/NNR.0b013e318216dfd3

Huang HT, Chang CM, Liu LF, Lin HS, Chen CH (2013) Trajectories and predictors of functional decline of hospitalised older patients. J Clin Nurs 22(9–10):1322–1331. https://doi.org/10.1111/jocn.12055

Hunter CL, Funderburk JS, Polaha J, Bauman D, Goodie JL, Hunter CM (2018) Primary care behavioral health (PCBH) model research: current state of the science and a call to action. J Clin Psychol Med Settings 25(2):127–156. https://doi.org/10.1007/s10880-017-9512-0

Lorig K (2015) Chronic disease self-management program: insights from the eye of the storm. Front Public Health 2:253. https://doi.org/10.3389/fpubh.2014.00253

Lynn J, Adamson DM (2003) Living well at the end-of-life: adapting health care to serious chronic illness in old age. Rand Health, Santa Monica, CA

Mackintosh N, Sandall J (2016) The social practice of rescue: the safety implications of acute illness trajectories and patient categorisation in medical and maternity settings. Soc Health Illness 38(2):252–269. https://doi.org/10.1111/1467-9566.12339

Martin C, Sturmberg J (2009) Complex adaptive chronic care. J Eval Clin Pract 15(3):571–577. https://doi.org/10.1111/j.1365-2753.2008.01022.x

McDonald KM, Sundaram V, Bravata DM, Lewis R, Lin N, Kraft SA et al (2007) AHRQ technical reviews. In: Closing the quality gap: a critical analysis of quality improvement strategies (Vol. 7: Care Coordination). Agency for Healthcare Research and Quality (US), Rockville, MD

Mitchell PM, Ferketich S, Jennings BM (1998) Quality health outcomes model. Image J Nurs Scholar 30(1):43–46

Montori VM (2019) Turning away from industrial health care toward careful and kind care. Acad Med 94(6):768–770. https://doi.org/10.1097/acm.0000000000002534

National Health Service Kidney Care End-of-Life Programme (2015) End-of-life care in advanced kidney disease. https://www.england.nhs.uk/improvement-hub/wp-content/uploads/sites/44/2017/11/Advanced-kidney-disease.pdf

Naylor MD, Brooten DA, Campbell RL, Maislin G, McCauley KM, Schwartz JS (2004) Transitional care of older adults hospitalized with heart failure: a randomized, controlled trial. J Am Geriatr Soc 52(5):675–684. https://doi.org/10.1111/j.1532-5415.2004.52202.x

Nuno R, Coleman K, Bengoa R, Sauto R (2012) Integrated care for chronic conditions: the contribution of the ICCC Framework. Health Policy 105(1):55–64. https://doi.org/10.1016/j.healthpol.2011.10.006

Oni T, McGrath N, BeLue R, Roderick P, Colagiuri S, May CR, Levitt NS (2014) Chronic diseases and multimorbidity—a conceptual modification to the WHO ICCC model for countries in health transition. BMC Public Health 14:575. https://doi.org/10.1186/1471-2458-14-575

Paradies Y, Ben J, Denson N, Elias A, Priest N, Pieterse A et al (2015) Racism as a determinant of health: a systematic review and meta-analysis. PLoS One 10(9):e0138511. https://doi.org/10.1371/journal.pone.0138511

Quiñones AR, Botoseneanu A, Markwardt S, Nagel CL, Newsom JT, Dorr DA, Allore HG (2019) Racial/ethnic differences in multimorbidity development and chronic disease accumulation for middle-aged adults. PLoS One 14(6):e0218462. https://doi.org/10.1371/journal.pone.0218462

Reed E, Corner J (2015) Defining the illness trajectory of metastatic breast cancer. BMJ Support Palliat Care 5(4):358–365. https://doi.org/10.1136/bmjspcare-2012-000415

Ruetsch C, Tkacz J, Kardel PG, Howe A, Pai H, Levitan B (2013) Trajectories of health care service utilization and differences in patient characteristics among adults with specific chronic pain: analysis of health plan member claims. J Pain Res 6:137–149. https://doi.org/10.2147/jpr.S38301

Schaink AK, Kuluski K, Lyons RF, Fortin M, Jadad AR, Upshur R, Wodchis WP (2012) A scoping review and thematic classification of patient complexity: offering a unifying framework. J Comorb 2:1–9

Serpa S, Ferreira CM (2019) Micro, meso, and macro levels of social analysis. Int J Soc Stud 7:3. https://doi.org/10.11114/ijsss.v7i3.4223

Sinnott C, Mc Hugh S, Boyce MB, Bradley CP (2015a) What to give the patient who has everything? A qualitative study of prescribing for multimorbidity in primary care. Br J Gen Pract 65(632):E184–E191. https://doi.org/10.3399/bjgp15X684001

Sinnott C, Mc Hugh S, Fitzgerald AP, Bradley CP, Kearney PM (2015b) Psychosocial complexity in multimorbidity: the legacy of adverse childhood experiences. Fam Pract 32(3):269–275. https://doi.org/10.1093/fampra/cmv016

The Lancet (2018) Making more of multimorbidity: an emerging priority. Lancet 391(10131):1637. https://doi.org/10.1016/S0140-6736(18)30941-3

van der Heide I, Poureslami I, Mitic W, Shum J, Rootman I, FitzGerald JM (2018) Health literacy in chronic disease management: a matter of interaction. J Clin Epidemiol 102:134–138. https://doi.org/10.1016/j.jclinepi.2018.05.010

Vermunt N, Westert GP, Rikkert M, Faber MJ (2018) Assessment of goals and priorities in patients with a chronic condition: a secondary quantitative analysis of determinants across 11 countries. Scand J Prim Health Care 36(1):80–88. https://doi.org/10.1080/02813432.2018.1426149

Wagner EH, Austin BT, Von Korff M (1996) Improving outcomes in chronic illness. Manag Care Quart 4(2):12–25. http://europepmc.org/abstract/MED/10157259

Webster F, Christian J, Mansfield E, Bhattacharyya O, Hawker G, Levinson W, Collaborative B (2015) Capturing the experiences of patients across multiple complex interventions: a meta-qualitative approach. BMJ Open 5(9):9. https://doi.org/10.1136/bmjopen-2015-007664

Zulman DM, Jenchura EC, Cohen DM, Lewis ET, Houston TK, Asch SM (2015) How can ehealth technology address challenges related to multimorbidity? Perspectives from patients with multiple chronic conditions. J Gen Intern Med 30(8):1063–1070. https://doi.org/10.1007/s11606-015-3222-9

Part V
Interventions

Nursing Care Processes

Terry L. Jones

Introduction

Healthcare professions have a social contract with the public as they exist for the sole purpose of serving the public good (ANA 2010). This contract requires that healthcare professions engage in self-regulation to ensure quality performance. Therefore, each discipline has a social mandate to evaluate the effect of their respective interventions on health outcomes. In the current value-based purchasing climate, reimbursement for services/interventions is tied to quality (see Chaps. 2 and 14). Thus, the healthcare disciplines also have an economic imperative to measure and evaluate the effect of interventions on health outcomes.

Nurses play a significant role in the delivery and coordination of care activities within and across healthcare teams. Consequently, there are few care elements that do not pass through nurses' hands, and few client outcomes that are not influenced by nursing care processes (Jones 2016). This chapter focuses on interventions and their measures that may help evaluate the unique nursing contribution to quality healthcare. The chapter begins with how nursing interventions are conceptualized within the QHOM (Mitchell et al. 1998), followed by discussions of the challenges in defining, measuring, and evaluating nursing interventions. System characteristics' effects on nursing intervention are described. Additionally, two exemplars of nursing interventions, nurse surveillance and symptom management, are discussed. Finally, implications and future directions are described.

T. L. Jones (✉)
School of Nursing, Virginia Commonwealth University, Richmond, VA, USA
e-mail: tjones69@vcu.edu

© Springer Nature Switzerland AG 2021
M. Baernholdt, D. K. Boyle (eds.), *Nurses Contributions to Quality Health Outcomes*, https://doi.org/10.1007/978-3-030-69063-2_9

Nursing Care Processes: Linkages to QHOM

The QHOM places nursing interventions as directed at the system, the client, or both to affect outcomes (Fig. 9.1). The proposed relationships in the QHOM are congruent with the theoretical perspectives reflected in ecological system frameworks (Bronfenbrenner 2005; Jones et al. 2019b, in press) and structuration theories (Baber 1991; Bodilica et al. 2015; Giddens 1984; Stone 2005). From the lens of an ecological system, nursing care is embedded within a multilevel system, e.g., macro-, meso-, and microlevels (Serpa and Ferreira 2019). Each system level may have multiple subsystems that affect and are affected by other subsystems. Moreover, the system is a social system comprised of social structures (i.e., rules, norms, policies, and relationships) within which individual nurses deliver care for clients or act to change the system. Adding to this view is social structures and human agency from a structuration framework (Giddens 1984). Social structures are created by human action, yet social structures also function to constrain or enable human action once created. Human agency involves intentional actions. Interdependent structure-agency relationships support multiple pathways of nursing intervention. Nurses may exert agency to deliver client-level interventions (individuals, families, and communities) to improve health outcomes. However, social structures across various subsystems may affect how the nurse enacts these interventions or how clients receive them. Nurses may also exert agency to deliver system-level

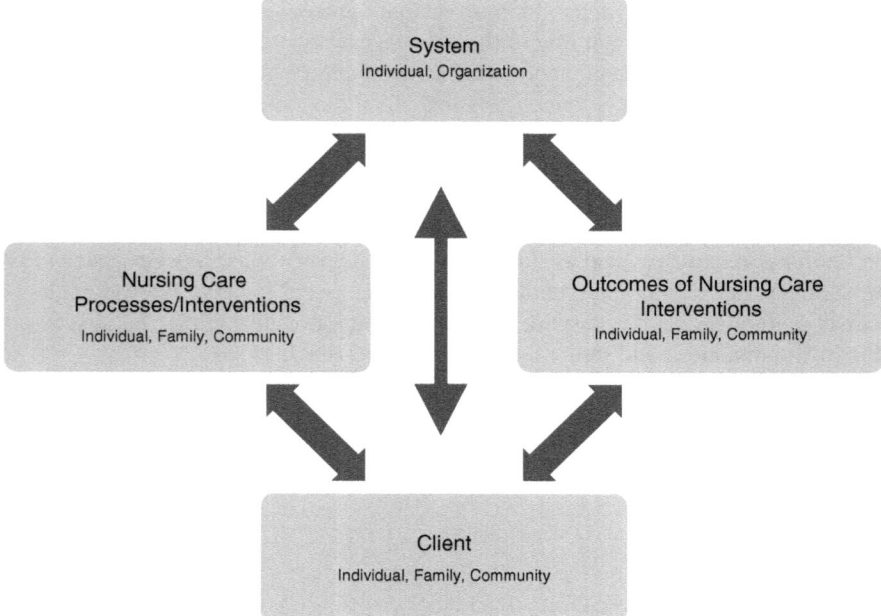

Fig. 9.1 Framework for nursing care processes/interventions

interventions. Through system-level interventions, nurses seek to create or adapt social structures to enable rather than constrain interventions related to health promotion, prevention of illness and injury, alleviation of suffering, and client advocacy. However, a first step is to define what nursing interventions are.

The Essence of Nursing Interventions

In the context of improvement initiatives related to nursing care quality, i.e., the extent to which nursing care improves patient outcomes, a discipline-specific definition of interventions or processes is needed. Such a definition must address what distinguishes a nursing intervention from the myriad of other interventions directed toward patients or the system of care from the healthcare team. The definition of a nursing intervention should ideally reflect the roles and responsibilities of nursing: (a) the *discipline of nursing* (i.e., the science of nursing—what nurses are educated to do), (b) the *profession of nursing* (i.e., the legal scope of nursing practice—what nurses are licensed to do), and (c) the *job of nursing* (i.e., the work of nursing—what nurses are paid to do). However, nursings' roles and responsibilities are continuously evolving, and these aspects of nursing are not always aligned. For example, in the current work environment, nurses may not be practicing at the full extent of their training and license. At the same time, they may be assigned and paid to perform activities that have nothing to do with the science or profession of nursing (e.g., clerical duties or passing meal trays). Moreover, as a result of scientific advancements and changes in delivery systems, nurses play an increasing role in monitoring physiologic health and coordinating services across settings. Therefore, the demarcation line between nursing and non-nursing interventions is not always clear and is never static.

Snyder et al. (1996) highlighted key challenges and contentious issues in defining nursing interventions in their review of national and international nursing intervention initiatives. The interrelated issues of active intervention and nurse autonomy have been points of disagreement within the discipline. In the 1990s, the International Council of Nursing (ICN) initiated the International Classification in Nursing Project (ICNP) and put forth the following statements regarding the definition of nursing interventions:

> Intervention means literally "a coming between" the patient and the problem in order to modify or influence the problem; the word implies active interference, and the phrase "nursing intervention" may therefore appear to be limited to treatments and procedures (ICN 1993, p. 110).

Other prominent scholars at the time similarly defined nursing interventions as actions performed by nurses to achieve patient outcomes (Gordon 1987; Snyder 1992; Snyder et al. 1996). Based on these statements, some argued that activities related to assessment and evaluation do not qualify as nursing interventions. The argument's basis was twofold: (1) assessment does not directly achieve an outcome and (2) many assessments are prescribed by physicians and therefore fall into the category of *delegated medical functions* (Snyder et al. 1996). In other words, just because a nurse does it does not make it *nursing* or an *intervention*. Moreover, this perspective limited nursing interventions to active treatments that can be autonomously initiated by nurses.

In contrast, a less restrictive definition emerged from the National Intervention Classification (NIC) project (McCloskey and Bulechek 1992). The following statements from the NIC project acknowledge autonomous and nonautonomous aspects of nursing practice:

> Any direct care treatment that a nurse performs on behalf of a client. Nursing interventions include nurse-initiated treatments and physician-initiated treatments (McCloskey and Bulechek 1992, p. xvii).

Despite the reference to *direct care treatment*, the inclusion of activities related to assessment and evaluation in the initial list of 332 nursing interventions suggests a liberal interpretation of the term *treatment*. The NIC definition has subsequently been refined as "*any* treatment, based upon clinical judgement and knowledge, that a nurse performs to enhance patient/client outcomes" (Butcher et al. 2018, p. xii). Notably, the current NIC taxonomy includes 565 nursing interventions that reflect all aspects of the nursing process, direct and indirect care activities (e.g., activities related to managing the environment and interdisciplinary collaboration), and elements of autonomous and nonautonomous practice.

Despite the absence of a universally accepted definition of a nursing intervention, there does seem to be some consensus around the idea that nurses function within three general role categories: dependent, independent, and interdependent (Table 9.1). The classification of nursing roles and functions into these categories is described further in the Nursing Role Effectiveness Model (NREM), first introduced by Irvine et al. (1998) and refined by Doran (2011). The types of interventions for which nursing is duty bound to measure and manage are inherent in the very definition of nursing, "*the protection, promotion, and optimization of health and abilities, prevention of illness and injury, alleviation of suffering through the*

Table 9.1 Broad categories of nursing interventions/processes

Independent nursing practice	Interdependent nursing practice	Dependent nursing practice
Role functions and responsibilities for which only nurses are held accountable	Role functions and responsibilities in which nurses engage that are partially or totally dependent on the functions of other healthcare professionals	Role functions and responsibilities associated with the implementation of medical orders and medical treatments
Examples include the activities of assessment, decision-making, intervention, and follow-up	Examples include coordination of care	Examples include implementation of standing orders

diagnosis and treatment of human response, and advocacy in the care of individuals, families, communities, and populations" (ANA 2010, p. 8). Therefore, nursing is accountable for and obligated to measure independent, interdependent, and dependent nursing practice interventions.

The Complexity of Nursing Interventions

Nursing interventions often fall into the category of complex interventions (MRC 2006). Interventions are considered complex when they have several interacting or interdependent components (Bleijenberg et al. 2018; Craig et al. 2013; MRC 2006). The presence of multiple interdependencies adds to the length and complexity of the causal chain that links the intervention to outcomes. Additional challenges that emerge from this complexity include the difficulty in standardizing the intervention's delivery and the significant influence of the local context (i.e., system and social structures). Consequently, it is often difficult to identify the active ingredients in complex interventions and evaluate their effectiveness. The implementation of rapid response teams (RRTs) is a prime example of an organization- or system-level nurse-driven complex intervention.

Example: Rapid Response Teams

The RRT is an intervention designed to improve detection and management of clinical deterioration for hospitalized patients outside the intensive care unit (ICU). The RRT intervention contains two primary arms that support the cognitive and behavioral aspects of nurse surveillance. The afferent arm, or active arm, of the RRT intervention includes collecting and interpreting data points predictive of clinical deterioration. The efferent or the response arm is the deployment of the RRT to the bedside of deteriorating patients and the subsequent diagnosis and management of those patients (Jones et al. 2011).

Multiple interdependencies (among activities and people) and active ingredients are involved in the RRT intervention. For example, appropriate activation of the response arm depends on accurate and timely identification of clinical deterioration in the active arm. Consequently, the RRT intervention includes at a minimum all of the following: timely collection and documentation of relevant assessment data; staff competent in clinical reasoning and pattern recognition; designated RRT members; a mechanism for rapid notification of the RRT; effective team communication; and structural empowerment of the RRT to order and execute interventions to reverse clinical deterioration once activated.

Each interdependency within the RRT intervention presents an area of vulnerability to breakdown and is potentially influenced by human factor limitations and system or social structures. For example, work overload, distractions, and disruptions may delay collecting and interpreting relevant data. In competitive and hierarchical cultures, staff may hesitate to activate the RRT for fear of being perceived as weak and incompetent or overstepping disciplinary boundaries. Moreover, biases toward quantitative data may cause nurses to delay activation of the RRT until significant vital sign changes emerge despite earlier changes in more qualitative cues, such as patient affect. Once the RRT is deployed to the bedside, treatment execution may be impeded by disagreements between the RRT and the patient's primary providers. Thus, the mechanism of action for the RRT intervention is long and convoluted. Timely data collection and interpretation by nurses in the afferent arm may not result in the activation of the efferent arm. Moreover, timely activation of the efferent arm may not result in timely clinical stabilization. In other words, a successful RRT intervention is contingent upon system characteristics.

System Characteristics' Effect on Nursing Interventions

The bidirectional interactions between the client, system, and interventions in the QHOM suggest that changes in one are contingent upon support or changes in the other. For example, client-level interventions are the product of social structures within the system, and system-level interventions are the mechanisms through which nurses transform the system. Therefore, the nature and effectiveness of client-level interventions are contingent upon system characteristics. Moreover, this contingency implies that client-level interventions cannot be improved without synergistic system-level interventions in many instances. These contingencies are evident in the Nursing Care Performance Framework proposed by Dubois et al. (2013) and empirically supported by the science of unfinished nursing care.

Unfinished Nursing Care

In the Nursing Care Performance Framework, Dubois et al. (2013) described three functional nursing subsystems to include: "(1) acquiring, deploying and maintaining nursing resources, (2) transforming nursing resources into nursing services, and (3) producing positive changes in a patient's condition as a result of nursing services" (p. 6). The first subsystem includes the structures and processes involved in generating the supply of nursing staff (e.g., volume and skill mix) and working conditions (e.g., workload and scheduling). The second subsystem includes individual nurses applying the nursing process to deliver client-level interventions. The output of the first subsystem (the supply of nurses) clearly serves as the second subsystem's input. When the supply of nurses is insufficient relative to care and work demands, nurses are unable to effectively execute client-level interventions. This phenomenon appears in the literature as *unfinished nursing care*. The output of the second subsystem (unfinished nursing care) subsequently functions as one input into the third subsystem and contributes to suboptimal patient outcomes.

The phenomenon of *unfinished nursing care* was first introduced in 2001 under the label *tasks left undone* (Aiken et al. 2001). By 2007, additional terms for the phenomenon began to appear in the literature with regularity to include *missed care* (Kalisch and Williams 2009) and *implicitly rationed care* (Schubert et al. 2007). The findings of an early state of the science review suggested that these terms were being used to reflect a common underlying phenomenon. The term *unfinished nursing care* was introduced to serve as a unifying umbrella term (Jones et al. 2015). The common phenomenon was defined as *"a problem of time scarcity that prompts nurses to engage in implicit rationing of care through the process of clinical prioritization that results in care left undone"* (Jones et al. 2015). Internationally, 55–98% of nursing staff surveyed report leaving one or more nursing care elements unfinished (Al-Kandari and Thomas 2009; Ausserhofer et al. 2013; Schubert et al. 2013). In other words, at least 55% of hospitalized clients may not receive all needed nursing interventions. Moreover, variations in levels of unfinished nursing care have been documented at the hospital and unit level across the United States (Jones 2014; Kalisch et al. 2011, 2012; Kalisch and Lee 2010). Time scarcity due to inadequate human resources remains the strongest identified predictor of unfinished nursing care.

Examples of Nursing Interventions

In the following section, two examples of crucial nursing interventions are reviewed, and potential performance measures useful for quality assessment and performance improvement are discussed. The two examples include surveillance and symptom management. Both represent essential and complex nursing interventions that are rarely provided entirely by a single nurse. Consequently, both are vulnerable to the effects of system characteristics. Therefore, both the client- and system-level aspects of the intervention are discussed.

Surveillance

Robust conceptualizations of surveillance as a nursing intervention are described by Titler (1992), Doughterty (1999), McCloskey and Bulechek (2000), Schoneman (2002), Kutney-Lee et al. (2009), Schmidt (2010), Kelly and Vincent (2010), Dresser (2012), and Pfrimmer et al. (2017). These conceptualizations are highly congruent with the following definition: "a process to primarily identify threats to patient health and safety through purposeful and ongoing acquisition, interpretation and synthesis of patient data for clinical decision making" (Kelly and Vincent 2010, p. 658). This definition underscores the applicability of the intervention of surveillance to all patient populations and care settings. Moreover, it suggests that surveillance is a precursor to clinical decision-making and, as such, may be foundational to all other interventions. Two published concept analyses (Dresser 2012; Kelly and Vincent 2010) clearly situate surveillance as a complex intervention. The intervention of nurse surveillance is designed to promote health and prevent injury through two primary mechanisms: early detection of clinical deterioration and early intervention.

Early detection of clinical deterioration begins with the timely acquisition of relevant patient data. Nurses may gather data by direct observation, communication with others (e.g., patients, family members, and other members of the care team), review of electronic and paper health records, and retrieval of data from electronic devices (e.g., medical equipment). Following data acquisition, nurses use cognitive processes (rational and intuitive thinking) to interpret the data and synthesize the information gleaned. Nurses then judge the meaning of the information in relation to the trajectory of the patient's clinical status (i.e., improving, unchanged, or deteriorating) and the degree of risk for injury. Based on their judgments, nurses make decisions related to the appropriate course of action (e.g., immediate intervention or continued surveillance).

System-Level Interventions to Support Surveillance

The complexity of today's healthcare environment presents many challenges to effective nurse surveillance. Advances in science and technology have significantly increased the volume of patient data available to support surveillance and the range of available treatment options for clinical deterioration. Nurse staffing is further constrained by economic imperatives to reduce costs, often resulting in increased workloads for individual nurses (see Chaps. 3, 4, and 13). Consequently, the human capacity for information processing is often insufficient to meet nurse surveillance's cognitive demands (Chap. 5). Moreover, healthcare teams have grown in size and diversity due to increased specialization and emerging delivery models. Thus, communication of information generated during the surveillance process to multiple team members can be cumbersome and time consuming. Therefore, system-level interventions involving the adoption of various tools and aids (protocols, information technology (IT), and rounding) are often used to overcome these challenges and improve client-level surveillance capacity.

Complication-specific screening and risk assessment tools are used to support the cognitive and behavioral components of surveillance. These tools typically contain a list of data elements required to assess the risk for specific complications. The lists serve as prompts for data gathering to ensure that the right data are collected, which reduces reliance on nurse memory and prior experience. Screening tools also include scoring systems developed with predictive analytics to facilitate the information processing required for timely and accurate interpretation of multiple data points. Often a single composite score is generated, and cut points indicate varying degrees of risk for specific complications. In some instances, treatment protocols are developed and standardized based on these risk scores. These system-level protocols guide the clinical decision-making and execution components of surveillance. The effectiveness of these tools is enhanced when they are embedded in health IT systems such as the electronic health record (EHR). Digital documentation combined with artificial intelligence algorithms supports the automatic computation of risk scores and the generation of evidence-based treatment recommendations.

Additional IT aids to support *remote* surveillance include electronic sensors and video monitoring equipment. These IT modalities support the data gathering component of surveillance by enabling continuous and automated client observation without a nurse's presence at the bedside, for example, beds equipped with electronic sensors that detect pressure changes associated with patients getting out of bed (Graham 2012; Hempel et al. 2013; Sahota et al. 2014) and cameras (Votruba et al. 2016). These surveillance technologies are also being deployed to care settings outside the acute care setting (Fisk 2015) (see Chap. 6).

Rounding is another system-level intervention often used to enhance nurse surveillance. Various types of rounding appear in the literature: intentional, proactive surveillance, and interprofessional. Rounding involves planned interactions for specific purposes. These planned interactions are routinized and habituated by creating social structures (e.g., policies, protocols, and documented workflows). Emphasis on early detection and early intervention to enhance patient safety and prevent adverse events is implicit in each type of rounding's definitions and descriptions. For example, intentional rounding (also known as hourly rounding, purposeful rounding, scripted rounding, and proactive nurse rounding) is described as regular checks of individual patients at set intervals to proactively assess and attend to patient needs (Al Danaf et al. 2017; Christiansen et al. 2018; Forde-Johnston 2014; Gonzolo et al. 2014; Harrington et al. 2013; Hutchinson et al. 2017; Mitchell et al. 2014; Sims et al. 2018).

Proactive surveillance rounding evolved as an adjunct to another system-level surveillance-related intervention, RRTs (Danesh et al. 2019). As described previously, RRTs were designed to facilitate early detection and intervention for clinical deterioration outside the ICU. Building on an RRT presence, a dedicated and centrally located surveillance team, often the same as the RRT, does proactive surveillance rounds. The surveillance team prospectively reviews the automated (and continuously updated) early warning scores for all patients in the organization. The team will be deployed to the bedside of patients with concerning risk profiles to intervene as indicated. Finally, interprofessional rounding is planned encounters between the care team members to discuss patient status and develop, evaluate, and revise the treatment plan. Emphasis is placed on shared information and shared decisions (Gonzalo et al. 2016; Henneman et al. 2012). In summary, protocols, IT, and rounding are system-level interventions used for client-level surveillance, but more needs to be done to improve patient health and safety.

Measuring and Evaluating Surveillance Interventions

The challenges to the empirical measurement of surveillance are similar to other complex interventions. Surveillance is not easily dichotomized as present or absent, or good or bad. In the purest sense, surveillance is present and good when the *five rights* of the process are present: right data, time, judgment, decision, and execution. Each of these rights is temporally and contextually dependent. Patients present with different risk profiles based on their health history (past and present), nursing and medical diagnoses, treatment regimens, genetic makeup, social support, and socioeconomic status. Consequently, they are at risk for different types of clinical deterioration and injury. Therefore, variation is expected in the type and frequency of data collection and the interpretation of data values across patients. For example, data requirements for a postoperative patient are different than for a woman in labor. Moreover, the correct judgment and decision about an elevated temperature on postoperative day 1 are different from postoperative day 7.

Patient data may be obtained and documented by multiple clinicians and technology aids. However, recording a data point does not guarantee that a nurse will see or interpret that data. Similarly, the sounding of an alarm or the flashing of an alert does not guarantee that risk is accurately or expediently recognized. Thus, a high quantity of recorded data and high alarm and alert utilization are not synonymous with good surveillance. Measuring data volume only captures one of the active ingredients of this complex intervention (Jones 2011). Good surveillance is contingent upon all of the active ingredients to include good judgment and decision-making. These cognitive processes reflect the mental work of nurses. A nurse may accurately interpret the gathered data, but unless the resulting judgment is communicated, this mental work remains invisible and unmeasurable.

Quantitative measures are reductionistic by nature and typically only capture a snapshot in time. A snapshot measure's timing may or may not accurately reflect the quality of a whole dynamic process. For example, a nurse may be quite vigilant in surveillance in the morning but less so in the afternoon. Similarly, multiple nurses provide surveillance for each patient during an episode of care, and they may do so with varying degrees of vigilance. Poor surveillance when a patient's condition is unchanged means something very different from poor surveillance when clinical deterioration is in progress. Poor surveillance can be the difference between a good and a bad outcome at any single point in time. Thus capturing the timing of surveillance is as crucial as the quantity of surveillance.

Because of the inherent measurement challenges, indirect or proxy measures for surveillance are often used. The Hospital Nurse Surveillance Capacity Profile (Kutney-Lee et al. 2009) is an example of a proxy measure for surveillance based on structural factors that theoretically influence nurse surveillance. As the name implies, it is not a measure of the *actual* volume or quality of nurse surveillance; instead, it measures an organization's *capacity* for nurse surveillance. The authors of the measure asserted that the cumulative and temporal aspects of surveillance preclude the ability to associate the surveillance effectiveness by a single nurse with a single patient's outcome. Moreover, they conceptualized surveillance as "a collective effort of interventions delivered by multiple nurses over time, as well as interventions by individual nurses" (Kutney-Lee et al. 2009, p. 219). Therefore, they developed an organization-level measure comprised of nurse characteristics (nurse staffing, nurse education, nurse clinical experience, and nurse experience) and practice environment. The variables included in the profile were selected based on previous evidence linking them to patient outcomes. Though nurse surveillance is often hypothesized to be part of the causal chain linking these variables to patient outcomes, these relationships have not been empirically validated.

Data required to compute the Hospital Nurse Surveillance Capacity Profile are obtained from self-reported nurse surveys. Survey data are aggregated at the hospital level, and hospitals are ranked separately for each variable. The final profile consists of the individual variable rankings and a composite score computed as the mean across the individual rankings. The authors demonstrated significant relationships between surveillance capacity scores and two adverse events (injury falls and nosocomial infections). The Hospital Nurse Surveillance Capacity Profile's intended uses include identifying areas for organizational improvement, tracking organizational performance over time, and benchmarking organizational performance against comparable institutions.

Examples of adverse patient outcomes commonly used as proxy measures for nurse surveillance in the acute care practice setting include failure to rescue (Clarke and Aiken 2003; Needleman and Buerhaus 2007) and care escalations (Danesh et al. 2019). Both outcomes are conceptually characterized as failures of early detection and intervention practices (Danesh et al. 2019; Mushta et al. 2018). Failure to rescue is endorsed by the National Quality Forum (NQF 2004) (see Chaps. 2 and 14). This measure is extracted from administrative databases that include diagnostic codes for complications and iatrogenic injury and discharge status. A care escalation is defined as the unplanned transfer from a lower level of care (e.g., acute care unit) to a higher level of care (e.g., intensive care unit) regardless of outcome (death or survival). Moreover, the care escalation measure does not require documentation of specific complications and can be extracted from administrative databases that include charge management fields related to bed type (Danesh et al. 2019).

High rates of failure to rescue and care escalation are presumed to result from poor surveillance; however, empirical evidence to validate this presumption is lacking. While consistent evidence links failure to rescue with care structures theoretically linked to surveillance (e.g., nurse staffing and the previously described surveillance capacity profile), a direct link to actual nurse surveillance has not been empirically established. Shever (2011) is credited with the most robust attempt to directly link nurse surveillance and failure to rescue. The empirical measure of nurse surveillance in this study was limited to the data gathering component of nurse surveillance. Specifically, the measure included the frequency of documented surveillance activities related to assessment and monitoring documented in the EHR. Propensity scores were used to match patients who received high doses of nurse surveillance (an average of 12 or more surveillance activities per day) with patients who received low doses of surveillance (an average of less than 12 surveillance activities per day). The results supported a significant difference in the risk of failure to rescue among the two groups. Specifically, patients in the high-dose group had reduced odds of failure to rescue by about 50% (OR = 0.52) compared to patients in the low-dose group. The findings of this single study are promising but have not been replicated.

Symptom Management

Symptom management is acknowledged as an important *nurse-sensitive performance measure* (Bolton et al. 2007; Sidani 2011). Symptoms are defined as subjective sensations or experiences, reflecting perceived changes or abnormalities in one's biopsychosocial functioning (Sidani 2011). Thus, symptoms are part of the human response to diseases and their treatments. Symptom management involves a constellation of activities applied to ameliorate symptoms. Symptoms often prompt individuals to seek healthcare and, if not managed effectively, contribute to the experience of suffering. Thus, symptom management is germane to nursing's role in alleviating suffering.

Any disease process can produce a high symptom burden and high symptom distress if uncontrolled. However, the risk for these and other associated adverse consequences is higher in patients with one or more chronic illnesses. An illness is considered chronic if it lasts more than 6 months, is not curable, and potentially limits activity (Bushor and Rowser 2015). In an acute illness, symptoms resolve with curative treatment, often during or shortly after the incident encounter (i.e., hospitalization or outpatient visit) under close clinician supervision. Thus, symptom management in acute illness is time limited and primarily falls under clinicians' purview in acute care settings. In contrast, patterns of recurring and remitting symptoms are an inherent aspect of chronic illness. Patients with chronic conditions experience symptom recurrence between traditional episodic care visits that are often separated by long stretches of time (see Chap. 8).

The symptom experience begins with symptom appraisal. In concert with the conscious awareness of one or more symptoms, individuals engage in an evaluation process to assign meaning to the experience. Meaning is derived based on a client's perceived symptom characteristics of severity, frequency, duration, timing, and impact on daily life. Responses to symptoms stem from the assigned meaning and include physiological (e.g., stress), emotional (e.g., anxiety), and behavioral components. The presence of a behavioral response signifies a transition from symptom experience to symptom management. During symptom management, clients act alone or in concert with others to "avert, delay, or minimize the symptom experience" (Humphreys et al. 2008, p. 144). Sidani (2011) described the range of symptom management strategies employed by clients as follows:

> Patients may ignore the symptom; assume a "wait and see" attitude; seek advice from laypersons (i.e., family members and friends), from available resources (e.g., the World Wide Web), or healthcare professionals; use commonly recommended strategies, home remedies, or alternative therapies; and apply self-initiated treatment based on common knowledge (e.g., over-the-counter medications), or previous experience (p. 134).

The outcomes or consequences of symptom management are multidimensional and interrelated. The most direct outcome is symptom status that reflects the degree of symptom control achieved. Symptoms may be completely controlled (i.e., eliminated and no longer experienced), partially controlled (i.e., reduced in frequency, severity, or impact), or uncontrolled (i.e., remaining the same or worsening in frequency, severity, or impact). Prolonged partially and uncontrolled symptoms have multiple adverse effects that may manifest as limited functional status, reduced health-related quality of life, comorbidity, symptom distress, symptom burden, increased healthcare utilization and costs, and mortality. Symptom status functions as a feedback loop to evaluate the effectiveness of symptom management.

Similar to surveillance intervention, early detection and early intervention are fundamental aspects of symptom management. Early detection of symptoms is comparable to the early detection of clinical deterioration as described for the surveillance intervention. Nurses use cognitive processes to determine which symptoms or symptom clusters are most relevant based on their knowledge of diseases, treatments, and client characteristics. Nurses then decide appropriate symptom management interventions and engage other cognitive and behavioral processes to execute the decisions. Symptom profiles vary by condition, and different symptoms require different preventive and management approaches. Moreover, clients present with varying levels of knowledge and motivation for self-care and self-management. Therefore, these actions must be tailored to each client's context.

System-Level Interventions to Support Symptom Management

The complexity of today's healthcare environment presents many challenges to effective symptom management in chronic illness. System characteristics that facilitate client-level symptom management are often inadequate. In response to reimbursement policies' economic constraints, increasingly more emphasis is placed on early discharge from inpatient encounters with the transition of more care to the post-acute setting. Although acute care nurses may be positioned to *initiate* symptom management, they cannot see this intervention through to fruition. For example, they may begin client education based on the initial symptom profile, but they are unlikely to evaluate symptom management behaviors before discharge. This evaluation should happen in the post-acute care setting. The handoff and communication processes for nursing care related to symptom management between acute and post-acute settings are suboptimal (see Chap. 11). In the post-acute care setting, patients with chronic illness often require treatment from multiple health professionals across multiple subspecialties. Roles and responsibilities for symptom management may not be clearly delineated, and nurses across settings may be unable to access each other's care documentation related to symptom management. This lack of access hinders continuity of symptom management care across practice settings. Moreover, in post-acute settings, staffing models do not always support sufficient nurse staffing and time allocation for symptom management activities (Jones et al. 2019a).

A variety of system-level interventions to better support symptom management continue to emerge. Examples of care delivery models that may provide improved support for symptom management include those with designated patient homes (Colligan et al. 2017; Kuntz et al. 2014), nurse-led disease management and symptom management clinics (Henry et al. 2013; Whitmer et al. 2011), nurse care coordinators (Mkanta et al. 2007), nurse navigators (Bellomo 2016; Hébert and Fillion 2011; Jeyathevan et al. 2017), and case managers (Aiken et al. 2006; Li et al. 2017). These models represent adaptations to larger system structures to enable improved care integration across settings and designated nurses for post-acute symptom management (see Chap. 11).

Access to provider documentation across settings related to symptom management is improved through the adoption of EHRs (Kallen et al. 2012; O'Malley et al. 2015). The impact of EHRs on symptom management is further enhanced by integrating standardized symptom surveillance surveys and evidence-based symptom management protocols. Patient-reported outcome measures (PROMs) are standardized measures of physical symptoms that providers can complete during history taking or by the patient before the provider encounter (Stover et al. 2019; Yang et al. 2018). These tools serve as prompts to ensure complete and consistent symptom appraisal and promote patient-clinician communication about symptom management strategies (Hinami et al. 2016; Santana and Feeny 2014). Moreover, longitudinal data from these tools provide feedback for clinicians and clients regarding the effectiveness of selected symptom management strategies.

Evidence-based symptom management protocols and practice guidelines help nurses identify best practices to manage specific symptoms and can be embedded in clinical decision support systems to expedite the process further. For example, pain management protocols may automatically pop up when the symptom of pain is documented in the EHR. Moreover, in conjunction with telehealth and mobile health technologies, such standardized protocols are used to support remote symptom management (Beck et al. 2017; Breen et al. 2015). In summary, new care delivery models, sharing of client data across care settings, and symptom management protocols are all system-level interventions that will improve client health if implemented widely.

Measuring Symptom Management

The challenges to the empirical measurement of symptom management are similar to other complex interventions, such as those described previously in this chapter. Moreover, symptom management is conceptualized as both process and outcome (Bolton et al. 2007; Richard and Shea 2011; Sidani 2011). Symptom management as a process includes the previously described activities related to symptom appraisal and behavioral response. Whereas symptom management as a health outcome is the extent to which symptoms are effectively managed, the process of symptom management is not easily dichotomized as present or absent, or good or bad. In the purest sense, symptom management is present and good when all of the active ingredients are performed correctly and timely. Ideally, measures of symptom management should address all components of the intervention. Symptom management strategies should be matched to symptom profiles. Therefore, a universal measure of symptom management for all patients is unlikely. Rather, population-specific measures may be more useful.

Implications and Future Directions

This chapter established system-level and client-level nursing interventions as foundational to the healthcare system and highlighted key interdependencies between them. Consequently, data about nurses, systems, and nursing interventions are essential to support robust quality assessment and performance improvement initiatives leading to improved healthcare outcomes. This chapter also established that nursing interventions are complex and associated with inherent challenges to standardization and measurement. Given the importance of robust nurse intervention measures to quality assessment and performance improvement, quality scholars must work strategically to overcome these challenges and develop a comprehensive set of valid and reliable nurse intervention measures to examine the nursing contribution to quality patient care. In order to achieve this goal, quality scholars must be skilled in the science of complex interventions. The Medical Research Council (MRC), based in the United Kingdom, is an excellent resource in this area. The MRC provides free access to many educational materials on their web site to include their widely referenced guidance, *Developing and Evaluating Complex Interventions* (MRC 2006). Scholars with skills in this area will be more equipped to identify the active ingredients for complex nursing interventions, explicate their mechanisms of action, and determine the system structures required for effective execution. These steps are foundational to the development of the interventions themselves and are also foundational to the development of associated empirical measures.

Quality scholars must also know the criteria for effective performance measures and the process for endorsement of measures by the National Quality Forum (NQF). NQF provides free access to related educational materials on their web site (https://www.qualityforum.org/Measures_Reports_Tools.aspx). Quality scholars with skills in this area will be more equipped to develop nurse intervention measures that provide meaningful data for quality assessment and performance improvement initiatives. Moreover, measures that achieve NQF endorsement criteria are more likely to be widely adopted. Wide adoption leads to increased measurement consistency and a more robust evidence base for performance evaluation and benchmarking across care settings.

Quality scholars must also be skilled in extracting data about nurses and nursing interventions in existing clinical and operational databases. Despite the lack of standardized nursing care intervention measures, increasingly more data about nurses and nursing care interventions are collected. However, these data are often not captured using standardized definitions. They reside in disparate databases designed to support local operational departments (e.g., human resources, payroll, health records and billing, finance, and EHRs) (Huber et al. 1992). The feasibility of using existing data is dependent upon access to data science resources. Therefore, quality scholars must include colleagues with data science skills to expand the capacity of improvement teams to efficiently extract meaningful information related to nursing interventions and health outcomes. These cross-functional teams must collaborate to develop and define quality metrics and implement strategies to standardize procedures for data collection, extraction, harmonization, and analysis. Without a substantial investment in data science resources across health systems, it is unlikely that a robust set of quality metrics sensitive to nursing care will be developed or adopted. Ultimately, this limits nursing's capacity for the meaningful examination of practice, self-regulation, and validation of our unique contribution to quality healthcare.

References

Aiken LH, Clarke SP, Sloane DM, Sochalski JA, Busse R, Clarke H et al (2001) Nurses' reports on hospital care in five countries. Health Aff 20(3):43–53. https://doi.org/10.1377/hlthaff.20.3.43

Aiken LS, Butner J, Lockhart CA, Volk-Craft BE, Hamilton G, Williams FG (2006) Outcome evaluation of a randomized trial of the PhoenixCare Intervention Program: program of case management and coordinated care for the seriously chronically ill. J Palliat Med 9(1):1–126

Al Danaf J, Chang BH, Shaear M, Johnson KM, Miller S, Nester L, Williams AW, Aboumatar HJ (2017) Surfacing and addressing hospital patients' needs: proactive nurse rounding as a tool. J Nurs Manag 26:540–547

Al-Kandari F, Thomas D (2009) Factors contributing to nursing task incompletion as perceived by nurses working in Kuwait general hospitals. J Clin Nurs 18:3430–3440. https://doi.org/10.1111/j.1365-2702.2009.02795

American Nurses Association (ANA) (2010) Nursing's social policy statement: the essence of the profession. Nursebooks.org, Silver Spring, MD

Ausserhofer D, Zander B, Busse R, Schubert M, Rafferty AM, Schwendiamann R (2013) Prevalence, patterns and predictors of nursing care left undone in European hospitals: results from the multicountry cross-sectional RN4CAST study. Br Med J Qual Saf 23:126–135. https://doi.org/10.1136/bmjqs-2013-002318

Baber Z (1991) Beyond the structure/agency dualism: an evaluation of Giddens' Theory of Structuration. Sociol Inq 61(2):219–230

Beck SL, Eaton LH, Echeverria C, Mooney KH (2017) SymptomCare@Home. Developing and integrated symptom monitoring and management system for outpatients receiving chemotherapy. CIN: Comput Informat Nurs 35(10):520–529

Bellomo C (2016) Oral chemotherapy: patient education and nursing intervention. J Oncol Nurs Soc Online 7(6):20–27

Bleijenberg N, de Man-van Ginkel JM, Trappenburg JCA, Ettema RGA, Sino CG, Heim N, Hafsteindóttir TB, Richards DA, Schuurmans MJ (2018) Increasing value and reducing waste by optimizing the development of complex interventions: enriching the development phase of the Medical Research Council (MRC) Framework. Int J Nurs Stud 79:86–93

Bodilica V, Spraggon M, Tofan G (2015) A structuration framework for bridging the macro-micro divide in healthcare governance. Health Expect 19:790–804

Bolton LB, Donaldson NE, Rutledge DN, Bennett C, Brown DS (2007) The impact of nursing interventions. Overview of effective interventions, outcomes, measures, and priorities for future research. Med Care 64(2):123S–143S

Breen S, Ritchie D, Scholfield P, Hsueh Y, Gough K, Santamaria N, Kamateros R, Maguire R, Kearney N, Arandia S (2015) The patient remote intervention and symptom management system (PRISMS)—a telehealth-mediated intervention enabling real-time monitoring of chemotherapy side-effects in patients with haematological malignancies: study protocol for a randomised controlled trial. Trials 16(472):1–17

Bronfenbrenner U (ed) (2005) Making human beings human: bioecological perspectives on human development. Sage Publications, Thousand Oaks, CA

Bushor L, Rowser M (2015) Symptom management of chronic illness in the adult outpatient setting. J Hosp Palliat Nurs 17(4):285–290

Butcher HK, Bulechek GM, Dochterman JM, Wagner CM (eds) (2018) Nursing interventions classification (NIC), 7th edn. Elsevier, St. Louis, MO

Christiansen A, Coventry L, Graham R, Jacob E, Twigg D, Whitehead L (2018) Intentional rounding in acute care adult healthcare settings: a systematic mixed methods review. J Clin Nurs 27:1759–1792

Clarke SP, Aiken LH (2003) Failure to rescue. Am J Nurs 103:42–47

Colligan EM, Ewald E, Keating NL, Parashuram S, Spafford M, Ruiz S, Moiduddin (2017) Two innovative cancer care programs have potential to reduce utilization and spending. Med Care 55:873–878

Craig P, Dieppe P, Macintyre S, Michie S, Nazareth I, Pettigrew M (2013) Developing and evaluating complex interventions: the new medical council guidance. Int J Nurs Stud 50:585–592

Danesh V, Neff D, Jones TL, Arorian K, Unruh L, Andrews D, Guerrier L, Venus SJ, Jimenez E (2019) Can proactive rapid response team rounding improve surveillance and reduce unplanned escalations in care? A controlled before and after study. Int J Nurs Stud 91:128–133

Doran DM (ed) (2011) Nursing outcomes. State of the science, 2nd edn. Jones & Bartlett Learning, Sudbury, MA

Doughtery DM (1999) Surveillance. In: Bulechek GM, McCloskey JC (eds) Nursing interventions: effective nursing treatments, 3rd edn. Saunders., Philadelphia, PA, pp 524–532

Dresser S (2012) The role of nursing surveillance in keeping patients safe. J Nurs Adm 42(7/8):361–368

Dubois CA, D'Amour D, Pomey MP, Girard F, Brault I (2013) Conceptualizing performance of nursing care as a prerequisite for better measurement: a systematic and interpretative review. BMC Nurs 12:7. https://doi.org/10.1186/1472-6955-12-7

Fisk MJ (2015) Surveillance technologies in care homes: seven principles for their use. Work Older People 19(2):51–59

Forde-Johnston C (2014) Intentional rounding: a review of the literature. Nurs Stand 28(32):37–42

Giddens A (1984) The constitution of society: introduction of the theory of structuration. University of California Press, Berkley, CA

Gonzalo JD, Himes J, McGillen B, Shifflet V, Lehrman E (2016) Interprofessional collaborative care characteristics and occurrence of bedside interprofessional rounds: a cross-sectional analysis. BMC Health Serv Res 16(459):1–9

Gonzolo JD, Kuperman E, Lehman E, Haidet P (2014) Bedside interprofessional rounds: perceptions of benefits and barriers by internal medicine nursing staff, attending physicians, and house staff physicians. J Hosp Med 9(10):646–651

Gordon M (1987) Nursing diagnoses. McGraw-Hill, New York

Graham BC (2012) Examining evidence-based interventions to prevent inpatient falls. Medsurg Nurs 21(5):267–270

Harrington A, Bradley S, Jeffers L, Linedale E, Kelman S, Killington G (2013) The implementation of intentional rounding using participatory action research. Int J Nurs Pract 19:523–529

Hébert J, Fillion L (2011) Gaining a better understanding of the support function of oncology nurse navigators from their own perspective and that of people living with cancer: Part I. Canad Oncol Nurs J Winter:33–38

Hempel S, Newberry S, Wang Z, Booth M, Shanman R, Johnson B, Shier V, Saliba D, Spector WD, Ganz DA (2013) Hospital fall prevention: a systematic review of implementation, components, adherence, and effectiveness. J Am Geriatr Soc 61:483–494

Henneman EA, Gawlinski A, Giuliano KK (2012) Surveillance: a strategy for improving patient safety in acute and critical care units. Crit Care Nurse 32(2):e9–e18

Henry PCL, Man CA, Fung YS (2013) Effectiveness of nurse-led disease management programs on health outcomes and health service utilization in adult patients with chronic obstructive pulmonary disease: a systematic review protocol. Joanna Briggs Inst Datab Syst Rev Implement Rep 11(1):307–328

Hinami K, Alkhalil A, Chouksey S, Chua J, Trick WE (2016) Clinical significance of physical symptom severity in standardized assessments of patient reported outcomes. Qual Life Res 26:2239–2243

Huber DG, Delaney C, Mehmert M et al (1992) A nursing management minimum data set. Significance and development. J Nurs Adm 22(78):35–40

Humphreys J, Lee KA, Carrieri-Kohlman V et al (2008) Theory of symptom management. In: Smith MJ, Liehr PR (eds) Middle range theory for nursing. Springer Publishing, New York, pp 145–158

Hutchinson M, Higson M, Jackson D (2017) Mapping trends in the concept of nurse rounding: a bibliometric analysis and research agenda. Int J Nurs Pract 23:1–9

International Council of Nurses (ICN) (1993) Nursing's next advance: an international classification for nursing practice (ICNP). Author, Geneva, Switzerland

Irvine D, Sidani S, Hall LM (1998) Finding value in nursing care: a framework for quality improvement and clinical evaluation. Nurs Econ 16(3):110–131

Jeyathevan G, Lemonde M, Brathwaite AC (2017) The role of oncology nurse navigators in enhancing patient empowerment within the diagnostic phase for adult patients with lung cancer. Canad Oncol Nurs J 27(2):164–177

Jones TL (2011) A retrospective exploration of patient-ventilator monitoring intensity, therapeutic intervention intensity, and compliance with lung protective guidelines in a cohort of patients with adult respiratory distress syndrome. World Views Evid Based Nurs 8(1):40–50

Jones T (2014) Validation of the perceived implicit rationing of nursing care (PIRNCA) instrument. Nurs Forum 49(2):77–78

Jones TL (2016) What nurses do when time is scarce—and why. J Nurs Adm 46(9):449–454. https://doi.org/10.1097/NNA.0000000000000374

Jones DA, DeVita MA, Bellomo R (2011) Rapid-response teams. N Engl J Med 365(2):139–146

Jones T, Hamilton P, Murry N (2015) Unfinished nursing care, missed care, and implicitly rationed car: state of the science review. Int J Nurs Stud 52(6):1121–1137. https://doi.org/10.1016/j.ijnstu.2015.02.012

Jones T, Willis E, Amorim-Lopes M, Drach-Zahavy A (2019a) Advancing the science of unfinished nursing care: exploring the benefits of cross-disciplinary knowledge exchange, knowledge integration and transdisciplinarity. J Adv Nurs 75:905–917

Jones TL, Yoder LH, Baernholdt M (2019b) Variation in academic preparation and progression of nurses across the continuum of care. Nurs Ourlook 67:381–392

Jones T, Drach-Zahavy A, Amorim-Lopes M, Wilis E (in press) Systems, economics and neoliberal politics: theories to understand missed nursing care. Nurs Health Sci

Kalisch BJ, Lee KH (2010) The impact of teamwork on missed nursing care. Nurs Outlook 58(5):233–241. https://doi.org/10.1016/j.outlook.2010.06.004

Kalisch BJ, Williams RA (2009) Development and psychometric testing of a tool to measure missed nursing care. J Nurs Adm 39(5):211–219

Kalisch BJ, Tschannen D, Lee KH (2011) Do staffing levels predict missed nursing care? Int J Qual Health Care 23(3):302–308

Kalisch BJ, Gosselin K, Choi SH (2012) A comparison of patient care units with high versus low levels of missed nursing care. Health Care Manag Rev 37(4):320–328. https://doi.org/10.1097/HMR.0b013e318249727e

Kallen MA, Yang D, Haas N (2012) A technical solution to improving palliative and hospice care. Support Care Cancer 20:167–174

Kelly L, Vincent D (2010) The dimensions of nursing surveillance: a concept analysis. J Adv Nurs 67(3):652–661

Kuntz G, Tozer JM, Snegosky J, Fox J, Neuman K (2014) Michigan oncology medical home demonstration project: first-year results. J Oncol Pract 10(5):294–297

Kutney-Lee A, Lake ET, Aiken LH (2009) Development of the hospital nurse surveillance capacity profile. Res Nurs Health 32:217–228

Li D, Elliott T, Klein G, Ur E, Tang TS (2017) Diabetes nurse case management in a Canadian tertiary care setting: results of a randomized controlled trial. Can J Diabetes 41:297–304

McCloskey JC, Bulechek GM (1992) Nursing interventions classification (NIC), 2nd edn. Mosby Year Book, St Louis, MO

McCloskey JC, Bulechek GM (2000) Nursing interventions classification (NIC), 3rd edn. Mosby Year Book, St Louis, MO

Medical Research Council (2006) Developing and evaluating complex interventions: new guidance. www.mrc.ac.uk/complexinterventionsguidance

Mitchell PH, Fertich S, Jennings BM (1998) Quality health outcomes model. Image J Nurs Sch 30(1):43–46

Mitchell MD, Trotta RL, Lavenberg JG, Umscheid CA (2014) Hourly rounding to improve nursing responsiveness. A systematic review. J Nurs Adm 44(9):462–472

Mkanta WN, Chumbler NR, Richardson LC, Kobb RF (2007) Age-related differences in quality of life in cancer patients. A pilot study of a cancer care coordination/home-telehealth program. Cancer Nurs 30(6):434–440

Mushta J, Rush KL, Andersen E (2018) Failure to rescue as a nurse-sensitive indicator. Nurs Forum 53:84–92

National Quality Forum (2004) National voluntary consensus standards for nursing-sensitive care: an initial performance measure set. A consensus report. Author, Washington, DC. https://www.qualityforum.org/Publications/2004/10/National_Voluntary_Consensus_Standards_for_Nursing-Sensitive_Care__An_Initial_Performance_Measure_Set.aspx

Needleman J, Buerhaus PI (2007) Failure to rescue: comparing definitions to measure quality of care. Med Care 45(10):913–915

O'Malley AS, Draper K, Gourevitch R, Cross DA, Scholle SH (2015) Electronic health records and support for primary care teamwork. J Am Informat Assoc 22:426–434

Pfrimmer DM, Johnson MR, Guthmiller ML, Lehman JL, Rhudy LM (2017) Surveillance: a nursing intervention for improving patient safety in critical care environment. Dimens Crit Care Nurs 36(1):45–52

Richard AA, Shea K (2011) Delineation of self-care and associated concepts. J Nurs Scholarsh 43(3):225–264

Sahota O, Drummond A, Kendrick D, Grainge MJ, Vass C, Sach T, Gladman J, Avis M (2014) REFINE (REducing Falls in In-patieNt Elderly) using bed and bedside chair pressure sensors linked to radio-pagers in acute hospital care: a randomised controlled trial. Age Aging 43:247–253

Santana M, Feeny D (2014) Framework to assess the effects of using patient-reported outcome measures in chronic care management. Qual Life Res 23:1505–1513

Schmidt LE (2010) Making sure: registered nurses watching over their patients. Nurs Res 59(6):400–405

Schoneman D (2002) The intervention of surveillance across classification systems. Int J Nurs Terminol Classif 13(4):137–147

Schubert M, Glass TR, Clarke SP, Schaffert-Witvliet B, De Geest S (2007) Validation of the Basel extent of rationing of nursing care instrument. Nurs Res 56(6):416–424

Schubert M, Ausserhofer D, Desmedt M, Schwendimann R, Lesaffre E, Li B, De Geest S (2013) Levels and correlates of implicit rationing of nursing care in Swiss acute care hospitals—A cross-sectional study. Int J Nurs Stud 50:230–239. https://doi.org/10.1016/j.ijnurstu.2012.09.016

Serpa S, Ferreira CM (2019) Micro, meso, and macro levels of social analysis. Int J Soc Stud 7:3. https://doi.org/10.11114/ijsss.v7i3.4223

Shever LL (2011) The impact of surveillance on failure to rescue. Res Theory Nurs Pract Int J 25(2):107–126

Sidani S (2011) Symptom management. In: Doran DM (ed) Nursing outcomes the state of the science, 2nd edn. Jones & Bartlett Learning, Ontario, Canada

Sims S, leamy M, Davies N, Schnitzler K, Levenson R, Mayer F, Grant R, Brearly S, Gourlay S, Ross F, Harris R (2018) Realist synthesis of intentional rounding in hospital wards: exploring the evidence of what works, for whom, in what circumstances and why. BMJ Qual Saf 27:743–757

Snyder M (1992) Independent nursing interventions, 2nd edn. Delmar, Albany, NY

Snyder M, Egan EC, Nojima Y (1996) Defining nursing interventions. Image J Nurs Sch 28(2):137–141

Stone R (2005) Structuration theory. Palgrave-MacMillan, London, UK

Stover AM, Stricker CT, Hammelef K, Hensen S, Carr P, Jansen J, Deal AM, Bennett AV, Basch EM (2019) Using stakeholder engagement to overcome barriers to implementing patient-reported outcomes (PROs) in cancer care delivery. Med Care 57:S92–S99

Titler MG (1992) Interventions related to surveillance. Nurs Clin N Am 27(2):495–502

Votruba L, Graham B, Wisinski J, Syed A (2016) Video monitoring to reduce falls and patient companion costs for adult inpatients. Nurs Econ 34(4):185–189

Whitmer K, Preumer J, Wilhelm C, McCraig L, Hester JDB (2011) Development of an outpatient oncology symptom management clinic. Clin J Oncol Nurs 15(2):175–179

Yang LY, Manhas DS, Howard AF, Olson RA (2018) Patient-reported outcome use in oncology: a systematic review of the impact on patient-clinician communication. Support Care Cancer 26:41–60

Interprofessional Practice and Education

10

Alan W. Dow, Deborah DiazGranados,
and Marianne Baernholdt

Introduction

Healthcare has been described as a complex, adaptive system (Lipsitz 2012). A complex system has multiple parts—in the case of healthcare: clients, their families, healthcare workers, facilities, technology, and medications, among others. With the proliferation of technology, medications, and ways of delivering care over recent decades, the healthcare system has become increasingly complex, perhaps best exemplified by the increasing number of people with a greater chronic disease burden (Hajat and Stein 2018). To function optimally, healthcare must remain adaptive to the needs of individual patients and broader communities. The parts of the complex system can interact in many different ways, and adaptation should be driven by individual clients and their families' needs. Better interprofessional practice is one of the key strategies for the healthcare system to manage this complexity and effectively adapt to patients' needs.

The benefits of enhanced interprofessional practice have been articulated for nearly 50 years (Institute of Medicine 1972). The negative consequences of poor interprofessional practice were identified as a leading cause of both harmful medical errors and overall gaps in health services' quality (IOM 2001). However, done

A. W. Dow (✉)
Medicine and Health Administration, Virginia Commonwealth University,
Richmond, VA, USA
e-mail: alan.dow@vcuhealth.org

D. DiazGranados
Wright Center for Clinical and Translational Research, School of Medicine, Virginia
Commonwealth University, Richmond, VA, USA
e-mail: diazgranados@vcu.edu

M. Baernholdt
School of Nursing, University of North Carolina at Chapel Hill, Chapel Hill, NC, USA
e-mail: marianne_baernholdt@unc.edu

© Springer Nature Switzerland AG 2021   177
M. Baernholdt, D. K. Boyle (eds.), *Nurses Contributions to Quality Health
Outcomes*, https://doi.org/10.1007/978-3-030-69063-2_10

well, effective interprofessional practice, through which healthcare workers in a complex adaptive system are continually working together to improve care, can create a learning health system that continually works to provide even better care (Institute of Medicine 2013). This aspiration has been embraced by the National Collaborative for Improving the Clinical Learning Environment (NCICLE), representing more than 30 professional organizations (NCICLE 2020). NCICLE was formed to promote the reciprocal relationship between clinical learning and patient safety, focusing on interprofessional relationships. Similarly, the correlation between the quality of interprofessional practice and the well-being and retention of healthcare practitioners has been emphasized (Dow et al. 2019; NAM 2019).

However, despite this policy basis for interprofessional practice, linking interventions to enhance interprofessional practice to improvements in patient outcomes has been challenging (Reeves et al. 2017). Changing professional interaction patterns is difficult, and targeted health outcomes often require a long period of follow-up. As such, frameworks, especially the QHOM (Mitchell et al. 1998), are needed that provide a more complete understanding of the relationship between interprofessional practice and improving health. Moreover, frameworks are needed to help develop, implement, and assess interventions to improve patients' care quality.

Interprofessional Practice: Linkages with the QHOM

Although Donabedian's structure-process-outcomes model (SPO) (Donabedian 1988) has long been the leading framework for understanding health outcomes, the QHOM provides a more complete framework for understanding the complexity inherent in how interprofessional practice affects health (see Fig. 10.1). The Donabedian model separates inputs and processes and describes them as linearly related to outcomes. In contrast, the QHOM model describes an interdependent relationship between the client and the system and the outcomes those interactions generate. Outcomes are not static but rather inputs as feedback to the client and the systems. This feedback is essential for adaptation in complex systems.

Unlike the Donabedian model, the QHOM model defines the role of interventions. Interventions capture a broad range of activities. Examples include a training program to improve interprofessional collaboration, adding a new health professional/discipline into a clinical environment, or changing how payment incentivizes care. Each of these may target the interprofessional team and could be seen as an intervention to change interprofessional practice. Importantly, in the QHOM, interventions do not lead to outcomes; instead, interventions work through the complexity of the healthcare system and clients' lives to impact outcomes. The QHOM helps us better understand the system.

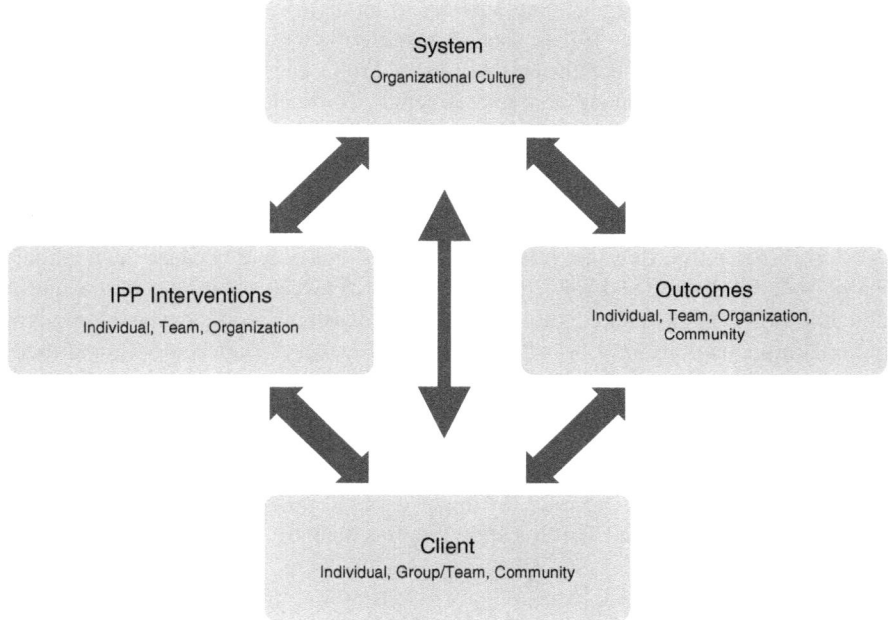

Fig. 10.1 Framework for interprofessional practice

Interprofessional Practice and Education Within a Complex System

What Is Interprofessional Practice?

All health professions adhere to a common value base, that is, improving the human condition. However, each profession has different professional traditions that are, in part, represented by different scopes of practice. Interprofessional practice sits at the intersection between a client's right to receive the best available healthcare and the profession-specific values and abilities each profession can bring to bear to help a client. This intersection can be a source of conflict or a synergy source, depending on the quality of interprofessional practice.

Nevertheless, how best to define interprofessional practice remains debated. The most commonly accepted definition from the World Health Organization (World Health Organization 2010) states that collaborative practice is: "… when multiple health workers from different professional backgrounds provide comprehensive services by working with patients, their families, carers and communities to deliver the highest quality of care across settings." This definition is functional but does not capture the power dynamics between professions or the influence of broader system forces such as payment and regulation on collaboration between different health professions.

In contrast, Fawcett argues that there are at least two views of what constitutes IPP/IPE. The first is that IPP is a team-based collaborative practice where "the members of each area of healthcare have distinct roles and role activities that do not overlap as they engage in collaborative practice" (Fawcett 2014, p. 178). The second view focuses on interprofessional practice, which is derived from the explorations of interdisciplinary research. In this view, "an integrative and reciprocally interactive approach that actualizes a synthesis of diverse disciplinary perspectives leading to a new level of thinking about … a topic or even a new discipline" (Fawcett 2013, p. 376). In this view, the roles and activities are unclear because the boundaries of specific discipline knowledge are blurred. Fawcett captures the tension in collaboration between shared knowledge and profession-specific expertise. Several national organizations have opined that the effectiveness of interprofessional practice is only optimized when all team members contribute fully and equally from their distinct disciplinary perspective (Hawkins et al. 2018; NAM 2013; Perlo et al. 2017). This opinion integrates Fawcett's second articulated perspective on interprofessional practice into the WHO definition. It begs the question of when does interprofessional interaction become of high enough quality to be described as interprofessional practice? This question remains unanswered.

Contrasting Interprofessional Education and Interprofessional Practice

Interprofessional education is defined by the WHO (World Health Organization 2010) as "… when two or more professions learn about, from and with each other to enable effective collaboration and improve health outcomes." Although both IPP and IPE require interaction between individuals from different professions, interventions to enhance IPP seek to improve health outcomes whereas IPE targets the learning of the individuals involved (Oandasan and Reeves 2005). Educators have delivered IPE activities in various venues, including classrooms, simulation centers, and clinical areas. Most impact assessments are short-term and focused on attitudinal changes rather than generalized and maintained behavior change that impacts patient outcomes (Abu-Rish et al. 2012). Whether IPE is effective and how best to deliver it are unknown (Reeves et al. 2013).

The effectiveness of IPP and IPE is thought to depend on the quality of collaboration between the healthcare professionals involved. Fawcett (2014) writes how IPP may be similar to team science, where there is a need for those involved to engage in knowledge integration. The process of knowledge integration requires that individuals be willing and capable of integrating knowledge from other professions (Cronin and Weingart 2007), consistent with both attitudinal and cognitive learning needs from IPE. For example, each team member should have a shared definition of the problem and patient case and how each profession fits into the patient's care. When a sense of sharedness is lacking, conflict or errors may occur (Mcgrath and Argote 2001).

Holmboe et al. (2016) suggested that IPE and IPP are implemented best through co-learning where a deliberate flattening of the hierarchy among professions and among teachers and students has occurred. On the one hand, more advanced learners may have already developed a strong professional attitudinal foundation that interferes with interprofessional collaboration. On the other hand, providing IPE to early learners may be challenging because they may not have mastered basic competence in their profession. Early learners may not be ready to actively participate in interprofessional practice as a representative of their profession. How best to time IPE so that it supports effective IPP is still in need of additional research.

Science that Informs IPP and IPE

IPP and IPE have several types of literature to draw from to inform their application and research agendas. For example, educational psychology and its theories of motivation, cognition, and engagement (Arkes and Garske 1977; Snow 1989; Tittle 1994) are critical for informing how activities are prepared and delivered, and most importantly, how IPE activities are framed to learners. Social psychology and research on social identity, self-categorization, and social comparison provide the underpinnings of what to consider when approaching training or education activities in IPE and IPP (Goethals 1986; Hogg and Terry 2000; Tajfel 1982). Organizational psychology informs IPP and IPE through research in team dynamics (Rosen et al. 2018), systems theory, or leadership and followership. In addition to these research areas, there is a growing literature base that is interdisciplinary in nature and can inform the work of IPP and IPE initiatives (Fiore 2008; Poole et al. 2004; Van Swol and Kane 2019).

Characteristics Important for Interprofessional Practice

One approach to conceptualize the factors impacting IPP or IPE is micro/meso/macro levels (Oandasan and Reeves 2005). Microlevel factors are at the level of the individual. These include psychological states such as attitudes toward collaboration and personal knowledge, such as understanding of different scopes of practice. IPE interventions typically target micro factors.

Meso-level factors span from the team level to the organizational level. These might include how an organization's leadership and chain of command are structured or how different professions are deployed to support optimal patient care and collaboration. IPE interventions at the meso level are often focused on training teams at the unit level. In comparison, IPP interventions may be broader and not even recognized as interventions that positively or negatively impact IPP.

Macro-level factors work at the societal and political level. Payment, licensure, and malpractice systems are macro-level approaches that can positively or negatively impact IPP. Recent work on accreditation standards for IPE is an example of

IPE interventions at a macro-level. Like meso-level interventions, the impact of a macro-level intervention in IPP in a discrete care setting may not be considered.

The QHOM helps consider how an intervention might be translated through these levels of impact. A macro-level intervention may have unanticipated micro-level effects for practitioners or clients, such as providing altering pathways to access care by changing payment. Conversely, macro-level change generally stems from problems identified at the micro and meso levels in providing optimal care to clients and communities. This complexity and interdependence are central to the QHOM.

Organizational Culture

Because the QHOM is grounded in systems theory, congruence is an important concept. Congruence theory (Nadler and Tushman 1980), a foundation for understanding systems theory, explains that when there is congruence or fit among tasks, interventions, people, structure, and culture, there is a higher level of effectiveness. One manifestation of a system is organizational culture. Organizational culture can be defined as the shared assumptions, values, and beliefs that characterize a setting and shape all work activities (Schneider et al. 2013). In healthcare, different cultures exist between organizations/hospital systems, clinical units, or even shifts. All work happens within an organizational system, and that system has, as its background culture.

For interventions intended to improve interprofessional practice, the system's culture defines the process of work, including how quickly and effectively an intervention can lead to change (Gale et al. 2014). Alternatively, an intervention might seek to change the system culture. Although defining and measuring culture are challenging, the QHOM, by embracing healthcare's complex interrelatedness, provides an illustration that may begin to help define cultural differences and the many ways culture may shape the quality and outcomes of care. This type of approach is being applied in the literature focused on interprofessional practice through the realist synthesis approach (Pawson et al. 2005; Pawson 2006) where the driving questions of research are not just "what works for whom" but "what works for whom in which context" (Rycroft-Malone et al. 2012). Drawing from implementation science, this approach has been gaining traction in the IPP/IPE literature; it is beginning to shed some light on how culture shapes work and the uptake of interventions (Hewitt et al. 2014). The QHOM articulates that interventions to improve interprofessional practice are impacted by culture even as they often seek to change the culture. For researchers and others interested in improving healthcare, the QHOM pushes us to question how to conceptualize an intervention.

Also, while studying interventions usually starts from the perspective of the intervention acting on the system and/or the client to lead to an outcome, the QHOM recognizes that the system and client act upon the intervention. For example, many interventions may target an improvement of a system's interprofessional collaboration. The modified collaboration may affect the fidelity of implementing the intervention, the satisfaction of healthcare workers with the intervention, and, ultimately, how the intervention interacts with clients and impacts outcomes. Interventions may succeed or fail based on qualities of interprofessional practice and may lead to unanticipated outcomes. The QHOM pushes us to embrace the system's complexity and interdependence and all parts of healthcare delivery.

Interprofessional Practice Interventions

Despite the importance of better interprofessional practice from the theoretical and policy perspectives, how best to improve interprofessional practice has been challenging. A Cochrane review of studies through November 2015 found only nine experimental studies of interventions to increase interprofessional practice (Reeves et al. 2017). These studies showed only mild evidence of benefit to patient outcomes. The authors also described the interventions and impact as heterogeneous and stated that it was difficult to draw generalizable conclusions. Unfortunately, even interventions that work within this complex, adaptive system and across micro, meso, and macro levels may take years to manifest benefit (especially for educational or workforce development interventions) and lead to change that is difficult to detect (IOM 2015; Oandasan and Reeves 2005). Controlled trials are often not feasible, are potentially unethical, and may bias findings (Zwarenstein and Treweek 2009). Instead, the complexity integral to these settings requires a more pragmatic approach that recognizes that interventions should be shaped by each patient's needs and the capacity of each setting.

Interventions to improve interprofessional practice seek to change interactions among the healthcare workers and clients in the system to enhance patient outcomes. Interventions that improve interprofessional practice fall into three main groups: interprofessional education, teamwork training, and implementing novel interprofessional care models. The implications of the QHOM to each will be discussed below.

Interprofessional Education

IPE was designated a high-priority area for health professions education in 2003 (IOM 2003). Subsequently, competencies were developed to guide curriculum development (Interprofessional Education Collaborative (IPEC) 2016), and accrediting standards for IPE have been implemented in nearly all health professions (Health Professions Accreditors Collaborative 2019; Zorek and Raehl 2013). IPE has become a global phenomenon, with educational programs developing many different approaches to meet these regulations and aspirations.

There is limited evidence for the benefit of IPE interventions on practice (Illingworth and Chelvanayagam 2017). A Cochrane review of interprofessional education found only 15 comparative studies which were generally positive, but were described in interventions, participants, and studied outcomes (Reeves et al. 2013). The authors stated that drawing generalizable conclusions was not possible. Meanwhile, most of the rapidly proliferating IPE programs focus on pre-licensure learners. Evaluation of these programs is generally short-term and focused on learner satisfaction or acceptability, often without comparison groups (Abu-Rish et al. 2012).

Why the limited evidence for IPE despite years of intensive investment? Framed within the QHOM, most IPE interventions are distant from the systems of practices and the clients who receive services. Although the need to link IPE activities closer to practice outcomes has been articulated by the National Academy of Medicine (IOM 2015), education and practice remain fundamentally separate despite being dependent on each other for future workforce and faculty (Frenk et al. 2010). The impact of IPE, as currently evaluated, is simply too distant from the challenges it hopes to affect.

How then to proceed with considering IPE under the QHOM? The real benefit of IPE may be in how it impacts systems and specific practitioners. For example, establishing a more complete professional identity for healthcare professionals anchored within an interprofessional approach to work may lead to healthcare workers who collaborate more effectively (Khalili et al. 2013). In turn, these individuals may change systems to support a culture of greater collaboration that can be measured both in measures of organizational cultures and benefits to patient outcomes (Dow and Thibault 2017). However, achieving these aspirations is far from certain despite the QHOM helping to frame this approach.

Team Training

Another approach to enhance interprofessional practice is team training. Team training effectively improves team performance in healthcare across several settings (Hughes et al. 2016). For example, the training of surgical teams has been shown to decrease mortality (Neily et al. 2010). In less acute settings, the benefit of team-building interventions is more mixed (Miller et al. 2018). However, interprofessional team training outperforms team training that is not interprofessional (Hughes et al. 2016). The most effective team training is based on competencies and matched to the clinical context's needs (Rosen et al. 2018). For example, in one study, 25 interprofessional teams from ambulatory, long-term care, hospital, and home health received training over a year to reduce falls (Eckstrom et al. 2016). The strategy adopted across sites differed; for example, adding Tai Chi classes was more likely in long-term care facilities, while ambulatory facilities were more likely to initiate fall screening. Although didactic lectures alone are not effective, workshops, simulations, and team performance reviews are all effective, with the most beneficial approach being uncertain (McEwan et al. 2017).

Nevertheless, team training also faces challenges to implementation in healthcare. As a manifestation of the complex adaptive system, teams form in response to a stimulus, usually the patient's needs. These teams are highly variable and often unpredictable (Dow et al. 2017; Yao et al. 2018). Also, the number of healthcare workers needed to meet an individual patient's needs is large, making training cumbersome if not impossible. Whereas training a surgical team with fixed members clearly has benefits, developing generalized competency in teamwork through team training may not be beneficial. For example, TeamSTEPPS, probably the most widely used model for team training in healthcare, has been applied to various settings with heterogeneous outcomes, which makes generalization about benefit challenging (Chen et al. 2019).

How then can the QHOM help us apply team training? Some interactions between clients and systems involve consistent, core groups of healthcare practitioners. These groups are promising targets for team training. Beyond surgical teams, outpatient clinics and rehabilitation settings may fit these criteria. In other settings, where team membership is more dynamic, system redesign, as mentioned below, can segment work processes to define fixed teams better and reap the benefits of team training (DiazGranados et al. 2018). When contrasted with pre-licensure interprofessional education, team training brings IPE concepts into the system and closer to the clients. Outcomes become easier to measure, including changes in the overall culture of an organization. Less certain is how a pre-licensure IPE foundation or team training in one setting may translate to a new setting or team.

System Redesign

A third approach to enhancing interprofessional practice is redesigning systems to support novel models of interprofessional work. With this approach, care is constructed differently, typically with professional responsibilities being redistributed across different professional roles with overlapping scopes of practice. For example, over a hundred comparative studies have been done on new collaboration models between pharmacists and primary care practitioners (de Barra et al. 2019). However, these models are not uniformly beneficial (de Barra et al. 2019), suggesting that they need to be shaped to best meet clients' needs in the system's context. Clients generally benefit from these models though the benefit is greatest for relatively specific outcomes, such as hypertension control, and less clear for more complex outcomes such as overall healthcare utilization. During the Asheville Project, a partnership between primary care, community pharmacists, local businesses, and government in Asheville, North Carolina, clients demonstrated improvements in diabetes and lipid control as well as cost savings (Cranor et al. 2003). Clients with the greatest need—type 1 diabetics and the most uncontrolled—benefitted the most (Cranor & Christensen 2003). However, context also mattered; employees of one company had better outcomes than employees from the rest of the companies.

Examining the integration of behavioral health practitioners in primary care tells a similar story. Formalized collaboration between mental health practitioners and primary care practitioners has been shown to improve clinical outcomes for depression (Bower et al. 2006; Thota et al. 2012) and anxiety disorders

(Muntingh et al. 2016). Yet, these models must be integrated into practice in a way that is acceptable to practitioners, clients, and others. Approaches have included shared visits, in-person connections to mental health practitioners known as "warm handoffs," and geographically separated locations for care with structured approaches to sharing care. Closer collaboration is more resource intensive and whether collaborative care is cost effective depends on multiple factors in the care environment, including the method of collaboration, how care is paid for, and whether the benefit is realized by the multiple parties involved, including clients, employers, and insurers (Grochtdreis 2015).

Example of an IPP Intervention in One Healthcare System

A Quality Scholars Program focused on improving care outcomes in a large Academic Medical Center ran for 2 years (Baernholdt et al. 2019). Interprofessional dyads of practitioners—usually but not always a nurse and a doctor—collaborated to tackle a quality issue. They were supported in this work by a didactic curriculum on quality improvement and leadership and project mentorship via a dedicated coach. Before enrolling in the program, each team defined a quality problem and committed to working on that issue over most of a year. What unfolded over the two iterations of the program demonstrates the challenges of interprofessional practice interventions and the utility of the QHOM.

Every team was able to implement changes in the system. From the perspective of implementing an intervention, all were successful. However, the majority of these interventions did not impact the system or clients as expected. Typically, they had no discernable benefit, and teams had to implement additional changes to improve the health outcome that was their focus area. However, some teams did have a demonstrable, beneficial impact on outcomes. For example, one team decreased intensive care unit length of stay, improved patient outcomes, and saved millions of dollars for the health system (National Academy of Medicine 2017). For every team, the system and clients' needs forced them to adapt the intervention they initially designed.

Moreover, which teams would be successful was not predictable from the beginning. Although good ideas, leadership, and dedication were necessary, they were not enough; successful implementation depended on the unit's preceding care patterns and willingness to adopt a new care approach. Teams needed to try many approaches and continue to adapt and measure impact as they discovered what worked within each individualized context.

As the QHOM illustrates, it is not just the outcomes that are important but the relationship between the components. A redesigned model of practice may not translate across different contexts and cultures. Similarly, benefits accrued to the system, such as improved interprofessional practice, may not always benefit clients or other stakeholders.

Summary and Future Directions

The utility of the QHOM for interprofessional practice helps us understand the relationship between interventions and the other model components within the complex adaptive system of healthcare. As interventions act on the system, client, or both, each component of the system shapes others bidirectionally and leads to outcomes at both the system and client level. Interventions, being distant from outcomes and shaped through the system culture and unique client characteristics, may have outcomes that are unpredictable and often challenging to measure.

The QHOM helps us appreciate healthcare complexity and the importance of asking how components interact and influence each other. The QHOM adds this complexity to the SPO model and admits that structures, processes, and outcomes are interdependent rather than static antecedents and results. Processes can change structures, and outcomes shape both. In terms of interprofessional practice, the QHOM identifies that our healthcare workers are always adapting to each other, clients' needs, and the setting's constraints. The QHOM provides the freedom to make these changes so that health outcomes can be best achieved based on the moment's capacity.

In the QHOM, moving interventions from being intermediaries between structures and outcomes to antecedents that impact both systems and clients to create outcomes—sometimes unexpected—changes the perspective. Leaders, researchers, or policymakers seek to "do" something. Framing this "doing" as an addition to the environment that impacts the system and the clients more accurately represents the approach to improvement.

All of this helps consider interprofessional practice differently. Applied to interventions that seek to increase interprofessional practice as a way of improving health outcomes, the QHOM offers these guiding principles:

1. Interventions with a long-time horizon for impact, such as interprofessional education, must be evaluated by how they impact the relationship between clients and systems that eventually lead to outcomes. As such, interprofessional education may be more about cultural change than changing a single individual's behaviors. Evaluating success through a sociological or organizational lens may be the most appropriate path.
2. The QHOM interrelationships exist within a cultural milieu that determines the capacity for an intervention to impact both the model's proximal and distal components. The needs of clients are both manifestations of this culture and shapers of this culture. As such, how best to meet clients' needs with an intervention depends on system factors that may not transfer from one setting to another. For example, as seen in team training research, the best approach may vary by context. Customization and ongoing evaluation of impact are necessary.
3. Tracking outcomes may offer some insight into a system's strengths and weaknesses and which interventions have a greater chance of success. Suppose a promising intervention fails to improve health outcomes. In that case, the relationship between the component parts and impact on each other should be areas

for troubleshooting how to revamp the intervention. Potentially, a failed intervention may still be beneficial if better adapted to the system.

These principles, stemming from the QHOM, help understand work and its impact on the work better. They move beyond the question of "Did it work?" to questions of "Who did it work for?" and "Why or why not?" The QHOM embraces healthcare complexity with all its interacting parts, especially the collaboration of healthcare workers. Improving healthcare is not simple, but it is work worth engaging to understand the work of healthcare better, how workers engage in it, and how that work can most benefit clients and their families.

The QHOM provides a way to understand the complex healthcare system and how interventions might succeed or fail. The work that has utilized the QHOM and research from psychology, sociology, and communications provides evidence for understanding how to develop practitioners, prepare organizations, and structure tasks for effective teamwork. However, additional work is needed to further our understanding. Primarily our recommendations focus on research that studies teamwork longitudinally and across boundaries in healthcare, studies the conflict across disciplines that may arise and its impact on IPP and IPE, and investigates the context that is the healthcare system and how it has implications for IPP and IPE.

First, there is a need for research to examine how IPP is conducted over time and across boundaries. Patient care often extends beyond discreet short time periods, such as a few hours, and across teams and boundaries, such as several teams of clinicians across different health systems. Therefore, additional research is needed to inform how clinicians' function in these complex systems. Some literature has identified how healthcare can be defined by more complex structures such as multiteam systems (DiazGranados et al. 2014, 2017) and the complexity of care provided to patients. Research needs to be conducted to understand the structures, competencies, and developmental needs of teams.

Second, research should continue to understand how professional identity impacts how teams engage in IPP, and also critically, this research could inform both IPE and IPP initiatives. Moreover, research in this area of how professional identity impacts processes and outcomes can inform training interventions. Might it be that the learners be taught that as they develop their professional identity? That it not only means they identify with being a nurse, for example but that they are also a part of a larger identity of being a healthcare practitioner?

Third, as we have mentioned throughout, healthcare is a complex system; additional research should consider the impact of context on educational and practice initiatives. At the writing of this chapter, the healthcare system had to reinvent providing care for patients during the COVID-19 pandemic. Systems have changed their care for patients to be completely reliant on telemedicine, something that had not been common practice; research is needed to understand the impact of technology on how teams interact. Moreover, technology such as electronic health records (EHR) (see Chap. 6) are central to how teams interact with one another. Additional research that can inform how to teach learners about the use of the EHR as a team member could benefit team dynamics in healthcare teams.

References

Abu-Rish E, Kim S, Choe L, Varpio L, Malik E, White AA, Zierler B (2012) Current trends in interprofessional education of health sciences students: a literature review. J Interprof Care 226(6):444–451. https://doi.org/10.3109/13561820.2012.715604

Arkes HR, Garske JP (1977) Psychological theories of motivation. Brooks, Cole

Baernholdt M, Feldman M, Davis-Ajami ML, Harvey LD, Mazmanian PE, Mobley D, Dow A (2019) An interprofessional quality improvement training program that improves educational and quality outcomes. Am J Med Qual 34(6):577–584. https://doi.org/10.1177/1062860618825306

Bower P, Gilbody S, Richards D, Fletcher J, Sutton A (2006) Collaborative care for depression in primary care. Making sense of a complex intervention: systematic review and meta-regression. Br J Psychiatry 189:484–493

Chen AS, Yau B, Revere L, Swails J (2019) Implementation, evaluation, and outcome of TeamSTEPPS in interprofessional education: a scoping review. J Interprof Care 33(6):795–804. https://doi.org/10.1080/13561820.2019.1594729

Cranor CW, Christensen DB (2003) The Asheville Project: short-term outcomes of a community pharmacy diabetes care program. J Am Pharm Assoc 52(6):838–850

Cranor CW, Bunting BA, Christensen DB (2003) The Asheville Project: long-term clinical and economic outcomes of a community pharmacy diabetes care program. J Am Pharm Assoc 43(2):173–184

Cronin MA, Weingart LR (2007) Representational gaps, information processing, and conflict in functionally diverse teams. Acad Manag Rev 32(3):761–773. https://doi.org/10.2307/20159333

de Barra M, Scott C, Johnston M, De Bruin M, Scott N, Matheson C, Bond C, Watson M (2019) Do pharmacy intervention reports adequately describe their interventions? A template for intervention description and replication analysis of reports included in a systematic review. BMJ Open 9(12):e025511

DiazGranados D, Dow AW, Perry SJ, Palesis JA (2014) Understanding patient care as a multiteam system. In: Shuffler ESML, Rico R (eds) Pushing the boundaries: multiteam systems in research and practice. Emerald Group Publishing Limited, Bradford, pp 95–113

DiazGranados D, Shuffler M, Savage N, Dow AW, Dhindsa HD (2017) Defining the prehospital care multiteam system. In: Keebler PMJR, Lazzara EH (eds) Human factors and ergonomics of prehospital emergency care. CRC Press, New York

DiazGranados D, Dow AW, Appelbaum N, Mazmanian PE, Retchin SM (2018) Interprofessional practice in different patient care settings: a qualitative exploration. J Interprof Care 32(2):151–159. https://doi.org/10.1080/13561820.2017.1383886

Donabedian A (1988) The quality of care. How can it be assessed? JAMA 260(12):1743–1748. https://doi.org/10.1001/jama.260.12.1743

Dow A, Thibault G (2017) Interprofessional education—A foundation for a new approach to health care. N Engl J Med 377(9):803–805. https://doi.org/10.1056/NEJMp1705665

Dow AW, Zhu X, Sewell D, Banas CA, Mishra V, Tu SP (2017) Teamwork on the rocks: rethinking interprofessional practice as networking. J Interprof Care 31(6):677–678. https://doi.org/10.1080/13561820.2017.1344048

Dow AW, Baernholdt M, Santen SA, Baker K, Sessler CN (2019) Practitioner well-being as an interprofessional imperative. J Interprof Care 33(6):577–584. https://doi.org/10.1080/1356182 0.2019.1673705

Eckstrom E, Neal MB, Cotrell V, Casey CM, McKenzie G, Morgove MW, Lasater K (2016) An interprofessional approach to reducing the risk of falls through enhanced collaborative practice. J Am Geriatr Soc 64(8):1701–1707. https://doi.org/10.1111/jgs.14178

Fawcett J (2013) Thoughts about multidisciplinary, interdisciplinary, and transdisciplinary research. Nurs Sci Q 26(4):376–379. https://doi.org/10.1177/0894318413500408

Fawcett J (2014) Thoughts about collaboration - Or is it capitulation? Nurs Sci Q 27(3):260–261. https://doi.org/10.1177/0894318414534493

Fiore SM (2008) Interdisciplinarity as teamwork. Small Group Res 39(3):251–277. https://doi.org/10.1177/1046496408317797

Frenk J, Chen L, Bhutta ZA, Cohen J, Crisp N, Evans T, Zurayk H (2010) Health professionals for a new century: transforming education to strengthen health systems in an interdependent world. Lancet 376(9756):1923–1958. https://doi.org/10.1016/S0140-6736(10)61854-5

Gale NK, Shapiro J, McLeod HST, Redwood S, Hewison A (2014) Patients-people-place: developing a framework for researching organizational culture during health service redesign and change. Implement Sci 9:106

Goethals GR (1986) Social comparison theory. Personal Soc Psychol Bull 12(3):261–278. https://doi.org/10.1177/0146167286123001

Grochtdreis T, Brettschneider C, Wegener A, Watzke B, Riedel-Heller S, Härter M, König HH (2015) Cost-effectiveness of collaborative care for the treatment of depressive disorders in primary care: a systematic review. PLoS One 10(5):e0123078

Hajat C, Stein E (2018) The global burden of multiple chronic conditions: a narrative review. Prev Med Rep 12:284–293. https://doi.org/10.1016/j.pmedr.2018.10.008

Hawkins R, Silvester JA, Passiment M, Riordan L, Weiss KB for the National Collaborative for Improving the Clinical Learning Environment IP-CLE Planning Group. (2018). Envisioning the optimal interprofessional clinical learning environment: Initial findings from an October 2017 NCICLE symposium. https://ncicle.org/interprofessional-cle. Accessed 23 Feb 2021

Health Professions Accreditors Collaborative (2019) Guidance on developing quality interprofessional education for the health professions. Chicago, IL. https://healthprofessionsaccreditors.org/wp-content/uploads/2019/02/HPACGuidance02-01-19.pdf. Accessed 10 Aug 2020

Hewitt G, Sims S, Harris R. (2014) Using realist synthesis to understand the mechanisms of interprofessional teamwork in health and social care. J Interprof Care 28(6):501–506

Hogg MA, Terry DJ (2000) Social identity and self-categorization processes in organizational contexts. Acad Manag Rev 25(10):123–140

Holmboe ES, Foster TC, Ogrinc G (2016) Co-creating quality in health care through learning and dissemination. J Contin Educ Heal Prof 36:S16–S18. https://doi.org/10.1097/CEH.0000000000000076

Hughes AM, Gregory ME, Joseph DL, Sonesh SC, Marlow SL, Lacerenza CN, Salas E (2016) Saving lives: a meta-analysis of team training in healthcare. J Appl Psychol 101(9):1266–1304. https://doi.org/10.1037/apl0000120

Illingworth P, Chelvanayagam S (2017) The benefits of interprofessional education 10 years on. Br J Nurs 26(14):813–818. https://doi.org/10.12968/bjon.2017.26.14.813

Institute of Medicine (1972) Educating for the health team. National Academies Press, Washington

Institute of Medicine (2001) Crossing the quality Chasm: a new health system for the 21st century. National Academies Press, Washington

Institute of Medicine (IOM) (2003) Health professions education. National Academies Press, Washington, DC. https://doi.org/10.17226/10681

Institute of Medicine (2013) Best care at lower cost: the path to continuously learning health care in America. National Academies Press. Washington

Institute of Medicine (IOM) (2015) Measuring the impact of interprofessional education on collaborative practice and patient outcomes. National Academies Press, Washington, DC

Interprofessional Education Collaborative (IPEC) (2016) Core competencies for interprofessional collaborative practice: 2016 update. https://aamc-meded.global.ssl.fastly.net/production/media/filer_public/70/9f/709fedd7-3c53-492c-b9f0-b13715d11cb6/core_competencies_for_collaborative_practice.pdf. Accessed 10 Aug 2020

Khalili H, Orchard C, Laschinger HKS, Farah R (2013) An interprofessional socialization framework for developing an interprofessional identity among health professions students. J Interprof Care 27(6):448–453. https://doi.org/10.3109/13561820.2013.804042

Lipsitz LA (2012) Understanding health care as a complex system. JAMA 308:243–244. https:// doi.org/10.1001/jama.2012.7551

McEwan D, Ruissen GR, Eys MA, Zumbo BD, Beauchamp MR (2017) The effectiveness of teamwork training on teamwork behaviors and team performance: a systematic review and meta-analysis of controlled interventions. PLoS One 12(1):e0169604. https://doi.org/10.1371/journal.pone.0169604

Mcgrath JE, Argote L (2001) Group processes in organizational contexts. In: Blackwell handbook of social psychology: group processes. Wiley Blackwell, Hoboken, pp 603–627. https://doi.org/10.1002/9780470998458.ch25

Miller CJ, Kim B, Silverman A, Bauer MS (2018) A systematic review of team-building interventions in non-acute healthcare settings. BMC Health Serv Res 18(1):146. https://doi.org/10.1186/s12913-018-2961-9

Mitchell PH, Ferketich S, Jennings BM (1998) Quality health outcomes model. Image J Nurs Scholar 30(1):43–46. https://doi.org/10.1111/j.1547-5069.1998.tb01234.x

Muntingh AD, van der Feltz-Cornelis CM, van Marwijk HW, Spinhoven P, van Balkom AJ (2016) Collaborative care for anxiety disorders in primary care: a systematic review and meta-analysis. BMC Fam Pract 17:62

Nadler D, Tushman M (1980) A model for diagnosing organizational behavior. Organ Dyn 9(2):35–51. https://doi.org/10.1016/0090-2616(80)90039-X

National Academies of Sciences, Engineering and Medicine (2017) Exploring a Business Case for High-Value Continuing Professional Development: Proceedings of a Workshop. Washington, DC: National Academies of Sciences, Engineering and Medicine; https://doi.org/10.17226/24911

National Acadamy of Medicine (NAM) (2019) Taking action against clinician burnout. National Academies Press, Washington. https://doi.org/10.17226/25521

National Academy of Medicine (2013) Interprofessional education for collaboration. National Academies Press, Washington. https://doi.org/10.17226/13486

National Collaborative for Improving the Clinical Learning Environment (NCICLE) (2020) About us. https://www.ncicle.org/about-us. Accessed 20 Aug 2020

Neily J, Mills PD, Young-Xu Y, Carney BT, West P, Berger DH, Bagian JP (2010) Association between implementation of a medical team training program and surgical mortality. JAMA 304(15):1693–1700. https://doi.org/10.1001/jama.2010.1506

Oandasan I, Reeves S (2005) Key elements of interprofessional education. Part 2. Factors, processes and outcomes. J Interprof Care 19(Sup 1):39–48. https://doi.org/10.1080/13561820500081703

Pawson R (2006) Evidence-based policy: a realist perspective. Sage, New York

Pawson R, Greenhalgh T, Harvey G, Walshe K (2005) Realist review—a new method of systematic review designed for complex policy interventions. J Health Service Res Policy 10(Suppl 1):21–34. https://doi.org/10.1258/1355819054308530

Perlo J, Balik B, Swensen S, Kabcenell A, Landsman J, Feeley D (2017) Institute for Healthcare Improvement: IHI Framework for Improving Joy in Work. http://www.ihi.org/resources/Pages/IHIWhitePapers/Framework-Improving-Joy-in-Work.aspx?utm_campaign=tw&utm_source=hs_email&utm_medium=email&utm_content=55030673&_hsenc=p2ANqtz-81WYx9owYr8B3iIcLYPLq2qX5nWyLRxULW6tkQGKso3L4ejG70rSzitCWJNGE5kZ3WOzIkkftXZfB9f. Accessed 15 Oct 2017

Poole MS, Hollingshead AB, McGrath JE, Moreland RL, Rohrbaugh J (2004) Interdisciplinary perspectives on small groups. Small Group Res 35(1):3–16. https://doi.org/10.1177/1046496403259753

Reeves S, Perrier L, Goldman J, Freeth D, Zwarenstein M (2013) Interprofessional education: effects on professional practice and healthcare outcomes (update). Cochrane Database Syst Rev 3:CD002213. https://doi.org/10.1002/14651858.CD002213.pub3

Reeves S, Pelone F, Harrison R, Goldman J, Zwarenstein M (2017) Interprofessional collaboration to improve professional practice and healthcare outcomes. Cochrane Database Syst Rev 6(6):CD000072. https://doi.org/10.1002/14651858.CD000072.pub3

Rosen MA, DiazGranados D, Dietz AS, Benishek LE, Thompson D, Pronovost PJ, Weaver SJ (2018) Teamwork in healthcare: key discoveries enabling safer, high-quality care. Am Psychol 73(4):433–450. https://doi.org/10.1037/amp0000298

Rycroft-Malone J, McCormack B, Hutchinson AM, DeCorby K, Bucknall TK, Kent B, Schultz A, Snelgrove-Clarke E, Stetler CB, Titler M, Wallin L, Wilson V (2012) Realist synthesis: illustrating the method for implementation research. Implement Sci 7:33

Schneider B, Ehrhart MG, Macey WH (2013) Organizational climate and culture. Annu Rev Psychol 64:361–388

Snow RE (1989) Toward Assessment of Cognitive and Conative Structures in Learning. Educ Res 18(9):8–14. https://doi.org/10.3102/0013189X018009008

Tajfel H (1982) Social Psychology of Intergroup Relations. Annu Rev Psychol 33(1):1–39. https://doi.org/10.1146/annurev.ps.33.020182.000245

Tittle CK (1994) Toward an educational psychology of assessment for teaching and learning: theories, contexts, and validation arguments. Educ Psychol 29(3):149–162. https://doi.org/10.1207/s15326985ep2903_4

Thota AB, Sipe TA, Byard GJ, Zometa CS, Hahn RA, McKnight-Eily LR, Chapman DP, Abraido-Lanza AF, Pearson JL, Anderson CW, Gelenberg AJ, Hennesy KD et al. (2012) Collaborative care to improve the management of depressive disorders: a community guide systematic review and meta-analysis. Am J Prev Med 42(5):525–538

Van Swol LM, Kane AA (2019) Language and group processes: an integrative, interdisciplinary review. Small Group Res 50(1):3–38. https://doi.org/10.1177/1046496418785019

World Health Organization (2010) Framework for action on interprofessional education. https://apps.who.int/iris/bitstream/handle/10665/70185/WHO_HRH_HPN_10.3_eng.pdf;jsessionid=FE268197110070DA9A1A2982DEA9316C?sequence=1. Accessed 10 Aug 2020

Yao N, Zhu X, Dow A, Mishra VK, Phillips A, Tu SP (2018) An exploratory study of networks constructed using access data from an electronic health record. J Interprof Care 32(6):666–673. https://doi.org/10.1080/13561820.2018.1496902

Zorek J, Raehl C (2013) Interprofessional education accreditation standards in the USA: a comparative analysis. J Interprof Care 27(2):123–130. https://doi.org/10.3109/13561820.2012.718295

Zwarenstein M, Treweek S (2009) What kind of randomised trials do patients and clinicians need? Evid Based Med 14(4):101–103

Care Coordination

Beth Ann Swan

Introduction

Definitions of care coordination have proliferated over the last decade. The most recent definition from the National Quality Forum's (NQF) Care Coordination Endorsement Maintenance Project 2016–2017 is "a multidimensional concept that includes effective communication among healthcare providers, patients, families, caregivers (regarding chronic conditions); safe care transitions; a longitudinal view of care that considers the past, while monitoring present delivery of care and anticipating future needs; and the facilitation of linkages between communities and the healthcare system to address medical, social, educational and other support needs that align with patient goals" (National Quality Forum 2017, paragraph 1). Earlier definitions from NQF and the Agency for Healthcare Research and Quality (AHRQ) are given in Table 11.1 to provide a historical perspective. The definition of care coordination evolved to include the purposeful nature of the intervention, requirement for two or more participants, and most importantly the need for organization and harmonization of activities.

In the United States, 60% of adults have a chronic illness, and four in ten adults have two or more chronic illnesses (see Chap. 8). Chronic diseases are the leading causes of death and disability and leading drivers of the nation's $3.3 trillion in annual healthcare costs (National Center for Chronic Disease Prevention and Health Promotion 2019). With such a large population of chronically ill, the need for improved care is evident. For individuals and families, the lack of coordination leads to fragmented, inconsistent, and poorly planned care. Medical errors, duplication of tests, and paper shuffling can occur, with results ranging from inconvenient to life-threatening. The lack of coordinating care can also lead to unnecessary emergency room visits and hospitalizations, avoidable readmissions, and excessive resource use. Conversely, effective care coordination supports achieving the

B. A. Swan (✉)
Nell Hodgson Woodruff School of Nursing, Emory University, Atlanta, GA, USA

© Springer Nature Switzerland AG 2021   193
M. Baernholdt, D. K. Boyle (eds.), *Nurses Contributions to Quality Health Outcomes*, https://doi.org/10.1007/978-3-030-69063-2_11

Table 11.1 Definitions of care coordination

National organization	Definition
National Quality Forum (NQF 2010, p. 2)	"Care coordination is defined as an information-rich, patient-centric endeavor that seeks to deliver the right care (and only the right care) to the right patient at the right time ... A function that helps ensure that the patient's needs and preferences for health services and information sharing across people, functions and sites are met over time ... Care coordination maximizes the value of services delivered to patients by facilitating beneficial efficient, safe and high-quality patient experiences and improved health care outcomes"
Agency for Healthcare Research and Quality (AHRQ 2014, Paragraph 1)	"Care coordination is the deliberate organization of patient care activities between two or more participants (including the patient) involved in a patient's care to facilitate the appropriate delivery of health care services. Organizing care involves the marshaling of personnel and other resources needed to carry out all required patient care activities and is often managed by exchanging information among participants responsible for different aspects of care."
National Quality Forum (NQF 2017, Paragraph 1)	Care coordination is: "... the deliberate synchronization of activities and information to improve health outcomes by ensuring that care recipients' and families' needs and preferences for healthcare and community services are met over time."

quadruple aim, improving the care experience for individuals, improving individual health, reducing costs, and improving healthcare providers' work-life (Bodenheimer and Sinsky 2014). Examining care coordination as an intervention is an essential first step in understanding all the activities/components that contribute to delivering quality and safe person-centered and system-level outcomes.

Care Coordination: Linkages to the QHOM

Care coordination is embedded in all components of the QHOM (Mitchell et al. 1998) with multidirectional relationships whereby nursing care coordination interventions act through client and system characteristics to improve health outcomes. Additionally, client and system interactions affect health outcomes. This chapter examines the characteristics of care coordination related to individuals, providers, and organizational perspectives and describes the multifocal relationships among these perspectives and nursing interventions and care coordination outcomes as depicted in Fig. 11.1.

System Characteristics of Care Coordination

Although the chapter focus is care coordination as an intervention, it is essential to explore this (a) in the context of the structure of care coordination, (b) from the clinician and organizational perspectives, and (c) to be cognizant that locations of care coordination by RNs include programs in primary care, acute care, ambulatory

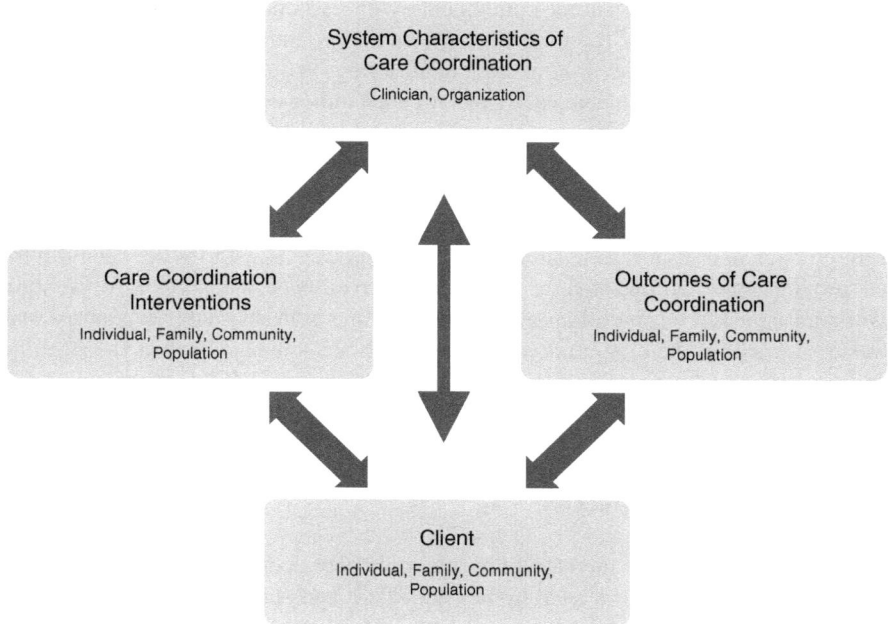

Fig. 11.1 Framework for care coordination

care, and home care; programs based in telehealth; and programs with remote monitoring (Conway et al. 2019).

Clinician Perspective

Care coordination requires a team to support the complex care and social support needs of individuals with chronic illnesses as they are typically high users of health, community, and social services (Heslop et al. 2014). While acknowledging care coordination is a part of the role for many healthcare professionals, this chapter focuses on the role of RNs in care coordination. Registered nurses are ideally positioned to be the point of accountability whether they are employed as care coordinators, in specific care coordinator roles, or whether they coordinate care in their everyday RN role.

The structural component of care coordination is found in the evidence-based dimensions and competencies of Care Coordination and Transition Management (CCTM) provided by RNs and includes (1) support for self-management, (2) education and engagement of individuals and families, (3) coaching and counseling of individuals and families, (4) advocacy, (5) population health management, (6) teamwork and collaboration, (7) cross-setting communication and transition, (8) person-centered care planning, and (9) nursing process (Haas et al. 2013). A logic model was developed to identify structural components with associated activities, processes, and outcomes in each of the nine Care Coordination and Transition Management dimensions. A logic model linking these relationships is depicted in Fig. 11.2.

The logic model has selected activities for each dimension listed, as well as specified outcomes. The logic model allows for RN contributions to be recognized and provides an estimate of RN value in care coordination and transition management, related to processes and outcomes of care (Haas and Swan 2014). These competencies relate to RNs in all settings across the healthcare continuum. They guide acute care practice and discharge teaching and planning, care transitions between different providers and settings of care, provision of surveillance, and support for persons with multiple chronic conditions as they live at home or in assisted living, or receive home care within the community, and cope with self-management of their health and healthcare (Swan et al. 2019). Consistent with the QHOM, these structural components link with interventions and resulting outcomes of care coordination.

Organizational Perspective

Healthcare systems have increased investment in care coordination service models such as patient-centered medical homes (PCMHs) and accountable care organizations (ACOs). Four examples of investment in care coordination services are the Serious Illness Care Program (Lakin et al. 2017), the Comprehensive Primary Care Initiative developed by the Centers for Medicare & Medicaid Services (CMS) (Peikes et al. 2018), a funded CMS innovation grant called COMPASS (Care of Mental, Physical, and Substance-Use Syndromes) (Katon and Unutzer 2006; Katon et al. 2005), and the Veterans Health Administration's Patient Aligned Care Teams (PACTs) providing interprofessional care coordination in primary care (Zulman et al. 2017). These programs are described in Table 11.2; however, the programs' common system characteristics are defined as care management, customized longitudinal care plans, and care coordination with other providers.

Client

From the individual and family perspective, people bring predisposing characteristics such as demographics, social structure, health beliefs, psychological characteristics, personal and family resources, individual's ability to access care, individual's self-perceived illness severity, and person-perceived need for care coordination (Vanderboom et al. 2017). Individuals needing care coordination may have multiple complex physical and social problems that are challenging to manage. The need for coordination is not defined by the number of diagnoses but by the complexity of health problems, the complexity of social situations, and the complexity manifested by frequent use of healthcare services (Vanderboom et al. 2015). Examples of challenges that exacerbate these complexities include (1) limited support from family and friends, limited social support, (2) limited financial resources, and (3) diverse language and cultural attributes (Vanderboom et al. 2015).

Program: The CCTM RN Model Logic Model

Situation: The Care Coordination Transition Management - Registered Nurse Model (CCTM RN) evolved to standardize work of all registered nurses using evidence from nursing and interprofessional literature on care coordination and transition management. The CCTM-RN Model specifies dimensions of CCTM and associated competencies - knowledge, skills, and attitudes - essential for the CCTM RN to meet the needs of individuals and families across the continuum of care. The preparation and work as an CCTM RN is recognized by a certification credential from the Medical Surgical Nursing Certification Board (MSNCB).

Inputs/Competencies	Outputs — Activities	Outputs — Participation	Outcomes — Short	Outcomes — Medium	Outcomes — Long
Support for Self Management	Enhance health literacy	CCTM RN, MD, APRN, Pharmacist, social worker	Baseline comprehensive needs assessment reflects individual values, preferences, goals	Solutions to most critical socioeconomic issues	Engaged, educated individual/family, increased ability to "cope" with care interventions
Advocacy	Negotiate & secure individual services; Coach person in self advocacy	CCTM RN, MD, APRN, Pharmacist, social worker	Individual/family concerns and goals heard, able to access providers, community services, medications	Individual/family compliance with treatment plan, medications	Keep primary care appointments, appointments in community agencies
Education and Engagement of Individual and Family	Assess readiness to learn/learning styles	CCTM RN, Pharmacist, social worker, dietician, psychologist	Individual/family can "teach back" info on care interventions	Increased engagement in preventative care and use of telehealth learning modalities	Engaged, educated individual/family
Cross Setting Communication and Transition	Coordination/collaboration between specialty and primary providers who develop and share the Individual Care Plan across settings	CCTM RN, MD, APRN, Pharmacist, social worker, dietician, psychologist, MD specialists, acute care, long-term care and home care RNs	Care Plan transmitted between setting, changes & updates communicated	Use of electronic Individual Care Plan for handoffs	Decreased errors, duplication, decreased costs
Coaching and Counseling of Individuals and Families	Answer questions individuals/families have before & after seeing provider visit	CCTM RN	Individuals/families come prepared with "Ask Me Three" questions to clinic or calls	Enhanced understanding of health care resources in the community and need to seek consultation prior to increased severity	Decreased ED use, increased ability to "cope" with care interventions
Nursing Process	Assess individual for knowledge understanding dx, needs, treatment, expected outcomes of treatment	CCTM RN	Best evidence used for interventions/outcomes; care plan is routinely updated	Electronic process indicators show compliance with EBP plan, short term EBP outcomes achieved	Long term EBP disease or health outcomes achieved at 80% level
Population Health Management	Expert use of population management tools (e.g. registries, analytics tools) to track and monitor select population characteristics	CCTM RN, MD, APRN, Pharmacist, social worker, dietician, MA, psychologist, MD specialists, acute care, long-term care and home care RNs	Maximize impact of visit or telehealth call regarding disease management, prevention & wellness through alerts	Enhanced process improvement; enhanced immunization rates, participation in wellness programming	Enhanced quality of care, achievement of benchmarks for prevention and wellness
Team Work and Collaboration	Inclusion of teamwork in orientation and continuing education	CCTM RN, MD, APRN, Pharmacist, social worker, dietician, MA, psychologist, MD specialists, acute care, long-term care and home care RNs	Enhanced understanding of interprofessional roles; communication techniques	Early collaboration when issue arises, team problem solving/planning	Less siloed care; engaged health care team; increased appreciation of team member contributions
Person-Centered Care Planning	Motivational interviewing; eliciting individual's goals and priorities	CCTM RN, MD, APRN, Pharmacist, social worker, dietician, MA, psychologist, MD specialists, acute care, long-term care and home care RNs	Individualized Care Plan; care planning activities transcend barriers/ transitions keeping the individual at the focus	Plan of care transparent for individual/family & perceive team is listening to their preferences/goals	Enhanced individual/family engagement & satisfaction with quality of care

Assumptions : Individuals will seek care across the continuum of care, individuals will access CCTM RN providers, individuals will be engaged in care processes. Providers will collaborate, work in teams, develop and use person-centered care plans. Organization will have EHR that operates across settings. Outcomes are shared by team, not discipline specific.

External Factors Slow development of interprofessional team education and practice; changes in reimbursement to value-based purchasing, slow implementation of EHRs that are operable across settings, and slow development of longitudinal plan of care that moves with individual between settings.

Fig. 11.2 Logic model for care coordination. Source: © 2018 by S. Haas & B.A. Swan. Reprinted with permission from Swan, B.A., Haas, S.A., Haynes, T.S., & Murray. (2019). Introduction. In S.A. Haas, B.A. Swan, & T.S. Haynes (Eds.), *Care coordination and transition management core curriculum* (pp. 14–16). American Academy of Ambulatory Care Nursing

Table 11.2 Organizational care coordination models and associated interventions and outcomes

Model	Interventions	Outcomes
Serious Illness Care Program (Lakin et al. 2017)	Integrated care management program coordinating care for chronically ill, medically complex individuals in primary care practices Focused on conversation and communication with individuals about their goals and values related to end-of-life care Nurse care coordinator-created customized care plan	Increase in communication and documentation in the EHR's advanced care planning module More comprehensive conversations covering more elements related to goals and values
COMPASS (Beck et al. 2018; Coleman et al. 2017; Rossom et al. 2017)	Defined care management process with a care team of at least one care manager, physician consultant, and psychiatrist Use of care management tracking system Monitoring of hospital and emergency department use	Reduces unnecessary hospital use and cost Reduces unnecessary emergency department use and cost Patient and provider satisfaction Patient Health Questionnaire (PHQ) less than 5 Systolic blood pressure less than 140, diastolic blood pressure less than 90 Hemoglobin A1c less than 8
PACTs (Zulman et al. 2017)	Interprofessional care team with four core members Comprehensive patient assessment Tracking of patient's health-related goals, priorities, and self-care challenges Assessment of physical function, cognitive impairment, social support, advance directives, medication adherence, and level of activation Frequent telephone contact Weekly team discussions of high-acuity patients Coordination of care with VA and non-VA providers	Satisfaction with model and each member of the care team Improved patient engagement Improved satisfaction with VA care Improved communication Improved activation levels
Comprehensive Primary Care Initiative (Peikes et al. 2018)	Enhanced access to and continuity of care Planned care for chronic conditions and preventive care Risk-stratified care management Patient and caregiver engagement Coordination of care with patients' other providers	Improved risk-stratified care management Improved access to appointments Improved access after-hours Improved care coordination after hospitalizations and emergency department visits

Effective care coordination by RNs occurs with different populations in a variety of settings. Populations include adults with diabetes; adults with dementia; adults with a terminal illness; children with special care needs; adults poststroke; adults with chronic obstructive pulmonary disease; adults with heart failure; disabled individuals with functional impairments; older adults in skilled nursing facilities; adults with chronic and complex illness and social needs; individuals with mental and physical health conditions; people living with cancer; persons at the end of life; older adults with multiple health, social, and nonmedical needs; and veterans (Breckenridge et al. 2019; Huitema et al. 2018; Kuo et al. 2018; Lee et al. 2018; Rentas et al. 2019; Rossom et al. 2017; Ruiz et al. 2017; Talley et al. 2018; Zulman et al. 2017).

Care Coordination Interventions

Care coordination is an effective intervention when working with various populations in many different settings, as described above. In the QHOM, RN care coordination can be a direct or indirect clinical process. For instance, a direct process would occur during a care visit, such as self-management education or teaching coping skills. An indirect clinical process would happen outside the care visit, such as telephone management of high-risk older adults at risk for hospitalization or facilitated communication between individual, family, and clinicians. Indirect care coordination focuses on activities such as administration, consultation, planning, and service development.

RN Clinical Processes: Direct Interventions

As a direct intervention, care coordination is delivered through a variety of activities. A systematic review of the nurse care coordinator role identified a range of in-person care coordination activities. These include developing plans of care, educating about disease and self-management using behavior change and health coaching principles, managing medications, performing comprehensive assessments, evidence-based care planning, and coaching for self-management (Conway et al. 2019).

Population care coordination utilizes principles from care coordination, case management, and population health to maximize health outcomes and resource utilization for populations and the individuals within them (Rushton 2015). There are many population-focused models using care coordination activities as an intervention. Two populations requiring ongoing, complex coordination are older adults and individuals living with cancer.

Care coordination for older adults is required in a variety of settings, including primary care and the community. Direct interventions in these models include assessing individual needs and goals; building and maintaining relationships; creating a plan of care; providing self-management support; providing transition management; linking individuals to community resources; coordinating medications; monitoring physical signs and symptoms; managing durable medical equipment; monitoring laboratory findings; communicating with primary care providers, pharmacists, caregivers, and community agencies; finding financial and community resources; and addressing complex physical, mental, social, and cultural needs (Kim et al. 2016; Scholz and Minaudo 2015; Vanderboom et al. 2015, 2017).

Complex cancer survivors require highly coordinated care to ensure optimal outcomes for their cancers, coexisting chronic conditions, and overall quality of life. Followed by oncologists with little or no care coordination with primary care providers, care is fragmented and providers are siloed, with suboptimal care quality (Lee et al. 2018). Care coordination interventions include both direct and indirect activities such as using an electronic health record-driven registry to facilitate individual's transitions between primary care and oncology care; co-locating an RN within a complex care team providing clinical care coordination, continuity, and transition management, and assisting individual self-management; registry review; and enhancing teamwork through coaching (Lee et al. 2018).

At the start of cancer treatment, individuals have an in-person meeting with the RN. During treatment, the RN tracks individuals to ascertain completion of initial cancer treatment, coordinates appointments and lab tests between primary care and specialty clinics weekly, and makes appointments with the social worker. At the end of the treatment, the RN provides treatment summary and follow-up guidelines, encourages interaction with primary care, recommends a transition to the care team posttreatment, tracks appointment results via the registry, synthesizes health and cancer history, educates on follow-up for cancer recurrence, educates on self-management for chronic diseases, educates on long-term effects of cancer treatment, and coordinates specialty care referrals including smoking cessation, health behaviors, and psychosocial counseling (Lee et al. 2018).

Additional population-based models requiring similar direct RN care coordination interventions include children with asthma (Garwick et al. 2015), individuals with pneumonia (Seldon et al. 2016), individuals living with diabetes (Talley et al. 2018), and individuals at the end of life (Ruiz et al. 2017). Successful care coordination not only requires direct interventions; indirect activities are just as critical.

RN Clinical Processes: Indirect Interventions

A systematic review of the nurse care coordinator role identified a range of indirect care coordination activities including arranging consultations with healthcare providers, arranging consultations with community service providers, monitoring medication adherence, collaborating with providers, educating about communicating with members of the healthcare team, ongoing contact with the individual over time, addressing transitions in care, identifying an action plan for situations of clinical deterioration, providing home-based case management, liaising with other providers and settings, providing case management services, supporting clinical visits with home telephone support, monitoring proactively, supporting caregivers, accessing community-based services, and providing navigator activities (Conway et al. 2019).

Outcomes of Care Coordination

Care coordination is a crucial strategy for addressing complex health and social issues and improving quality outcomes and performance measures. Care coordination models have been developed, recognizing that coordinating care for individuals with chronic conditions and complex healthcare needs requires new ways to provide care. Care coordination is intended to prevent costly consequences of poor management and improve short- and long-term quality for individuals, families, communities, and populations. The body of evidence linking care coordination to important quality outcomes is described below.

Person-centered outcomes resulting from care coordination as an intervention include quality of life, decreased symptom severity both physical and mental (depression, cognition), greater symptom control, concerns and problems, self-efficacy, knowledge about disease and self-management, continuity of care, treatment adherence, individual satisfaction with care, family satisfaction with care, and morbidity (Conway et al. 2019).

Organizational or system-centered outcomes resulting from care coordination as an intervention include decreased preventable hospitalizations and rehospitalization; resource use during hospitalization; length of stay; and inappropriate use of the following services: emergency department, outpatient clinic, home visit, hospice, physician visits, community service, physical therapy, occupational therapy, and rehabilitation. Further, care coordination can improve the number of patients receiving appropriate care, who have no treatment delays, and who go for follow-up appointments. Finally, organizations' throughput, costs, clinician satisfaction, and understanding of the care coordination role can all improve with care coordination (Conway et al. 2019).

Outcome Measures for RN Care Coordination

While the above quality outcomes are important, the creation of quality outcomes and performance measures that uniquely appraise the contribution of RNs to care coordination is critical. There is growing work by Start et al. (2018) in collaboration with Collaborative Alliance for Nursing Outcomes (CALNOC) that has led to developing outcome metrics for nine care coordination and transition management RN dimensions displayed in Table 11.3.

When implemented, these metrics will provide the data to track the outcomes of RN care coordination. Data will be even more robust when RN care coordination interventions are coded in SNOMED CT and tracked and linked to the outcomes

Table 11.3 Care coordination and transition management dimensions and validated outcome measures

Dimensions	Outcome measures
Support for self-management	1. Pain
Education and engagement of patient and family	2. HTN
	3. Community falls
Cross-setting communication and transition	4. BMI
Coaching and counseling of patients and family	5. Depression
	6. DM HCG A 1 C Rates and Targets Achieved (prioritized)
Nursing process: assessment, plan, intervention, evaluation	7. Opioid misuse
	8. Advanced planning
Teamwork and collaboration	9. Comprehensive DM/HgH1c
Patient-centered planning	Process:
Population health management	10. Risk assessment and follow-up plans
Advocacy	11. Interprofessional team engagement
	12. Reassessment
	Outcomes:
	13. Admission
	14. Readmission

Source: © 2019 by D. Brown & R. Start. Reprinted with permission from Austin, R., Mercier, N., Kennedy, R., Bouyer-Ferullo, S., Start, R., & Storer-Brown, D. (2019). Informatics competencies to support nursing practice. In S.A. Haas, B.A. Swan, & T.S. Haynes (Eds.), *Care coordination and transition management core curriculum* (p. 274). American Academy of Ambulatory Care Nursing

achieved. Two articles discuss how to discover value in the care coordination work of RNs across the care continuum and track the impact of care coordination done by other members of the interprofessional team (Haas and Swan 2014; Haas et al. 2016).

Summary

The QHOM provides a framework to describe and discuss the structural characteristics, interventions, and outcomes of nursing care coordination in the context of client—individual, family, community, and population. This chapter examined system characteristics of care coordination related to clinicians and organizational perspectives and described the multifocal relationships among these perspectives and nursing interventions and care coordination outcomes. RNs are increasingly looked to for leadership in the transformation of healthcare. Leveraging the RN role in care coordination is a strategy aimed at increasing the value for individuals, families, communities, and populations across the care continuum. It requires a commitment from nursing to lead and facilitate performance improvement that focuses on quality and safety and enhanced care delivery.

References

Agency for Healthcare Research and Quality (2014) What is care coordination? In: Care coordination measures atlas update. AHRQ, Rockville, MD. https://www.ahrq.gov/ncepcr/care/coordination/atlas/chapter2.html

Beck A, Boggs JM, Alem A, Coleman KJ, Rossom RC, Neely C, Solberg LI (2018) Large-scale implementation of collaborative care management for depression and diabetes and/or cardiovascular disease. J Am Board Fam Med 31(5):702–711. https://doi.org/10.3122/jabfm.2018.05.170102

Bodenheimer T, Sinsky C (2014) From triple to quadruple aim: care of the patient requires care of the provider. Ann Fam Med 12(6):573–576. https://doi.org/10.1370/afm.1713

Breckenridge ED, Kite B, Wells R, Sunbury TM (2019) Effect of patient care coordination on hospital encounters and related costs. Populat Health Manag 22:406–414. https://doi.org/10.1089/pop.2018.0176

Coleman KJ, Magnan S, Neely C, Solberg L, Beck A, Trevis J, Williams S (2017) The COMPASS initiative: description of a nationwide collaborative approach to the care of patients with depression and diabetes and/or cardiovascular disease. Gen Hosp Psychiatry 44:69–76

Conway A, O'Donnell C, Yates P (2019) The effectiveness of the nurse care coordinator role on patient-reported and health service outcomes: a systematic review. Evaluat Health Profess 42:263–296. https://doi.org/10.1177/0163278717734610

Garwick AW, Svavarsdottir EK, Seppelt AM, Looman WS, Anderson LS, Orlygsdottir B (2015) Development of an international school nurse asthma care coordination model. J Adv Nurs 71(3):535–546. https://doi.org/10.1111/jan.12522

Haas S, Swan BA (2014) Developing the value proposition for the role of the registered nurse in care coordination and transition management in ambulatory care settings. Nurs Econ 32:70–79

Haas S, Swan BA, Haynes T (2013) Developing ambulatory care registered nurse competencies for care coordination and transition management. Nurs Econ 31(1):44–47

Haas SA, Vlasses F, Havey J (2016) Developing staffing models to support population health management and quality outcomes in ambulatory care settings. Nurs Econ 34(3):126–133

Heslop L, Power R, Cranwell K (2014) Building workforce capacity for complex care coordination: a function analysis of workflow activity. Hum Resour Health 12:52-4491-12-52. https://doi.org/10.1186/1478-4491-12-52

Huitema AA, Harkness K, Heckman GA, McKelvie RS (2018) The spoke-hub-and-node model of integrated heart failure care. Canadian J Cardiol 34(7):863–870

Katon W, Unutzer J (2006) Collaborative care models for depression: time to move from evidence to practice. Arch Intern Med 166(21):2304–2306. https://doi.org/10.1001/archinte.166.21.2304

Katon WJ, Schoenbaum M, Fan MY, Callahan CM, Williams J Jr, Hunkeler E, Unutzer J (2005) Cost-effectiveness of improving primary care treatment of late-life depression. Arch Gen Psychiatry 62(12):1313–1320. https://doi.org/10.1001/archpsyc.62.12.1313

Kim TY, Marek KD, Coenen A (2016) Identifying care coordination interventions provided to community-dwelling older adults using electronic health records. Comput Informat Nurs CIN 34(7):303–311. https://doi.org/10.1097/CIN.0000000000000232

Kuo DZ, McAllister JW, Rossignol L, Turchi RM, Stille CJ (2018) Care coordination for children with medical complexity: whose care is it, anyway? Pediatrics 141(Suppl 3):S224–S232. https://doi.org/10.1542/peds.2017-1284G

Lakin JR, Koritsanszky LA, Cunningham R, Maloney FL, Neal BJ, Paladino J, Bernacki RE (2017) A systematic intervention to improve serious illness communication in primary care. Health Affairs (Project Hope) 36(7):1258–1264. https://doi.org/10.1377/hlthaff.2017.0219

Lee SJC, Jetelina KK, Marks E, Shaw E, Oeffinger K, Cohen D, Balasubramanian BA (2018) Care coordination for complex cancer survivors in an integrated safety-net system: a study protocol. BMC Cancer 18(1):1204-018-5118-7. https://doi.org/10.1186/s12885-018-5118-7

Mitchell PH, Ferketich S, Jennings BM (1998) Quality Health Outcomes Model. Image J Nurs Sch 30(1):43–46

National Center for Chronic Disease Prevention and Health Promotion (2019) Chronic diseases in America. https://www.cdc.gov/chronicdisease/resources/infographic/chronic-diseases.htm

National Quality Forum (2010) Care coordination. Retrieved from http://www.qualityforum.org/Publications/2010/10/Quality_Connections__Care_Coordination.aspx

National Quality Forum (2017) Care coordination endorsement maintenance project 2016–2017. http://www.qualityforum.org/ProjectDescription.aspx?projectID=83375

Peikes D, Dale S, Ghosh A, Taylor EF, Swankoski K, O'Malley AS, Brown RS (2018) The comprehensive primary care initiative: effects on spending, quality, patients, and physicians. Health Affairs (Project Hope) 37(6):890–899. https://doi.org/10.1377/hlthaff.2017.1678

Rentas KG, Buckley L, Wiest D, Bruno CA (2019) Characteristics and behavioral health needs of patients with patterns of high hospital use: implications for primary care providers. BMC Health Serv Res 19(1):81-019-3894-7. https://doi.org/10.1186/s12913-019-3894-7

Rossom RC, Solberg LI, Magnan S, Crain AL, Beck A, Coleman KJ, Unutzer J (2017) Impact of a national collaborative care initiative for patients with depression and diabetes or cardiovascular disease. Gen Hosp Psychiatry 44:77–85

Ruiz S, Snyder LP, Giuriceo K, Lynn J, Ewald E, Branand B, Bysshe T (2017) Innovative models for high-risk patients use care coordination and palliative supports to reduce end-of-life utilization and spending. Innov Aging 1(2):igx021. https://doi.org/10.1093/geroni/igx021

Rushton S (2015) The population care coordination process. Profess Case Manag 20(5):230–238; quiz 239-40. https://doi.org/10.1097/NCM.0000000000000105

Scholz J, Minaudo J (2015) Registered nurse care coordination: creating a preferred future for older adults with multimorbidity. Online J Issues Nurs 20(3):4

Seldon LE, McDonough K, Turner B, Simmons LA (2016) Evaluation of a hospital-based pneumonia nurse navigator program. J Nurs Adm 46(12):654–661. https://doi.org/10.1097/NNA.0000000000000422

Start R, Matlock AM, Brown D, Aronow H, Soban L (2018) Realizing momentum and synergy: benchmarking meaningful ambulatory care nurse-sensitive indicators. Nurs Econ 36:246–251

Swan BA, Conway-Phillips R, Haas S, De La Pena L (2019) Optimizing strategies for care coordination and transition management: recommendations for nursing education. Nurs Econ 37(2):77–85

Talley MH, Polancich S, Williamson JB, Frank JS, Curry W, Russell JF, Selleck C (2018) Improving population health among uninsured patients with diabetes. Populat Health Manag 21(5):373–377. https://doi.org/10.1089/pop.2017.0170

Vanderboom CE, Thackeray NL, Rhudy LM (2015) Key factors in patient-centered care coordination in ambulatory care: nurse care coordinators' perspectives. Appl Nurs Res ANR 28(1):18–24. https://doi.org/10.1016/j.apnr.2014.03.004

Vanderboom CE, Holland DE, Mandrekar J, Lohse CM, Witwer SG, Hunt VL (2017) Predicting use of nurse care coordination by older adults with chronic conditions. West J Nurs Res 39(7):862–885. https://doi.org/10.1177/0193945916673999

Zulman DM, Pal Chee C, Ezeji-Okoye SC, Shaw JG, Holmes TH, Kahn JS, Asch SM (2017) Effect of an intensive outpatient program to augment primary care for high-need Veterans Affairs patients: a randomized clinical trial. JAMA Intern Med 177(2):166–175. https://doi.org/10.1001/jamainternmed.2016.8021

Part VI
Outcomes

Client and Family Outcomes: Experiences of Care

12

Stefanie Bachnick and Michael Simon

Introduction

Among patient-reported outcomes, patient and family experience of care has become an indicator of quality healthcare delivery (Goodrich and Cornwell 2008). One way of assuring optimal patient and family experiences is through the delivery of person-centered care (PCC), which is "care that is (1) respectful of and responsive to individual patients' preferences, needs, and values and (2) ensuring that patients' values guide all decisions" (Institute of Medicine 2001, p. 49). Although this is a clear definition of PCC, its conceptualization is less clear. There is a proliferation of terms used to describe PCC, such as negotiated and individualized care, patient-centered care, people-centered care, person-focused care, or whole-person-centered care (De Silva 2014). Additionally, PCC and patient satisfaction often are used interchangeably. However, patient satisfaction is an outcome of PCC (Dwamena et al. 2012; McMillan et al. 2013; Rathert et al. 2013) and should not be confused with the multidimensional concept of PCC.

A 2015 Delphi study identified five PCC dimensions: (1) patient as a unique person, (2) patient involvement in care, (3) patient information, (4) clinician-patient communication, and (5) patient empowerment (Zill et al. 2015). Although further dimensions can be added, these five core dimensions are the most consistently described in the literature. This chapter uses the above National Academy of

S. Bachnick (✉)
Department of Public Health, Institute of Nursing Science, University of Basel, Basel, Switzerland
e-mail: stefanie.bachnick@unibas.ch

M. Simon
Department of Public Health, Institute of Nursing Science, University of Basel, Basel, Switzerland

Nursing Research Unit, Inselspital University Hospital, Bern, Switzerland
e-mail: m.simon@unibas.ch

© Springer Nature Switzerland AG 2021
M. Baernholdt, D. K. Boyle (eds.), *Nurses Contributions to Quality Health Outcomes*, https://doi.org/10.1007/978-3-030-69063-2_12

Medicine (NAM) definition of PCC (Institute of Medicine 2001) and the five core dimensions (Zill et al. 2015) while changing the word patient to person to use PCC's newest terminology (National Academies of Sciences 2018).

The concept of PCC can be applied to all settings (e.g., hospitals, nursing homes), service lines (e.g., medical, geriatric, pediatric, or psychiatric), and stages of care provision (e.g., admission, discharge). Patients with different diseases and various healthcare settings benefit from PCC, for instance, patients in rehabilitation care (Yun and Choi 2019) and patients with substance-use disorder (Marchand et al. 2019). However, due to PCC's multidimensional nature, its provision is broadly recognized as challenging (De Silva 2014; Luxford et al. 2010). PCC is a crucial intervention to assure that quality care is delivered (Berwick 2009) and should be an essential part of quality improvement strategies. This chapter first links PCC to the QHOM and then discusses PCC interventions at different healthcare system levels. Outcomes impacted by PCC interventions are discussed. Further, client, family, and system characteristics are described. Challenges in measuring PCC are included, followed by implications and future directions.

Person-Centered Care: Linkages with the QHOM

In the QHOM, PCC is an intervention that primarily impacts client and family outcomes, an essential part of delivering healthcare. PCC does not directly impact client and family outcomes but influences outcomes through system characteristics and client and family characteristics (see Fig. 12.1). There are bidirectional relationships between outcomes and client, family, and system characteristics and between these characteristics and the PCC interventions. Thus, continuous feedback loops are in place. Another unique feature is the multilevel dimensions of the QHOM. Through client, family, and system characteristics, PCC will influence not only client and family outcomes at the individual (micro) level, such as clients' health status, but also outcomes at the system (macro) level, such as efficiency, responsiveness, and financial outcomes (National Academies of Sciences 2018).

Person-Centered Care Interventions

PCC interventions can be implemented at different levels of the healthcare system. The World Health Organization (WHO) suggests using micro, meso, and macro levels (World Health Organization 2002). Although each of the levels interacts with one another, each has a distinct definition: micro is the patient or client level, meso is the organization or system level, and macro is the policy or environment level (Serpa and Ferreira 2019). In this section, interventions at the micro and macro levels are discussed. Meso-level system characteristics and interventions are discussed in Chap. 4, including adequate staffing, resources, and leadership.

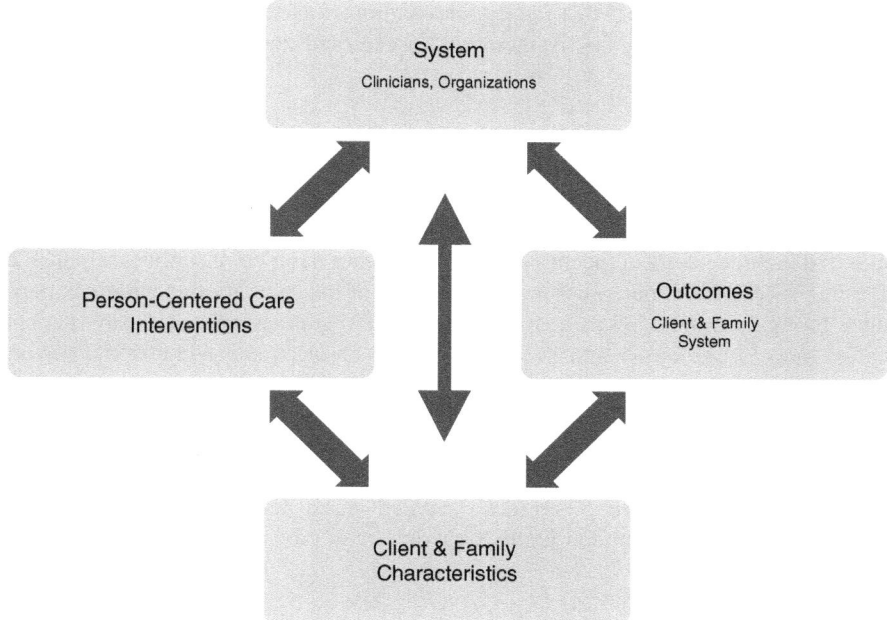

Fig. 12.1 Framework for person-centered care

Micro-level Interventions

Micro-level interventions that focus on the client and family address either a single PCC dimension or multiple dimensions. The multiple dimensions of PCC are mutually dependent. The dimensions *patient involvement in care* (dimension 2), *patient information* (dimension 3), and *clinician-patient communication* (dimension 4) can be viewed separately, but the three dimensions are also interconnected. Clients need information about diagnoses, treatment options, or alternative care processes to be involved in care. The information provides knowledge to be tailored to the clients' care needs. Therefore, *clinician-patient communication* (dimension 4) that acknowledges the value of verbal and nonverbal communication skills plays an important role (Zill et al. 2015). Moreover, the four dimensions together are prerequisites for the PCC dimension, *patient empowerment* (dimension 5), which encourages self-management and self-care (Gerteis et al. 1991; Zill et al. 2015).

A recent review of systematic reviews investigated PCC interventions for clients and families (Park et al. 2018). Twenty-one reviews investigated client interventions; nine interventions targeted family members. The most common interventions for clients were focused on client empowerment, client information, and physical support (Park et al. 2018). Intervention for clients' empowerment targeted clients' motivation to take part in self-care and disease self-management. Other interventions were directed towards clients' knowledge and skill development, such as risk factors and coping skills. Most family interventions focused on providing information and involvement of family members in care and decision-making processes (Park et al. 2018).

Macro-level Interventions

At the macro level, PCC interventions are mainly driven by broader healthcare policies and include payment incentives or penalties. For payment incentives, client and family processes and outcomes are often used. For instance, routine patient experience ratings are included in hospital performance comparisons alongside patient safety rates (see Chaps. 2 and 14 for more detail on incentives and hospital performance). Twenty-five percent of hospitals' total performance scores are based on patient experiences (Medicare.gov. n.d.), which subsequently determines 1.75% of overall hospital payments from the Centers for Medicare & Medicaid Services (Papanicolas et al. 2017). The better the hospital ratings from patients, the more the revenue hospitals receive. Therefore, one can argue that payment policies that include evaluating patient and family experiences of care are PCC interventions at the macro level.

Client and Family Characteristics

Client and family characteristics play a crucial role in PCC provision because they determine how interventions should be tailored to specific populations and, therefore, influence client and family outcomes. Demographic characteristics (e.g., age, gender, educational level) and clinical information (e.g., level of care dependency, type of disease) influence PCC outcomes. Further, both demographic and clinical data shape clients' and families' care preferences and care expectations, which are complex individual characteristics based on clients' and families' beliefs, values, and needs (Bowling and Rowe 2014). However, findings on what characteristics are important are inconclusive. For example, in one study, older patients tend to have fewer unmet expectations than younger patients (Shawa et al. 2017). In another study, Krupat et al. (2001) found that patients who were aged 60 and older, who were male, and who had a high school degree or less experienced less patient-centered care compared to younger, more educated, and female patients (Krupat et al. 2001). Whatever clients' expectations are, though, the more expectations are met, the more positively they rate their experiences with care (Abdel Maqsood et al. 2012; Bowling et al. 2013).

Client and family culture also plays a role. A German cross-sectional study investigated the factors influencing patients' perceptions of person-centered nursing care. Better self-rated health status and educational level of less than 9 years were associated with higher PCC ratings (Koberich et al. 2016). However, in an American secondary data analysis of patient PCC perceptions using the Oncology Patients' Perceptions of the Quality of Nursing Care Scale, there were no associations between gender or age and nursing care ratings. At the same time, a lower educational level was associated with higher PCC ratings in oncology (Radwin 2003). Client characteristics have the potential to influence not only PCC interventions but also system characteristics. For example, patient acuity and care dependency level can influence nurse work environment elements, such as job stress, perceived workload, and care left undone (Wynendaele et al. 2019), which are all part of system characteristics.

System Characteristics

System or organizational characteristics affect how PCC interventions impact client and family outcomes. These characteristics include setting, as well as organizational barriers and facilitators. Healthcare settings (e.g., hospitals, nursing homes) and service lines (e.g., medicine, geriatric, pediatric, psychiatric) contribute to the heterogeneity and complexity of PCC interventions. For example, in hospital units caring for patients with dementia, PCC interventions differ substantially from those in pediatric acute care units. Although the core dimensions of PCC, (1) patient as a unique person, (2) person involvement in care, (3) person information, (4) clinician-person communication, and (5) person empowerment, are represented in both examples, care principles and processes will vary.

System characteristics have the potential to affect PCC interventions as both a barrier and a facilitator. Examples of barriers are traditional organizational practices and structures such as clinicians not having the ability to work autonomously, lack of rooms for private communication between clinician and client, and time constraints in the provision and education of PCC interventions. Other barriers are organizational and clinician attitudes, including lack of continuous attention and engagement with PCC routines, lack of client involvement and engagement in care and decisions, and lack of seeing the client as a whole person (Dellenborg et al. 2019; Gondek et al. 2017; Moore et al. 2017; Nkrumah and Abekah-Nkrumah 2019). Studies have shown the importance of appropriate organizational leadership (Bachnick et al. 2018; Bokhour et al. 2018; Gabutti et al. 2017), sufficient teamwork (Gabutti et al. 2017), and adequate staffing and resources (Bachnick et al. 2018; Jarrar et al. 2018; Zhu et al. 2018) for improvement of PCC provision and clients' ratings of their experience.

However, organizational characteristics can also facilitate PCC interventions. For example, work environments that enable PCC interventions include strong leadership and management as role models for implementing PCC interventions. Additionally, continuous training opportunities that ensure that the organization has well-trained clinicians with a genuine knowledge of PCC interventions are essential for PCC interventions to succeed (Dellenborg et al. 2019; Gondek et al. 2017; Moore et al. 2017; Nkrumah and Abekah-Nkrumah 2019). Training should include approaches of clinicians whereby they emphasize PCC values, working practices, and interprofessional teamwork.

Outcomes Associated with Person-Centered Care Interventions

The heterogeneity and complexity of PCC interventions affect outcomes. Depending on the intervention's focus (e.g., on one or more PCC dimensions), the outcomes naturally vary for both client and family outcomes and system outcomes.

Client and Family Outcomes

For PCC interventions, improved client and family outcomes are the goal. PCC interventions' impact on client and family outcomes was examined in systematic reviews (Park et al. 2018). The findings suggested that although the PCC interventions were diverse, positive effects were found across many outcomes, including clients' increased quality of life, satisfaction, confidence, and well-being and reduced levels of depression, burden, stress, and anxiety. For family members, the interventions improved knowledge, care skills, and confidence levels and lowered levels of stress, anxiety, and depression (Park et al. 2018). In studies investigating specific client outcomes, the evidence is inconsistent. For example, studies with type 2 diabetes and acute coronary syndrome populations found improvements in self-efficacy (Cheng et al. 2017; Okrainec et al. 2017; Pirhonen et al. 2017). In contrast, studies with broadly defined patient populations did not show improved self-efficacy following PCC provision (Chiang et al. 2018).

System Outcomes

Inconsistent results are also typical with regard to system outcomes (i.e., clinical and economic). On the one hand, systematic reviews and individual studies assessing the effects of PCC interventions on system outcomes find reductions in unplanned visits and readmission rates in groups that received PCC interventions (Anhang Price et al. 2014; Bertakis and Azari 2011; Deek et al. 2016; Fiorio et al. 2018; Okrainec et al. 2017). On the other hand, studies correlating PCC with mortality rates have produced varying results (Chiang et al. 2018; Fiorio et al. 2018; Goldfarb et al. 2017). Because clinical outcomes influence economic outcomes, the evidence is similarly inconclusive regarding PCC interventions' relationship with cost-effectiveness: some studies report that cost reductions accompany PCC interventions (Anhang Price et al. 2014; Fiorio et al. 2018; Stone 2008) while other studies found no effect (Olsson et al. 2013; Uittenbroek et al. 2018). A reason for the inconsistent evidence is not only the heterogeneity of the PCC interventions but also related to client, family, and system characteristics.

Challenges Measuring Person-Centered Care

Due to its multidimensional nature, the assessment, provision, and measurement of PCC are broadly recognized as challenging (De Silva 2014: Luxford et al. 2010). Challenges arise in the measurement of PCC with diverse instruments and methods but also its methodological weaknesses.

PCC Measures

A standard PCC measure does not exist (De Silva 2014), and available assessment instruments suffer from methodological weaknesses due to conceptualization issues and psychometric properties. Instruments claim to measure PCC experiences from patients' perspective (Davis et al. 2008; Jenkinson et al. 2002; Suhonen et al. 2012b; Tzelepis et al. 2015), clinician's perspectives (Sullivan et al. 2013), or a combination of both patient and clinician perspectives (De Silva 2014; Suhonen et al. 2012a). Additionally, some instruments measure the overall concept of PCC (Charalambous et al. 2012; Davis et al. 2008), whereas others measure only specific dimensions (De Silva 2014; Hudon et al. 2011; Phillips et al. 2015).

Regardless of the extent PCC dimensions are covered in an instrument, no widely used instrument accounts for patient preferences (Bachnick et al. 2021; Coulter and Cleary 2001). Patient preferences are a key element in the NAM definition of PCC, which is care that is "respectful of and responsive to individual patients' preferences, needs, and values" (Institute of Medicine 2001, p. 49). Evaluating whether patients' preferences are met requires two elements: assessing their preferences and ratings of the care they actually received to meet those preferences. Today there are no measures of either of those two elements in standard PCC instruments.

Many of the existing instruments measuring whether PCC is present have been tested psychometrically in specific settings, populations, and countries and therefore require adaptions in order to be used in other settings, populations, and countries (Cheng et al. 2017; Edvardsson et al. 2008; Radwin 2003; Suhonen et al. 2010). In the UK, the most commonly accepted patient experience instrument is the National Health Service (NHS) Adult Inpatient Survey, which is based on the Picker Patient Experience Questionnaire (PPE-15) (De Courcy et al. 2012; Jenkinson et al. 2002; Leatherman and Sutherland 2007). In Switzerland, it is common for PCC instruments to include items from the PPE-15 and the Hospital Consumer Assessment of Healthcare Providers and Systems (HCAHPS) instrument (Ausserhofer et al. 2013; Bachnick et al. 2018; Bovier et al. 2004). The HCAHPS instrument was developed in the United States to measure patients' general experience and satisfaction with care in various settings (AHRQ n.d.). Some argue that the HCAHPS is a PCC instrument (Cleary 2016), even though it only includes one of the five vital PCC dimensions: communication with clinicians.

Methodological Challenges

Questionnaire surveys are the most used method to measure PCC across different healthcare settings. The majority of PCC surveys have been developed by clinicians and researchers, with little or no patient involvement (Wiering et al. 2017). A scoping review of 190 studies found insufficient patient participation across studies. Not a single study involved patients in determining which outcomes should be measured (Wiering et al. 2017). However, nearly 60% of the studies involved patients in specific item development, most often through focus groups and interviews. To test comprehensibility, only half of the studies used cognitive interviews or other methods involving patients (Wiering et al. 2017). The findings support the position that outcome assessments such as the HCAHPS and the NHS instruments do not address elements important to clients. Similar results were found for Germany. A recently published Delphi study confirmed different opinions between clinicians and clients regarding the relevance of PCC dimensions (Zeh et al. 2019). These findings strengthen the argument that clients need to be involved in the development of PCC measures.

Indeed, lacking involvement of patients in the development of PCC measures might lead to measures with little or no actionable relevance for clinical practice or system redesigns. Another methodological challenge is that current PCC measures are challenging to utilize for benchmarking across healthcare organizations. For example, since 2009, the Swiss National Association for Quality Development in Hospitals (ANQ 2017) measure has been used to assess patients' hospital stay experience. However, results show neither trends nor significant changes; with few exceptions, hospitals receive extremely high patient experience ratings (ANQ 2017). Such low variability can be explained in two ways. Swiss hospitals across the board deliver high-quality care, or the measure is not sufficiently sensitive to detect between-hospital differences. The latter explanation is most likely and indicates that the measure requires improvement.

Aside from the problem of distinguishing low- from high-performing organizations, a further question exists regarding the uneven influence of client and organizational characteristics, which are usually handled by using risk adjustment in comparisons (Abel et al. 2014; Orindi et al. 2016). Existing guidelines for risk adjustment recommend reporting both crude and adjusted values (AHRQ n.d.; NHS England Analytical Team (Medical and Nursing Analytical Unit) 2017; Swiss Academy of Medical Sciences (SAMS) 2009). However, there are variations in what and how risk adjustments are applied. A study from 2014 reviewed 142 organizations' benchmark reports (115 hospitals and 27 physicians) and assessed whether each report specified the comparison methods used (Damberg et al. 2014). The level of detail varied widely, for instance, designation of the risk adjustment methods used (Damberg et al. 2014). Methods should be clearly stated to increase transparency, reliability, and overall credibility and discern whether differences are due to real differences in performance (van Dishoeck et al. 2011), for example, PCC interventions provided.

In summary, several systematic reviews have evaluated the evidence of PCC interventions and measurements. In general, the majority of studies were of low quality with methodological flaws including insufficient sample sizes (Rathert et al. 2013; Segers et al. 2019; Yun and Choi 2019), a wide diversity of measurements and interventions (Park et al. 2018; Rathert et al. 2013), inconsistent results (Yun and Choi 2019), and limited study comparison and generalizability (Barbosa et al. 2015; Dwamena et al. 2012; McMillan et al. 2013; Rathert et al. 2013). Although dozens of PCC studies are available, PCC assessment, implementation, and influence on outcomes remain unclear. Perhaps most importantly regarding PCC provision, the current conceptualization of PCC is too vague, resulting in unclear measures and, therefore, limited use for benchmark comparisons.

Implications and Future Directions

PCC is one key element of quality of care and affects all components of the QHOM. The provision of PCC interventions aims to improve client and family outcomes through client, family, and system characteristics. However, several client, family, and system characteristics influence how interventions affect client and family outcomes. Moreover, there are several challenges in the provision of PCC due to PCC's complexity; heterogeneity of populations, interventions, and healthcare settings; and methodological challenges regarding PCC measures. The next steps in providing PCC interventions are the need to focus on both the interactions between PCC interventions and system characteristics and the methodological challenges, including developing appropriate PCC measures and common ways of measuring PCC.

When improving PCC provision through system characteristics, one must first identify where there are possibilities for change (Berwick et al. 2003). Therefore, future research has to focus on assessing system structures and processes that influence PCC delivery and clients' experience of care. Such evidence will be crucial to inform quality improvement strategies and interventional research on facilitating factors or eliminating barriers to implementing PCC in healthcare settings.

Finally, in order to improve PCC, the methodological challenges surrounding PCC have to be acknowledged. For the current PCC measures, this includes how they are measured and how they are used. A starting point is to engage clients and families in measure development, and then assess what their preferences are and their ratings of the received care (Bachnick 2018). A balance between these two parameters indicates the provision of high levels of PCC; a gap indicates that patient preferences were not met, in other words, that lower levels of PCC were delivered. As this approach allows individual clients to register their preferences, its use will shed light on core PCC dimensions and, therefore, correct a significant shortcoming of current PCC conceptualizations. Only when PCC interventions are measured correctly can it be determined how clients' and families' care experience is optimized.

References

Abdel Maqsood AS, Oweis AI, Hasna FS (2012) Differences between patients' expectations and satisfaction with nursing care in a private hospital in Jordan. Int J Nurs Pract 18(2):140–146. https://doi.org/10.1111/j.1440-172X.2012.02008.x

Abel GA, Saunders CL, Lyratzopoulos G (2014) Cancer patient experience, hospital performance and case mix: evidence from England. Future Oncol 10(9):1589–1598. https://doi.org/10.2217/fon.13.266

Agency for Healthcare Reseach and Quality (n.d.) CAHPS Hospital Survey (H-CAHPS). https://www.cahps.ahrq.gov/

Anhang Price R, Elliott MN, Zaslavsky AM, Hays RD, Lehrman WG, Rybowski L, Cleary PD (2014) Examining the role of patient experience surveys in measuring health care quality. Med Care Res Rev 71(5):522–554. https://doi.org/10.1177/1077558714541480

ANQ, Nationaler Verein für Qualitätsentwicklung in Spitälern und Kliniken (2017) Patientenzufriedenheit Akutsomatik, Erwachsene Nationaler Vergleichsbericht Messung 2016. https://www.anq.ch/wp-content/uploads/2018/09/ANQ_Akut_Patientenzufriedenheit_Erwachsene_Nationaler-Vergleichsbericht_2017.pdf

Ausserhofer D, Schubert M, Desmedt M, Blegen MA, De Geest S, Schwendimann R (2013) The association of patient safety climate and nurse-related organizational factors with selected patient outcomes: a cross-sectional survey. Int J Nurs Stud 50(2):240–252. https://doi.org/10.1016/j.ijnurstu.2012.04.007

Bachnick S (2018) Patient-centered care in Swiss acute care hospitals: addressing challenges in patient experience measurement and provider profiling. (PhD Nursing Science). University of Basel, Basel, Switzerland. https://edoc.unibas.ch/66825/1/Dissertation_S.Bachnick.pdf

Bachnick S, Ausserhofer D, Baernholdt M, Simon M, Match^{RN} Study group (2018) Patient-centered care, nurse work environment and implicit rationing of nursing care in Swiss acute care hospitals: a cross-sectional multi-center study. Int J Nurs Stud 81:98–106. https://doi.org/10.1016/j.ijnurstu.2017.11.007

Bachnick S, Ausserhofer D, Baernholdt M, Simon M (2021) Preferences matter when measuring patient experiences with hospital care—a cross-sectional multi-center study. [Manuscript in Preparation]

Barbosa A, Sousa L, Nolan M, Figueiredo D (2015) Effects of person-centered care approaches to dementia care on staff: a systematic review. Am J Alzheim Dis Other Dement 30(8):713–722. https://doi.org/10.1177/1533317513520213

Bertakis KD, Azari R (2011) Patient-centered care is associated with decreased health care utilization. J Am Board Fam Med 24(3):229–239. https://doi.org/10.3122/jabfm.2011.03.100170

Berwick DM (2009) What 'patient-centered' should mean: confessions of an extremist. Health Aff 28(4):w555–w565. https://doi.org/10.1377/hlthaff.28.4.w555

Berwick DM, James B, Coye MJ (2003) Connections between quality measurement and improvement. Med Care 41(1 Suppl):30–38

Bokhour BG, Fix GM, Mueller NM, Barker AM, Lavela SL, Hill JN, Lukas CV (2018) How can healthcare organizations implement patient-centered care? Examining a large-scale cultural transformation. BMC Health Serv Res 18(1):168. https://doi.org/10.1186/s12913-018-2949-5

Bovier PA, Charvet A, Cleopas A, Vogt N, Perneger TV (2004) Self-reported management of pain in hospitalized patients: link between process and outcome. Am J Med 117(8):569–574. https://doi.org/10.1016/j.amjmed.2004.05.020

Bowling A, Rowe G (2014) Psychometric properties of the new patients' expectations questionnaire. Pat Exp J 1(1):111–130

Bowling A, Rowe G, McKee M (2013) Patients' experiences of their healthcare in relation to their expectations and satisfaction: a population survey. J R Soc Med 106(4):143–149. https://doi.org/10.1258/jrsm.2012.120147

Charalambous A, Chappell NL, Katajisto J, Suhonen R (2012) The conceptualization and measurement of individualized care. Geriatr Nurs 33(1):17–27. https://doi.org/10.1016/j.gerinurse.2011.10.001

Cheng L, Sit JWH, Choi KC, Chair SY, Li X, Wu Y, Tao M (2017) Effectiveness of a patient-centred, empowerment-based intervention programme among patients with poorly controlled type 2 diabetes: a randomised controlled trial. Int J Nurs Stud 79:43–51. https://doi.org/10.1016/j.ijnurstu.2017.10.021

Chiang CY, Choi KC, Ho KM, Yu SF (2018) Effectiveness of nurse-led patient-centered care behavioral risk modification on secondary prevention of coronary heart disease: a systematic review. Int J Nurs Stud 84:28–39. https://doi.org/10.1016/j.ijnurstu.2018.04.012

Cleary PD (2016) Evolving concepts of patient-centered care and the assessment of patient care experiences: optimism and opposition. J Health Polit Policy Law 41(4):675–696. https://doi.org/10.1215/03616878-3620881

Coulter A, Cleary PD (2001) Patients' experiences with hospital care in five countries. Health Aff 20(3):244–252. https://doi.org/10.1377/hlthaff.20.3.244

Damberg CL, Sorbero ME, Lovejoy SL, Martsolf GR, Raaen L, Mandel D (2014) Measuring success in health care value-based purchasing programs: findings from an environmental scan, literature review, and expert panel discussions. Rand Health Quart 4(3):9. https://www.ncbi.nlm.nih.gov/pubmed/28083347

Davis S, Byers S, Walsh F (2008) Measuring person-centred care in a sub-acute health care setting. Aust Health Rev 32(3):496–504. https://doi.org/10.1071/ah080496. http://www.publish.csiro.au/?act=view_file&file_id=AH080496.pdf

De Courcy A, West E, Barron D (2012) The national adult inpatient survey conducted in the English National Health Service from 2002 to 2009: how have the data been used and what do we know as a result? BMC Health Serv Res 12:71. https://doi.org/10.1186/1472-6963-12-71

De Silva D (2014) Helping measure person-centred care: a review of evidence about commonly used approaches and tools used to help measure person-centred care. https://www.swselfmanagement.ca/uploads/ResourceTools/Helping%20measure%20person-centred%20care.pdf

Deek H, Hamilton S, Brown N, Inglis SC, Digiacomo M, Newton PJ, Investigators FP (2016) Family-centred approaches to healthcare interventions in chronic diseases in adults: a quantitative systematic review. J Adv Nurs 72(5):968–979. https://doi.org/10.1111/jan.12885

Dellenborg L, Wikstrom E, Andersson Erichsen A (2019) Factors that may promote the learning of person-centred care: an ethnographic study of an implementation programme for healthcare professionals in a medical emergency ward in Sweden. Adv Health Sci Educ Theory Pract 24(2):353–381. https://doi.org/10.1007/s10459-018-09869-y

Dwamena F, Holmes-Rovner M, Gaulden CM, Jorgenson S, Sadigh G, Sikorskii A, Olomu A (2012) Interventions for providers to promote a patient-centred approach in clinical consultations. Cochrane Database Syst Rev 12:CD003267. https://doi.org/10.1002/14651858.CD003267.pub2

Edvardsson D, Sandman PO, Rasmussen B (2008) Swedish language Person-centred Climate Questionnaire—patient version: construction and psychometric evaluation. J Adv Nurs 63(3):302–309. https://doi.org/10.1111/j.1365-2648.2008.04709.x

Fiorio CV, Gorli M, Verzillo S (2018) Evaluating organizational change in health care: the patient-centered hospital model. BMC Health Serv Res 18(1):95. https://doi.org/10.1186/s12913-018-2877-4

Gabutti I, Mascia D, Cicchetti A (2017) Exploring "patient-centered" hospitals: a systematic review to understand change. BMC Health Serv Res 17(1):364. https://doi.org/10.1186/s12913-017-2306-0

Gerteis M, Edgman-Levitan DJ, Delbanco TL (1991) Introduction: medicine and health from the patient's perspective. In: Through the patient's eyes: understanding and promoting patient-centered care. Jossey-Bass Publishers, San Francisco, pp 1–13

Goldfarb MJ, Bibas L, Bartlett V, Jones H, Khan N (2017) Outcomes of patient- and family-centered care interventions in the ICU: a systematic review and meta-analysis. Crit Care Med 45(10):1751–1761. https://doi.org/10.1097/CCM.0000000000002624

Gondek D, Edbrooke-Childs J, Velikonja T, Chapman L, Saunders F, Hayes D, Wolpert M (2017) Facilitators and barriers to person-centred care in child and young people mental health services: a systematic review. Clin Psycholol Psychother 24(4):870–886. https://doi.org/10.1002/cpp.2052

Goodrich J, Cornwell J (2008) Seeing the person in the patient: the point of care review paper. https://www.kingsfund.org.uk/sites/default/files/Seeing-the-person-in-the-patient-The-Point-of-Care-review-paper-Goodrich-Cornwell-Kings-Fund-December-2008.pdf

Hudon C, Fortin M, Haggerty JL, Lambert M, Poitras ME (2011) Measuring patients' perceptions of patient-centered care: a systematic review of tools for family medicine. Ann Fam Med 9(2):155–164. https://doi.org/10.1370/afm.1226

Institute of Medicine (2001) Crossing the quality chasm: a new health system for the 21st century. National Academy Press, Washington, DC

Jarrar M, Rahman HA, Minai MS, AbuMadini MS, Larbi M (2018) The function of patient-centered care in mitigating the effect of nursing shortage on the outcomes of care. Int J Health Plann Manag 33(2):e464–e473. https://doi.org/10.1002/hpm.2491. https://pubmed.ncbi.nlm.nih.gov/29380909/

Jenkinson C, Coulter A, Bruster S (2002) The Picker Patient Experience Questionnaire: development and validation using data from in-patient surveys in five countries. Int J Qual Health Care 14(5):353–358. https://www.ncbi.nlm.nih.gov/pubmed/12389801

Koberich S, Feuchtinger J, Farin E (2016) Factors influencing hospitalized patients' perception of individualized nursing care: a cross-sectional study. BMC Nurs 15:14. https://doi.org/10.1186/s12912-016-0137-7

Krupat E, Bell RA, Kravitz RL, Thom D, Azari R (2001) When physicians and patients think alike: patient-centered beliefs and their impact on satisfaction and trust. J Family Pract 50(12):1057–1062. https://www.ncbi.nlm.nih.gov/pubmed/11742607

Leatherman S, Sutherland K (2007) A quality chartbook: patient and public experience in the NHS. The Health Foundation, New York

Luxford K, Piper D, Dunbar N, Poole N (2010) Patient-centred care: improving quality and safety by focusing care on patients and consumers discussion paper draft for public consultation. https://www.safetyandquality.gov.au/sites/default/files/migrated/PCCC-DiscussPaper.pdf

Marchand K, Beaumont S, Westfall J, MacDonald S, Harrison S, Marsh DC, Oviedo-Joekes E (2019) Conceptualizing patient-centered care for substance use disorder treatment: findings from a systematic scoping review. Substan Abuse Treat Prevent Policy 14(1):37. https://doi.org/10.1186/s13011-019-0227-0

McMillan SS, Kendall E, Sav A, King MA, Whitty JA, Kelly F, Wheeler AJ (2013) Patient-centered approaches to health care: a systematic review of randomized controlled trials. Med Care Res Rev 70(6):567–596. https://doi.org/10.1177/1077558713496318

Medicare.gov (n.d.) Hospital Compare. https://www.medicare.gov/hospitalcompare/search.html

Moore L, Britten N, Lydahl D, Naldemirci O, Elam M, Wolf A (2017) Barriers and facilitators to the implementation of person-centred care in different healthcare contexts. Scand J Caring Sci 31(4):662–673. https://doi.org/10.1111/scs.12376

National Academies of Sciences, Engineering, & Medicine (2018) Crossing the global quality chasm: improving health care worldwide. Washington, DC. https://www.nap.edu/catalog/25152/crossing-the-global-quality-chasm-improving-health-care-worldwide

NHS England Analytical Team (Medical and Nursing Analytical Unit) (2017) Statistical bulletin: overall patient experience scores; 2016 adult inpatient survey update. https://www.england.nhs.uk/statistics/2017/05/31/overall-patient-experience-scores-2016-adult-inpatient-survey-update/

Nkrumah J, Abekah-Nkrumah G (2019) Facilitators and barriers of patient-centered care at the organizational-level: a study of three district hospitals in the central region of Ghana. BMC Health Serv Res 19(1):900. https://doi.org/10.1186/s12913-019-4748-z

Okrainec K, Lau D, Abrams HB, Hahn-Goldberg S, Brahmbhatt R, Huynh T, Bell CM (2017) Impact of patient-centered discharge tools: a systematic review. J Hosp Med 12(2):110–117. https://doi.org/10.12788/jhm.2692

Olsson LE, Jakobsson Ung E, Swedberg K, Ekman I (2013) Efficacy of person-centred care as an intervention in controlled trials—a systematic review. J Clin Nurs 22(3-4):456–465. https://doi.org/10.1111/jocn.12039

Orindi BO, Lesaffre E, Sermeus W, Bruyneel L (2016) Impact of cross-level measurement nonin-variance on hospital rankings based on patient experiences with care in 7 European countries. Med Care 55(12):e150–e157. https://doi.org/10.1097/MLR.0000000000000580

Papanicolas I, Figueroa JF, Orav EJ, Jha AK (2017) Patient hospital experience improved modestly, but no evidence Medicare incentives promoted meaningful gains. Health Aff 36(1):133–140. https://doi.org/10.1377/hlthaff.2016.0808

Park M, Giap TT, Lee M, Jeong H, Jeong M, Go Y (2018) Patient- and family-centered care interventions for improving the quality of health care: a review of systematic reviews. Int J Nurs Stud 87:69–83. https://doi.org/10.1016/j.ijnurstu.2018.07.006

Phillips NM, Street M, Haesler E (2015) A systematic review of reliable and valid tools for the measurement of patient participation in healthcare. BMJ Qual Saf 25:130–131. https://doi.org/10.1136/bmjqs-2015-004357

Pirhonen L, Olofsson EH, Fors A, Ekman I, Bolin K (2017) Effects of person-centred care on health outcomes - A randomized controlled trial in patients with acute coronary syndrome. Health Policy 121(2):169–179. https://doi.org/10.1016/j.healthpol.2016.12.003

Radwin LE (2003) Cancer patients' demographic characteristics and ratings of patient-centered nursing care. J Nurs Scholarsh 35(4):365–370. https://doi.org/10.1111/j.1547-5069.2003.00365.x

Rathert C, Wyrwich MD, Boren SA (2013) Patient-centered care and outcomes: a systematic review of the literature. Med Care Res Rev 70(4):351–379. https://doi.org/10.1177/1077558712465774

Segers E, Ockhuijsen H, Baarendse P, van Eerden I, van den Hoogen A (2019) The impact of family centred care interventions in a neonatal or paediatric intensive care unit on parents' satisfaction and length of stay: a systematic review. Intens Crit Care Nurs 50:63–70. https://doi.org/10.1016/j.iccn.2018.08.008

Serpa S, Ferreira CM (2019) Micro, meso, and macro levels of social analysis. Int J Soc Stud 7:3. https://doi.org/10.11114/ijsss.v7i3.4223

Shawa E, Omondi L, Mbakaya BC (2017) Examining surgical patients' expectations of nursing care at Kenyatta National Hospital in Nairobi, Kenya. Eur Sci J 13(24)

Stone S (2008) A retrospective evaluation of the impact of the Planetree patient-centered model of care on inpatient quality outcomes. HERD 1(4):55–69. https://doi.org/10.1177/193758670800100406

Suhonen R, Berg A, Idvall E, Kalafati M, Katajisto J, Land L, Leino-Kilpi H (2010) Adapting the individualized care scale for cross-cultural comparison. Scand J Caring Sci 24(2):392–403. https://doi.org/10.1111/j.1471-6712.2009.00712.x

Suhonen R, Efstathiou G, Tsangari H, Jarosova D, Leino-Kilpi H, Patiraki E, Papastavrou E (2012a) Patients' and nurses' perceptions of individualised care: an international comparative study. J Clin Nurs 21(7-8):1155–1167. https://doi.org/10.1111/j.1365-2702.2011.03833.x

Suhonen R, Papastavrou E, Efstathiou G, Tsangari H, Jarosova D, Leino-Kilpi H, Merkouris A (2012b) Patient satisfaction as an outcome of individualised nursing care. Scand J Caring Sci 26(2):372–380. https://doi.org/10.1111/j.1471-6712.2011.00943.x

Sullivan JL, Meterko M, Baker E, Stolzmann K, Adjognon O, Ballah K, Parker VA (2013) Reliability and validity of a person-centered care staff survey in veterans health administration community living centers. Gerontologist 53(4):596–607. https://doi.org/10.1093/geront/gns140

Swiss Academy of Medical Sciences (SAMS) (2009) Erhebung, Analyse und Veröffentlichung von Daten über die medizinische Behandlungsqualität: empfehlungen [The collection, analysis and publication of data about quality of medical treatment: recommendations]. Schweizerische Ärztezeitung 90(26/27):1044–1054

Tzelepis F, Sanson-Fisher RW, Zucca AC, Fradgley EA (2015) Measuring the quality of patient-centered care: why patient-reported measures are critical to reliable assessment. Pat Prefer Adher 9:831–835. https://doi.org/10.2147/PPA.S81975

Uittenbroek RJ, van Asselt ADI, Spoorenberg SLW, Kremer HPH, Wynia K, Reijneveld SA (2018) Integrated and person-centered care for community-living older adults: a cost-effectiveness study. Health Serv Res 53(5):3471–3494. https://doi.org/10.1111/1475-6773.12853

van Dishoeck AM, Lingsma HF, Mackenbach JP, Steyerberg EW (2011) Random variation and rankability of hospitals using outcome indicators. BMJ Qual Saf 20(10):869–874. https://doi.org/10.1136/bmjqs.2010.048058

Wiering B, de Boer D, Delnoij D (2017) Patient involvement in the development of patient-reported outcome measures: a scoping review. Health Expect 20(1):11–23. https://doi.org/10.1111/hex.12442

World Health Organization (2002) Innovative care for chronic conditions: building blocks for action. https://www.who.int/chp/knowledge/publications/icccreport/en/

Wynendaele H, Willems R, Trybou J (2019) Systematic review: association between the patient-nurse ratio and nurse outcomes in acute care hospitals. J Nurs Manag 27(5):896–917. https://doi.org/10.1111/jonm.12764

Yun D, Choi J (2019) Person-centered rehabilitation care and outcomes: a systematic literature review. Int J Nurs Stud 93:74–83. https://doi.org/10.1016/j.ijnurstu.2019.02.012

Zeh S, Christalle E, Hahlweg P, Harter M, Scholl I (2019) Assessing the relevance and implementation of patient-centredness from the patients' perspective in Germany: results of a Delphi study. BMJ Open 9(12):e031741. https://doi.org/10.1136/bmjopen-2019-031741

Zhu J, Dy SM, Wenzel J, Wu AW (2018) Association of magnet status and nurse staffing with improvements in patient experience with hospital care, 2008–2015. Med Care 56(2):111–120. https://doi.org/10.1097/MLR.0000000000000854

Zill JM, Scholl I, Harter M, Dirmaier J (2015) Which dimensions of patient-centeredness matter?—results of a web-based expert Delphi survey. PLoS One 10(11):e0141978. https://doi.org/10.1371/journal.pone.0141978

Nurse Outcomes: Burnout, Engagement, and Job Satisfaction

13

Peter Van Bogaert and Erik Franck

Introduction

What makes nurses like their job as proud and engaged professionals and as clinically competent and critical thinkers? What makes nurses open-minded and eager to learn about continuous change focused on improved care delivery and patient outcomes? An empowered nurse workforce is one of the critical components for positive nurse outcomes. Additionally, the system characteristics of a healthy nurse work environment (NWE) are essential. System questions should address: What makes teams at the unit and organizational level perform beyond expectations with energy and creativity to innovate and underpin solutions for patients' and organizations' continuously changing needs?

Successful healthcare delivery creates value for a host of stakeholder groups: patients, healthcare professionals, management, policymakers, and society as a whole. It is imperative to recognize and attend to all stakeholders' interests. In the past few decades, healthcare organizations have been challenged by constant changes: budget constraints, an aging workforce, an aging patient population, more complex and chronic patient problems, a higher need for inter-professional collaboration and practice, and safe patient outcomes. Organizations and healthcare professionals, including nurses, are challenged to adapt in flexible ways that often lead to detrimental outcomes (e.g., burnout) for the healthcare professional and the patients in their care. The burnout literature spans 30 or so years (Dow et al. 2019). Thus, currently, there is a focus on healthcare professionals' well-being in general (Brigham et al. 2018).

In this chapter, nurse outcomes are explored using the QHOM, specifically, how nurse outcomes are affected by interventions at the individual nurse and system

P. V. Bogaert (✉) · E. Franck
Department of Nursing and Midwifery Science, Centre for Research and Innovation in Care (CRIC), University of Antwerp, Antwerpen, Belgium
e-mail: peter.vanbogaert@uantwerpen.be; erik.franck@uantwerpen.be

© Springer Nature Switzerland AG 2021
M. Baernholdt, D. K. Boyle (eds.), *Nurses Contributions to Quality Health Outcomes*, https://doi.org/10.1007/978-3-030-69063-2_13

levels. First, the nurse outcomes of engagement, burnout, job satisfaction, and turnover intentions are described briefly. Second, interventions at the individual level, such as personal leadership development, are discussed. Third, successful system interventions are discussed, including Magnet designation, to improve NWEs. In turn, improved NWEs improve nurse outcomes and ultimately improve patient safety and quality of care. Finally, an example from a program of research focused on nurse outcomes is provided. In this research example, favorable assessed NWE aspects such as nurse-physician relations, unit-level nurse management, hospital management, and organizational support were found to be strongly associated with balanced nurse work characteristics such as social capital, decision latitude, and workload. These three work characteristics are closely related to empowerment. In turn, balanced nurse work characteristics were associated with favorable nurse outcomes such as high engagement levels or low levels of burnout, job satisfaction, and organizational outcome of favorably assessed quality of care. Conclusions and future directions are provided. Overall, it is argued that both hospitals and nurses bear a responsibility to achieve optimal nurse outcomes that subsequently lead to better organizational and patient outcomes.

Nurse Outcomes: Linkages with the QHOM

For almost four decades, an international multitude of practitioners and researchers have been providing a body of knowledge that links system characteristics, interventions, client (nurse) characteristics, and nurse outcomes at the individual, team, and organizational levels as described in the QHOM (Mitchell et al. 1998). In the QHOM, nurse outcomes include nurses' well-being: engagement vs. burnout and job satisfaction, as well as attraction and retention to the profession and their employer. Outcomes are affected by interventions *that work through* the client and system (Fig. 13.1). In this chapter, the client is the nurse. It is understood (but not discussed in this chapter) that nurse outcomes are strongly linked with patient outcomes. Interventions that influence nurse outcomes via the nurse (client) include the development of personal leadership skills. Interventions that act through the system to improve NWEs include the Magnet Recognition Program (ANCC n.d.-a). Thus, individual- and system-level interventions can empower nurses to deal with the continuous challenges and changes in healthcare organizations that confront them daily. In other words, systems that implement such interventions have a culture where learning is implemented and encouraged. A learning culture is imperative for positive nurse outcomes and excellent patient care. Systems or organizations that manage to create such a professional development learning culture and embrace and prioritize organizational effectiveness will ensure their long-term sustainability and success.

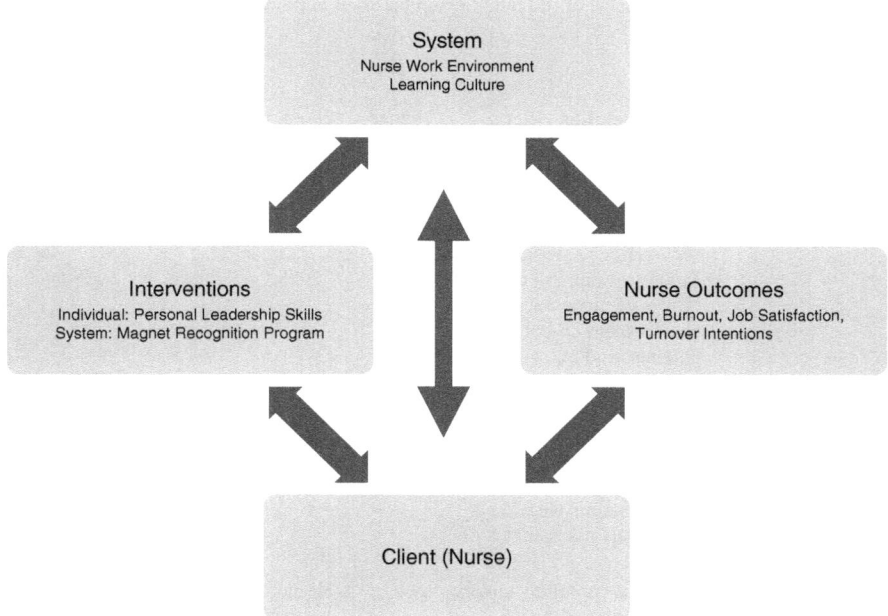

Fig. 13.1 Framework for nurse outcomes

Nurse Outcomes

The study of nurse outcomes is almost as old as the profession itself. The outcomes of job satisfaction and turnover or turnover intention have been studied extensively, followed by burnout and engagement. Nurse outcomes are related to patient outcomes—better nurse outcomes are associated with higher care quality ratings and patient safety. Thus, an understanding of what predicts nurse outcomes is essential (Van Bogaert and Clarke 2018a).

Several systematic reviews have examined the relationship between various aspects of the NWE and nurse outcomes (see Table 13.1). Review results show that the nurse outcomes most consistently associated with better hospital NWEs are lower burnout, lower emotional strains, or better psychological health (Copanitsanou et al. 2017; Halm 2019; Lake et al. 2019; Wei et al. 2018); higher job satisfaction or lower job dissatisfaction (Copanitsanou et al. 2017; Halm 2019; Lake et al. 2019; Petit Dit Dariel and Regnaux 2015; Wei et al. 2018); and higher intent to stay or lower turnover (Lake et al. 2019; Petit Dit Dariel and Regnaux 2015; Wei et al. 2018).

Table 13.1 Systematic reviews of the relationship between nurse work environments and nurse outcomes

Authors Date published, type of review	Review inclusion criteria	Studies in review	Nurse outcomes
Copanitsanou et al. (2017) Systematic review	• Years 1999–2014 • Studies in English • Research studies (prospective, cross-sectional, or retrospective) • Studies examining the effects of nurses' work environment on both patients' and nurses' outcomes • Studies in which both patients and nurses participated • Studies in which only questionnaires were used for the self-assessments of outcomes	10	Lower burnout and higher job satisfaction
Halm (2019) Critical evidence review	• Search of cumulative index • To Nursing and Allied Health Literature and MEDLINE • Key words: nurse, staffing, patient outcomes, Magnet hospitals, nursing excellence, and practice or work environments • Original research in the past 10 years	14	Higher quality of care and safety ratings; less job dissatisfaction and burnout
Lake et al. (2019) Meta-analysis	• July 2002–September 2018 • Use of the PES-NWI to measure work environment • Reported odds ratios (ORs) and 95% confidence intervals from regression models of four outcome classes: nurse job outcomes, safety and quality ratings, patient outcomes, and patient satisfaction	17	28–32% lower odds of job dissatisfaction, burnout, or intention to leave; 23–51% lower odds of rating nursing unit quality and safety as fair or poor; 22% lower odds of reporting that they were not confident that patients could manage care after discharge
Petit Dit Dariel and Regnaux (2015) Systematic review	• 1994–2014 • Quantitative studies comparing nurse and patient outcomes in Magnet-accredited hospitals with those in non-Magnet hospitals	10	Higher job satisfaction, lower intent to leave and turnover

Table 13.1 (continued)

Authors Date published, type of review	Review inclusion criteria	Studies in review	Nurse outcomes
Wei et al. (2018) Systematic review	• January 2005–December 2007 • Primary research studies with empirical data • Focused on nurse work environment • Written in English in the USA	54	Better psychological health and lower emotional strains; lower burnout; lower incivility; higher job satisfaction and retention; higher perceptions of autonomy, control over practice, nurse-physician relationships, and organizational support; higher new graduate 3-year retention rates

Predictors of Job Satisfaction and Turnover

Two predictors of job satisfaction and turnover are structural and psychological empowerment. Structural empowerment is the extent to which nurses have (a) formal and informal power in care delivery, (b) access to information and opportunities to improve personal development, and (c) supportive relations with subordinates, peers, and superiors (Kanter 1993). These conditions are linked with job satisfaction, engagement, productivity, and burnout (Laschinger et al. 2003, 2004; Laschinger and Finegan 2005). Psychological empowerment is the psychological response to work conditions and the extent to which a nurse experiences meaning, competence, self-determination, and impact (Eo et al. 2014; Laschinger et al. 2001; Spreitzer 1995; Wagner et al. 2013; Yang et al. 2013). However, a third concept, authentic leadership, plays a mediating role between nurse empowerment and job satisfaction (Dahinten et al. 2014; MacPhee and Bouthillette 2008; MacPhee et al. 2012, 2014).

Burnout and Engagement

In the first decade of this millennium, the Nurses' Early Exit Study (NEXT-Study) performed a comprehensive study in ten European countries to investigate the reasons, circumstances, and consequences of nurses' premature departure from their healthcare institution or the nursing profession (Hasselhorn et al. 2005). The most predictive factors for leaving nursing were burnout and poor-quality teamwork. Both are associated with NWEs. The study results showed that units with more nurses who perceived adequate staffing, good administrative support for nursing care, and good relations with physicians had better outcomes than those nurses who did not work on units with these characteristics. Further, nurses reported lower burnout, and patients were more than twice as likely to be satisfied with their care (Estryn-Béhar et al. 2007; Hasselhorn et al. 2005).

The NEXT-Study findings are closely related to the research that started more than 35 years earlier. This research investigated a phenomenon in human service professionals, whereby enthusiastic service providers in close contact with service users become emotionally drained, cynical, and not confident in their abilities. This phenomenon is identified as *burnout* and has three dimensions: emotional exhaustion, depersonalization, and personal accomplishment (Maslach et al. 2001). Research reveals that burnout is a critical mediator between areas of work-life or work environment and nurses' intention to leave their job (Leiter and Maslach 2009). From these studies on burnout, the opposite or positive concept was developed: *work engagement* (Maslach and Leiter 2008). Work engagement is a positive, fulfilled work-related state of mind characterized by (a) *vigor* or high levels of energy and mental resilience at work, (b) *dedication* or strong involvement in one's work accompanied by feelings of enthusiasm and significance, and (c) *absorption* or being fully engrossed in one's work and having difficulties detaching oneself from it (Schaufeli and Bakker 2003). Some researchers argue that work engagement is an independent, distinct, albeit related, concept negatively correlated with burnout (Bakker et al. 2011; Schaufeli and Salonova 2011). However, both burnout and engagement are linked to the concepts of job demand and job control (JDC-model). In the JDC model, high demand and low control are potential risks for job strain, psychological distress, and illness (burnout), whereas high demand and high control are linked with high engagement because they increase motivation and learning (Bakker and Demerouti 2007, 2017). Also, job control and job resources act as buffers for high demands' negative consequences (Adriaenssens et al. 2017; Ibrahim and Ohtsuka 2014). To improve nurse outcomes, both individual and system interventions are needed.

Interventions: Client (Nurse)

In the QHOM, interventions can target the client or individual nurse and the system or organization. For the individual nurse, interventions focus on developing *personal leadership skills*, with three key components: self-knowledge, self-awareness, and self-control.

Self-Knowledge

Self-knowledge is knowing who you are (or self-concept) and what motivates you in terms of values and purpose. According to Gottfredson (1981), occupational selection is influenced by two factors: the image the individual holds of a particular occupation and the individual's self-concept. Research about the motivations of people who enter professional nursing revealed that they are influenced by three groups of factors: restrictive factors such as financial or family responsibilities, attractive factors such as having positive role models in their surroundings, and internal motivation factors such as altruism and the desire to meet someone else's personal or emotional needs (Zysberg and Berry 2005). The third factor has been investigated less frequently. When asked why they entered the nursing profession, many nurses would answer "because I wanted to be of help to others" (Mimura et al. 2009, p. 604). However, when probed further why they wanted to help others, many nurses cannot answer that question. Because of the importance of self-concept, one possible explanation is that they want to help others compensate for negative self-concepts such as low self-esteem. Research findings show that nursing students have significantly lower self-esteem than medical students (Braspenning and Franck 2013). In turn, low self-esteem has been related to altruistic behavior (Schutz 1998). These findings suggest that nurses may unconsciously try to compensate for their lower self-esteem by caring for others. Therefore, developing self-knowledge, such as knowing who you are and what motivates you in terms of values and purpose, is the first step towards increasing self-knowledge.

Talent and Passion

Part of self-knowledge is being aware of one's talent and passion. In most healthcare organizations, nurses have specific job descriptions and are expected to perform the description's functions. However, assuming that everyone with the same functions has the same talent is erroneous. When *talent* is defined as the ability to do something(s) better, faster, and with less effort (Debisschop 2017), focusing on talent(s) alone ignores the fact that certain behaviors and competencies have a motivational component too. *Passion* is the strong inclination towards a self-defining activity that people like and in which they invest time and energy regularly (Vallerand 2012). Passion is the energy source that keeps someone moving towards goals. Some will argue that it is essential for nurses to know and develop talent and competencies, and passion(s) for their jobs. One way of doing so is by using the golden circle philosophy (Sinek 2009).

The golden circle (Sinek 2009) consists of three concentric circles with the outer circle defined as the WHAT, which has two components. The first is: What have you achieved? This achievement is one's resumé or curriculum vitae. For example, I am a certified ER nurse. The second WHAT is: What do you want to achieve? These are the goals one pursues. For example, I want to specialize as an advanced critical care nurse practitioner. In the nursing literature, this is also defined as a professional legacy, which answers the question: What in healthcare is better because of my efforts (Hinds et al. 2015)? Knowing what one wants to achieve or declare a professional legacy helps to maintain a focus on the meaning of an experience in the process of reaching a goal (Hinds et al. 2015). The middle circle is the HOW. Here, the question is: What experience, behavior, or competencies do you have that will help you reach your goal? For example, I am very good at active listening or in taking care of infected wounds. The inner circle in the model is defined as the WHY, also called the INNER WHY. Here one has to answer: What drives you as a nurse? From which values do you deliver patient care? Why did you become a nurse? Research indicates that the INNER WHY of an individual is linked to the more emotional limbic system of the human brain, whereas the WHAT questions are associated with higher order cognitive functions located in the neocortex of the brain (Sinek 2009).

Passion can thus be situated in a person's INNER WHY, whereas talent can be attributed to both the HOW and the INNER WHY. Many newer nurses start with a particular view on WHY they want to become a nurse. Moreover, some nurses seem to lose contact with their INNER WHY during their first years in clinical practice due to a non-supportive or unhealthy work environment. In a healthcare environment where system characteristics are rapidly evolving, knowing one's INNER WHY and HOW, passion, and talents is essential to staying aligned to one's WHAT or goals in the short and longer terms. Individual nurses can develop their self-knowledge by reflecting on the components of the golden circle.

Self-Awareness

Self-knowledge alone is not enough to achieve one's goals. The second step in expressing personal leadership is self-awareness, defined as the process of being aware of what triggers you and what and how this results in certain behaviors and effects in your immediate environment. Sometimes circumstances will trigger us, resulting in immediate emotions and emotionally driven or ineffective behaviors. An illustrative example is when a multidisciplinary surgical team in an academic medical center was observed with cameras and microphones installed in the operating room (Franck et al. 2016). At a certain point during a complicated surgical procedure, the surgeon was confronted with an unexpected problem. The workload increased, and the surgeon experienced a loss of control. He raised his voice and reacted emotionally towards the team members. The effects were clearly observed: communication processes froze for several minutes, and team members no longer felt safe to speak up, cross-check, or communicate otherwise.

One's self-awareness is influenced by both the hierarchical healthcare system and one's emotions. Hospitals are, by tradition, hierarchical, with the physician at the top. Hierarchy, or authority gradients, can create an unsafe environment for team members, inhibiting them from speaking up (Leonard et al. 2004). In turn, unnecessarily high risks result. Shifting from top-down organizational culture to a more team-oriented, bottom-up culture is challenging. A team-oriented culture is a crucial component in improving nurses' well-being, patient safety, and quality of care in healthcare organizations (Franck et al. 2018; Van Bogaert and Clarke 2018b). In addition to the organizational culture, communication is also influenced by factors intrinsic to individual healthcare professionals, such as speaking and listening skills, conflict resolution techniques, and appropriate assertion and advocacy instead of leading with one's emotions. Healthcare professionals work in emotionally charged settings, and evidence to date suggests that emotions play an integral role in patient safety (Heyhoe et al. 2016). In organizational psychology, the powerful impact of emotions on behavior is widely accepted. However, other than limited education around burnout and patient-centered care, healthcare professionals do not learn to recognize and anticipate the impact of their behavior in real time.

Self-Control

The third step in personal leadership is self-control. It refers to a dispositional capacity to regulate immediate dominant responses or tendencies, thoughts, behaviors, and emotions for a more delayed but desirable outcome, thereby promoting task completion (De Ridder et al. 2012). It is the ability to prioritize long-term over short-term goals, even when the latter are immediately gratifying. Research has found that self-control represents a key predictor of well-being by inhibiting undesired behaviors and fostering goal attainment and positive emotions (De Ridder and Gillebaart 2016). Emerging evidence shows that not using self-control, in other words, emotional reactivity (emotionally driven behavior) and ineffective coping strategies, impacts patient safety outcomes (Heyhoe et al. 2016) through less-than-optimal teamwork. Research examining self-control has demonstrated that lower self-control levels are associated with counterproductive work behaviors (Bolton et al. 2012). However, to achieve long-term changes in self-control and, therefore, work behaviors, recognizing the processes that will produce such changes is essential (Singleton et al. 2015).

The Interpersonal Circumplex Model

A model to guide all three personal leadership skills, self-knowledge, self-awareness, and self-control, is the interpersonal circumplex (IPC) model (Kiesler and Auerbach 2003). The IPC maps peoples' interpersonal behavior around two axes that indicate agency (dominant vs. submissive behavior) and communion (hostile vs. friendly behavior) (Redeker et al. 2012). Thus formulated, every form of interpersonal behavior is determined, on the one hand, by the degree of affiliation one bears to another in a relationship and, on the other hand, by the position of power one assumes towards the other. Such a circumplex model consists of categories of interpersonal behavior in relation to the communion axis and the agency axis. These categories are

- Directive and authoritarian behaviors are in the dominant-hostile quadrant.
- Distrustful and withdrawn behaviors are in the submissive-hostile quadrant.
- Inspiring and coaching behaviors are in the dominant-friendly quadrant.
- Participative and yielding behaviors are in the submissive-friendly quadrant (Gurtman 2009; Redeker et al. 2012).

The IPC model can be used as an outcome measure to map someone's interpersonal effectiveness and as a feedback instrument in an intervention to improve someone's interpersonal effectiveness or personal leadership skills.

Research guided by the IPC model investigated the combination of personality and interpersonal behavior of 587 staff nurses in general hospitals concerning burnout (Geuens et al. 2017). On average, nurses displayed a friendly-submissive interpersonal behavior (between participative and yielding). In another study, Braspenning and Franck (2013) compared nursing and medical students in their first and last years of education. Although both groups displayed submissive-friendly behavior, nursing students' interpersonal behavior in their first and last years of education was significantly more submissive than that of medical students. Given that higher levels of burnout are associated with more submissive behavior (Geuens et al. 2017), nurses need to know where they are on the submissive-dominant spectrum. They must also work to be less submissive individually and collectively—a process that has to start during basic nursing education (Geuens et al. 2017).

In summary, individual healthcare professionals are influenced by many cultural perspectives, personal values, assumptions, beliefs, and disciplinary perspectives that will influence their work (Singleton et al. 2015). Without personal leadership—self-knowledge, self-awareness, and self-control—interactions between nurses and patients and within multidisciplinary healthcare teams will not reach its full potential. Healthcare organizations need to be aware and invest in the personal development of their healthcare practitioners. Nurse managers of today need to coach their team members to cope with the continuous changes in healthcare by highlighting the purpose of changes, making contact with nurses' intrinsic motivation, and investing in training for individual nurses to develop personal leadership skills. However, as part of the health administration team, nurse managers also need to push for changes at the system level to improve nurse outcomes.

Interventions: System

System interventions that improve NWEs and, in turn, improve nurse outcomes resulted from studies of Magnet hospital attributes. The original magnet research study performed in the early 1980s focused on what makes nurses want to work or stay in certain hospitals, hence the term magnet (McClure et al. 2002). Despite periodic nursing shortages, some hospitals could attract and retain nurses far better than other hospitals. This initial study scrutinized potential generalizable aspects that attract and retain nurses (Kramer and Schmalenberg 2002; McClure and Hinshaw 2002). Further, the link of magnet hospitals with care quality was set from the beginning (Kramer and Hafner 1989). Two concepts were born: the *Forces of Magnetism* translated in the American Nurses Credentialing Center (ANCC) Magnet Recognition® program (ANCC n.d.-a; Urden and Monarch 2002) and *the nurse work environment* or *practice environment*. The work environment is measured most often in the Practice Environment Scale of the Nursing Work Index Revised (PES-NWI) (Lake 2002), the Essentials of Magnetism II (EOMII) (Schmalenberg and Kramer 2008), and the Healthy Work Environments Assessment Tool (AACN 2016). See Chap. 4 for details on these three measures.

Magnet Recognition Program

In 1990, ANCC (n.d.-a) instituted the Magnet Recognition Program as an accreditation process, with 14 *Forces of Magnetism* and 5 *Magnet Model Components*. The five components are transformation leadership; structural empowerment; exemplary professional practice; empirical quality results; and new knowledge, innovation, and improvement. These five components are key for better NWEs, leading to better nurse and patient outcomes. The Magnet program requires resources that not all hospitals have, so in 2007, the Pathway to Excellence Program (PTE) was initiated (ANCC n.d.-b) to assure accessibility to an NWE recognition program for all hospitals, regardless of size. The PTE program will not be discussed in this chapter. See Chap. 4 for a more detailed description of the Magnet and Pathway to Excellence Recognition Programs.

Research indicates that Magnet hospitals are associated with lower levels of burnout and turnover and greater job satisfaction in nurses (Aiken et al. 2008; Kelly et al. 2012; Kutney-Lee et al. 2015), as well as higher nurse-reported care quality (Stimpfel et al. 2014). Other studies related to team processes and outcomes identified three Forces of Magnetism as primary priorities for team performance. The three priorities are (a) a flat organizational structure where team-based decision-making prevails, (b) strong inter-professional relations, and (c) supportive managers and leaders who guide processes of aligned goals within units and at all levels within the organization (Van Bogaert et al. 2014a; Wolf and Greenhouse 2006). These three primary forces were associated with responsive teams. Responsive teams can handle situations effectively, are supported by staff cohesiveness, have members who follow the rules, are focused on achieving goals, and are feeling trust and optimism. In contrast, reactive teams work in crisis mode, in small cliques, focusing on survival, often feeling paranoia, distrust, and pessimism. More responsive teams supported by the Forces of Magnetism are essential to creating a healthy and positive work environment with positive nurse outcomes. These teams can also improve care delivery, continuously focused on better patient outcomes.

The RN4CAST study demonstrated how hospital organizational features impacted nurse recruitment and retention, and patient outcomes (Sermeus et al. 2011). This study found that favorable ratings of the NWE and staffing were associated with patients' ratings of their hospital as excellent (Aiken et al. 2017). In other words, nurses' ratings of the NWE are linked with independently made patient assessments. In summary, it is well documented that system-level interventions can use the Magnet Model and Forces of Magnetism in the NWE to improve nurse and patient outcomes.

Example of Nurse Outcome Program of Research

In this section, the association of individual and system characteristics with nurse outcomes is discussed using several studies from the Van Bogaert and colleagues' research program (Van Bogaert and Clarke 2018a). The research is guided by the

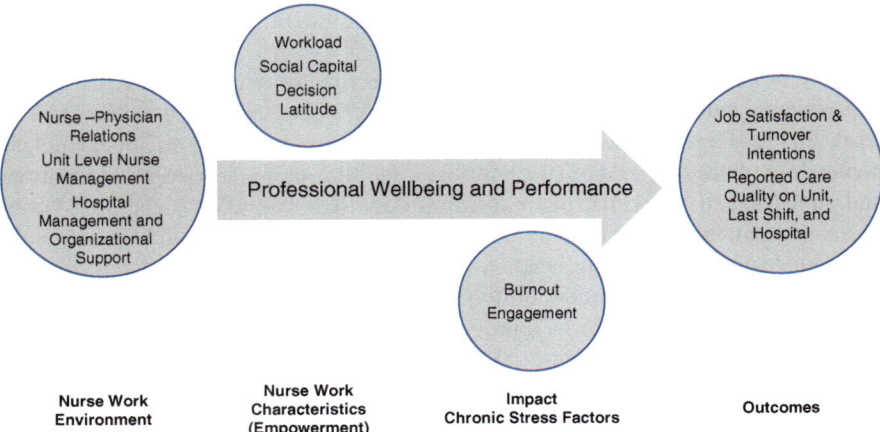

Fig. 13.2 Burnout and engagement model

Burnout and Engagement Model (Fig. 13.2). In the model, the NWE is measured using three dimensions of the Nursing Work Index-Revised Scale (Aiken and Patrician 2000): nurse-physician relations, nurse management at the unit level, and hospital management and organizational support. The work environment directly predicts empowerment and indirectly predicts burnout or engagement (Van Bogaert and Clarke 2018b; Van Bogaert et al. 2017b). Empowerment is described as nurse characteristics such as workload (or job demands), social capital (or experiences of peer support, shared values, and mutual trust), and decision latitude (or abilities to make decisions and the capacity to use and develop professional and personal skills). Also, NWE characteristics predict the nurse outcomes of job satisfaction and turnover intentions.

In the first study, strong direct predictors of all nurse outcomes are nurse management at the unit level and the nurse work characteristic, workload. Nurses experience outcomes personally and within teams, as shown by multilevel studies at the unit level (Van Bogaert et al. 2009, 2010, 2013, 2014a). In a second study, the identified associations were confirmed and extended in qualitative studies of staff nurses and nurse managers (Van Bogaert et al. 2017a). Nurses reported that they were concerned about the effect of high and prolonged job demands on care quality and patient safety. Moreover, respondents were concerned that they might overlook relevant patient signs and symptoms and neglect patients' mental and emotional needs. Further, both staff nurses and nurse managers reported staff nurses' feelings of sadness and querulousness.

These results of studies one and two were confirmed in a third study using a longitudinal design over 5 years. Findings were that unfavorably perceived hospital management and organizational support, along with unbalanced work characteristics such as unfavorable workload, social capital, and decision latitude, predicted higher burnout (Van Bogaert and Clarke 2018b). The study confirmed that poor nursing conditions were related to lower empowerment that, in turn, predicted high levels of burnout and low levels of work engagement. Consequently, nurses experienced job dissatisfaction and turnover intentions and reported low quality of care (Van Bogaert and Clarke 2018b). These findings were confirmed in a fourth study that included physicians. Good staff outcomes and assessed quality of care were associated with balanced work characteristics such as favorably perceived workload, social capital, and decision latitude in both nursing and medical staff (Van Bogaert et al. 2018).

In the final study, staff in one hospital implemented a quality improvement (QI) project. The hospital had Magnet designation and thus had invested significantly in the NWE (Van Bogaert et al. 2014b, 2017a). The hospital implemented the Productive Ward: Releasing Time to Care™ program developed by the National Health Service in the United Kingdom, to eliminate waste in care processes and increase added value for patients by providing increased time for staff nurses to deliver care (White et al. 2014; Van Bogaert et al. 2014b). This large-scale quality improvement project was supported by hospital management and leadership, who were strong drivers in aligning healthcare teams' goals. The study found a favorable impact on healthcare staff's perceptions of social capital and decision latitude (Van Bogaert and Clarke 2018a; Van Bogaert et al. 2017b). The overall program of research suggests that balanced nurse work characteristics are essential and robust indicators for nurse outcomes and quality of care. Therefore, nurse work characteristics can be used to monitor and evaluate interventions and changes in organizations.

Implications and Future Directions

System characteristics (NWE), interventions, client (nurse) characteristics, and outcomes are linked at the individual, team, and organizational levels described in the QHOM. The relationships are supported by almost four decades of growing knowledge and insights. Current and future challenges are how to provide and sustain healthcare professionals' capacity, such as staff nurses and their teams to improve care delivery continuously focused on better patient outcomes.

Training about personal leadership skills in self-knowledge, self-awareness, and self-control may help individual nurses cope with the complex challenges in healthcare settings. Future research is needed to investigate further the relationships among purpose, emotions, self-control, and patient safety. Interventions from positive psychology seem promising in influencing personal resilience and enhancing self-control. However, it might be difficult to justify human resource development in light of practical and financial demands on the healthcare system. However, one cannot afford not to invest in individual skills and system-level interventions. The managerial challenges of integrating these principles into a departmental or organizational culture (or colloquially, making them part of a unit's, team's, or organization's shared mental models) are not to be underestimated. The existing organization or departmental culture may produce counterpressures to changing ways of working and thus the work environment. Therefore, the entire hospital management needs to operate from a shared mental model to promote culture change that shifts the emphasis from individual performance to nonhierarchical teamwork to provide safer healthcare (Chap. 10).

Future challenges will be to create and sustain balanced work environments and work systems, focusing on stakeholders such as patients' and their family's needs, as well as healthcare practitioners and leadership needs, roles, and responsibilities. Work environments that are resilient to changes and demands focusing on developments and improvements are essential to creating a healthcare delivery system that provides high-quality care from nurses with high well-being.

References

Adriaenssens J, Hamelink A, Van Bogaert P (2017) Predictors of occupational stress and wellbeing in first-line nurse managers: a cross-sectional survey study. Int J Nurs Stud 73:85–92

Aiken LH, Patrician PA (2000) Measuring organizational traits of hospitals: the revised nursing work index. Nurs Res 49:146–153

Aiken LH, Clarke SP, Sloane DM, Lake ET, Cheney T (2008) Effects of hospital care environment on patient mortality and nurse outcomes. J Nurs Adm 38:223–229

Aiken LH, Sloane D, Griffiths P, RN4CAST Consortium (2017) Nursing skill mix in European hospitals: cross-sectional study of the association with mortality, patient ratings, and quality of care. BMJ Qual Saf 26:559–568. https://doi.org/10.1136/bmjqs-2016-005567

American Association of Critical-Care Nurses (2016) AACN healthy work environment assessment tool. https://www.aacn.org/nursing-excellence/healthy-work-environments/aacn-healthy-work-environment-assessment-tool

American Nurses Credentialing Center (n.d.-a) ANCC Magnet Recognition Program. https://www.nursingworld.org/organizational-programs/magnet/

American Nurses Credentialing Center (n.d.-b) ANCC pathway to excellence program. https://www.nursingworld.org/organizational-programs/pathway/

Bakker AB, Demerouti E (2007) The job demands-resources model: state of the art. J Managerial Psych 22:309–328

Bakker AB, Demerouti E (2017) Job demands-resources theory: taking stock and looking forward. J Occup Health Psychol 22:273–285

Bakker AB, Albrecht SL, Leiter MP (2011) Key questions regarding work engagement. Eur J Work Organiz Psychol 20:4–28

Bolton LR, Harvey RD, Grawitch MJ, Barber LK (2012) Counterproductive work behaviours in response to emotional exhaustion: a moderated mediational approach. Stress Health 28:222–233

Braspenning M, Franck E (2013) Personality and interpersonal behavior. A cross-sectional study in nursing and medicine students. [Unpublished masters thesis]

Brigham T, Barden C, Dopp AL, Hengerer A, Kaplan J, Malone B, Martin C, McHugh M, Nora LM (2018) A journey to construct an all-encompassing conceptual model of factors affecting clinician well-being and resilience. NAM Perspectives. Discussion Paper. National Academy of Medicine, Washington, DC. https://doi.org/10.31478/201801b. https://nam.edu/journey-construct-encompassing-conceptual-model-factors-affecting-clinician-well-resilience/

Copanitsanou P, Fotos N, Brokalaki H (2017) Effects of work environment on patient and nurse outcomes. Br J Nurs 26(3):172–176. https://doi.org/10.12968/bjon.2017.26.3.172

Dahinten VS, Macphee M, Hejazi S et al (2014) Testing the effects of an empowerment-based leadership development programme: part 2—staff outcomes. J Nurs Manag 22:16–28

De Ridder D, Gillebaart M (2016) Lessons learned from trait self-control in well-being: making the case for routines and initiation as important components of trait self-control. Health Psychol Rev 11:1–29. https://doi.org/10.1080/17437199.2016.1266275

De Ridder D, Lensvelt-Mulders G, Finkenauer C, Stok M, Baumeister R (2012) Taking stock of self-control: a meta-analysis of how trait self-control relates to a wide range of behaviors. Personal Soc Psychol Rev 16:76–99. https://doi.org/10.1177/1088868311418749

Debisschop M (2017) Along with passion and talent: study, work and life from the "Inner Why". (Dutch title: Vertrekken met passie en talent. Studeren, werken en leven vanuit het 'inner why') Pelckmans

Dow WA, Baernholdt M, Santen AS, Baker K, Sessler CN (2019) Practitioner well-being as an interprofessional outcome. J Interprofess Care 33(6):603–607. https://doi.org/10.108 0/13561820.2019.1673705

Eo Y, Kim YH, Lee NY (2014) Path analysis of empowerment and work effectiveness among staff nurses. Asian Nurs Res 8:42–48

Estryn-Béhar M, Van der Heijden BI, Ogińska H et al (2007) The impact of social work environment, teamwork characteristics, burnout, and personal factors upon intent to leave among European nurses. Med Care 45:939–950

Franck E, Depauw R, Vanmechelen M (2016) Team resource Management in Antwerp University Hospital Operation Theatre. [Unpublished report]

Franck E, Roes L, De Schepper S, Timmermans O (2018) Team resource management and quality of care. In: Van Bogaert P, Clarke S (eds) The organizational context of nursing practice. Concepts, evidence, and interventions for improvement. Springer International Publishing, New York

Geuens N, Van Bogaert P, Franck E (2017) Vulnerability to burnout within the nursing workforce—the role of personality and interpersonal behavior. J Clin Nurs 26:23–24. https://doi.org/10.1111/jocn.13808

Gottfredson LS (1981) Circumscription and compromise: a developmental theory of occupational aspirations. J Counsell Psychol Monogr 6:545–579

Gurtman MB (2009) Exploring personality with the interpersonal circumplex. Soc Personal Psychol Compass 3:601–619

Halm M (2019) The influence of appropriate staffing and healthy work environments on patient and nurse outcomes. Am J Crit Care 28:152–156. https://doi.org/10.4037/ajcc2019938

Hasselhorn HM, Tackenberg P, Muller BH (2005) Nurses early exit (NEXT) scientific report. University of Wuppertal NEXT-study coordination. www.next-study.net

Heyhoe J, Birks Y, Harrison R, O'Hara JK, Cracknell A, Lawton R (2016) The role of emotion in patient safety: are we brave enough to scratch beneath the surface? J R Soc Med 109(2):52–58. https://doi.org/10.1177/0141076815620614

Hinds PS, Britton DR, Coleman L, Engh E, Kunze Humbel T, Keller S et al (2015) Creating a career legacy map to help assure meaningful work in nursing. Nurs Outlook 63:211–218. https://doi.org/10.1016/j.outlook.2014.08.002

Ibrahim RZAR, Ohtsuka K (2014) Review of the job demand-control and job demand-control-support models: elusive moderating predictor effects and cultural implications. Southeast Asia Psychol J 1:10–21

Kanter RM (1993) Men and women of the corporation, 2nd edn. Basis books, New York

Kelly LA, McHugh MD, Aiken LH (2012) Nurse outcomes in Magnet® and non-Magnet hospitals. J Nurs Adm 42:S44–S49

Kiesler DJ, Auerbach SM (2003) Integrating measurement of control and affiliation in studies of physician-patient interaction: the interpersonal circumplex. Soc Sci Med 57(9):1707–1722. https://doi.org/10.1016/S0277-9536(02)00558-0

Kramer M, Hafner LP (1989) Shared values: impact on staff nurse job satisfaction and perceived productivity. Nurs Res 38:172–177

Kramer M, Schmalenberg C (2002) Staff identify essentials of magnetism. In: McClure ML, Hinshaw AS (eds) Magnet hospitals revisited: attraction and retention of professional nurses. American Nurses Association Publishing, Washington, pp 25–59

Kutney-Lee A, Stimpfel AW, Sloane DM, Cimiotti JP, Quinn LW, Aiken LH (2015) Changes in patient and nurse outcomes associated with magnet hospital recognition. Med Care 53:550–557. https://doi.org/10.1097/MLR.0000000000000355

Lake ET (2002) Development of the practice environment scale of the nursing work index. Res Nurs Health 25:176–188

Lake ET, Sanders J, Duan R, Riman KA, Schoenauer KM, Chen Y (2019) A meta-analysis of the associations between the nurse work environment in hospitals and 4 sets of outcomes. Med Care 57:353–361. https://doi.org/10.1097/MLR.0000000000001109

Laschinger HK, Finegan J (2005) Empowering nurses for work engagement and health in hospital settings. J Nurs Adm 35:439–449

Laschinger HK, Finegan J, Shamian J, Wilk P (2001) Impact of structural and psychological empowerment on job strain in nursing work settings: expanding Kanter's model. J Nurs Adm 31:260–272

Laschinger HK, Almost J, Tuer-Hodes D (2003) Workplace empowerment and magnet hospital characteristics: making the link. J Nurs Adm 33:410–422

Laschinger HK, Finegan JE, Shamian J, Wilk P (2004) A longitudinal analysis of the impact of workplace empowerment on work satisfaction. J Organ Behav 25:527–545

Leiter MP, Maslach C (2009) Nurse turnover: the mediating role of burnout. J Nurs Manag 3:331–339

Leonard M, Graham S, Bonacum D (2004) The human factor: the critical importance of effective teamwork and communication in providing safe care. Qual Saf Health Care 13(suppl 1):85–90

MacPhee M, Bouthillette F (2008) Developing leadership in nurse managers: the British Columbia nursing leadership institute. Nurs Leadersh 21:64–75

MacPhee M, Skelton-Green J, Bouthillette F, Suryaprakash N (2012) An empowerment framework for nursing leadership development: supporting evidence. J Adv Nurs 68:159–169

MacPhee M, Dahinten VS, Hejazi S et al (2014) Testing the effects of an empowerment-based leadership development programme: part 1—leader outcomes. J Nurs Manag 22:4–15

Maslach C, Leiter MP (2008) Early predictors of job burnout and engagement. J Appl Psychol 93:498–512

Maslach C, Schaufeli WB, Leiter MP (2001) Job burnout. Annu Rev Psychol 52:397–422

McClure ML, Hinshaw AS (2002) Magnet hospitals revisited: attraction and retention of professional nurses. American Nurses Association Publishing, Washington

McClure ML, Poulin MA, Sovie MD, Wandelt MA (2002) Magnet hospitals: attraction and retention of professional nurses (the Original Study). In: McClure ML, Hinshaw AS (eds) Magnet hospitals revisited: attraction and retention of professional nurses. American Nurses Association Publishing, Washington, pp 1–24

Mimura C, Griffiths P, Norman I (2009) Editorial: what motivates people to enter professional nursing? Int J Nurs Stud 46:603–605

Mitchell PH, Ferketich S, Jennings BM (1998) Quality Health Outcomes Model. Image J Nurs Sch 30(1):43–46

Petit Dit Dariel O, Regnaux JP (2015) Do Magnet®-accredited hospitals show improvements in nurse and patient outcomes compared to non-Magnet hospitals: a systematic review. JBI Database System Rev Implement Rep 13(6):168–219. https://doi.org/10.11124/jbisrir-2015-2262

Redeker M, de Vries R, Rouckhout D, Vermeren P, De Fruyt F (2012) Integrating leadership: the leadership circumplex. Eur J Work Organiz Psychol 23:435–455. https://doi.org/10.108 0/1359432X.2012.738671

Schaufeli W, Bakker A (2003) Utrecht work engagement scale: preliminary manual. Department of Psychology, Utrecht University Utrecht the Netherlands, Utrecht

Schaufeli WB, Salonova M (2011) Work engagement: on how to better catch a slippery concept. Eur J Work Organiz Psychol 20:39–46

Schmalenberg C, Kramer M (2008) Essentials of a productive nurse work environment. Nurs Res 57:2–13. https://doi.org/10.1097/01.NNR.0000280657.04008.2a

Schutz A (1998) Autobiographical narratives of good and bad deeds: defensive and favourable self-description moderated by trait self-esteem. J Soc Clin Psychol 17(4):466–475

Sermeus W, Aiken LH, Van den Heede K et al (2011) Nurse forecasting in Europe (RN4CAST): rationale, design and methodology. BMC Nurs 10:6. https://doi.org/10.1186/1472-6955-10-6

Sinek S (2009) How great leaders inspire action [Video]. TED Conferences. https://www.ted.com/talks/simon_sinek_how_great_leaders_inspire_action

Singleton JK, Santomasino M, Slyer JT (2015) A team process to support interprofessional care. J Interprofessional Educ Pract 1(1):28–31. https://doi.org/10.1016/j.xjep.2015.03.005

Spreitzer GM (1995) Psychological empowerment in the workplace: dimensions, measurement, and validation. Acad Manag J 38:1442–1465

Stimpfel AW, Rosen JE, McHugh MD (2014) Understanding the role of the professional practice environment on quality of care in Magnet® and non-Magnet hospitals. J Nurs Administr 44:10–16. https://doi.org/10.1097/NNA.0000000000000015

Urden LD, Monarch K (2002) The ANCC magnet recognition program converting research findings into action. In: McClure ML, Hinshaw AS (eds) Magnet hospitals revisited: attraction and retention of professional nurses. American Nurses Association Publishing, Washington, pp 103–115

Vallerand RJ (2012) The role of passion in sustainable psychological well-being. Psychol Well-Being: Theory Res Pract 2:1–21

Van Bogaert P, Clarke S (2018a) Concepts: organization of nursing work and the psychosocial experience of nurses. In: Van Bogaert P, Clarke S (eds) The organizational context of nursing practice: concepts; evidence and Interventions for improvements. Springer, New York, pp 5–47

Van Bogaert P, Clarke S (2018b) Organizational predictors and determinants of nurses' reported outcomes: evidence from a 10-year program of research. In: Van Bogaert P, Clarke S (eds) The organizational context of nursing practice: concepts; evidence and Interventions for improvements. Springer, New York, pp 49–100

Van Bogaert P, Clarke S, Vermeyen K, Meulemans H, Van de Heyning P (2009) Practice environments and their associations with nurse-reported outcomes in Belgian hospitals: development and preliminary validation of a Dutch adaptation of the Revised Nursing Work Index. Int J Nurs Stud 46:54–64

Van Bogaert P, Clarke S, Roelant E, Meulemans H, Van de Heyning P (2010) Impacts of unit-level nurse practice environment and burnout on nurse-reported outcomes: a multilevel modelling approach. J Clin Nurs 19:1664–1674

Van Bogaert P, Clarke S, Wouters K, Franck E, Willems R, Mondelaers M (2013) Impacts of unit-level nurse practice environment, workload and burnout on nurse-reported outcomes in psychiatric hospitals: a multilevel modelling approach. Int J Nurs Stud 50:357–365

Van Bogaert P, Timmermans O, Weeks SM, van Heusden D, Wouters K, Franck E (2014a) Nursing unit teams matter: impact of unit-level nurse practice environment, nurse work characteristics, and burnout on nurse reported job outcomes, and quality of care, and patient adverse events—a cross-sectional survey. Int J Nurs Stud 51:1123–1134

Van Bogaert P, Van Heusden D, Somers A et al (2014b) The Productive Ward program™: a longitudinal multilevel study of nurse perceived practice environment, burnout, and nurse-reported quality of care and job outcomes. J Nurs Adm 44:452–461

Van Bogaert P, Peremans L, Van Heusden D et al (2017a) Predictors of burnout, work engagement and nurse reported job outcomes and quality of care: a mixed method study. BMC Nurs 16:5

Van Bogaert P, Van Heusden D, Verspuy M et al (2017b) The Productive Ward Program™: a two-year implementation impact review using a longitudinal multilevel study. Can J Nurs Res 49:28–38

Van Bogaert P, Van Heusden D, Slootmans S et al (2018) Staff empowerment and engagement in a Magnet® recognized and joint commission international accredited academic centre in Belgium: a cross-sectional survey. BMC Health Serv Res 2018(18):756

Wagner JL, Warren S, Cummings G, Smith DL, Olson JK (2013) Resonant leadership, workplace empowerment, and "spirit at work": impact on RN job satisfaction and organizational commitment. Can J Nurs Res 45:108–128

Wei H, Sewell KA, Woody G, Rose MA (2018) The state of the science of nurse work environments in the United States: a systematic review. Int J Nurs Sci 5:287–300. https://doi.org/10.1016/j.ijnss.2018.04.010

White M, Wells JS, Butterworth T (2014) The productive ward: releasing time to care(™)—what we can learn from the literature for implementation. J Nurs Manag 22(7):914–923

Wolf GA, Greenhouse PK (2006) A road map for creating a Magnet work environment. J Nurs Adm 36:458–462

Yang J, Liu Y, Huang C, Zhu L (2013) Impact of empowerment on professional practice environments and organizational commitment among nurses: a structural equation approach. International journal of nursing practice. Int J Nurs Pract 19:44–55

Zysberg L, Berry DM (2005) Gender and students' vocational choices in entering the field of nursing. Nurs Outlook 53:193–198

Organizational Outcomes: Financial and Quality Measures

Nancy Dunton and Amenda Fisher

Introduction

In the two decades since the release of the National Institute of Medicine's report *To Err is Human: Building a Safer Health System* (1999), the nation has been focusing on improving patient care safety in hospitals, nursing homes, and other healthcare organizations. Improvement efforts include quality indicator (measure) development and utilization, assessment of the patient experience of care, identification and implementation of best practices, and assessment and promotion of a supportive practice environment (Bodenheimer and Sinsky 2014; Sikka et al. 2015). Measures of patient safety and care quality have made the continuing problem of patient safety visible to all stakeholders: patients, providers, payers, and policymakers. Policy mechanisms were implemented to improve patient care, including the use of comparison data in performance reports, public reporting, and payment incentives. These initiatives have had financial and reputational consequences (outcomes) for healthcare organizations.

This chapter addresses healthcare organization outcomes as an essential component of the QHOM. The chapter briefly reviews the history of policy initiatives and trends in organizational quality outcomes and concludes by discussing current issues in measuring and reporting organizational outcomes.

N. Dunton (✉)
Center for Healthcare Quality Research, School of Nursing, University of Kansas, Kansas City, KS, USA
e-mail: ndunton@kumc.edu

A. Fisher
Health & Well-Being, Walmart Inc., Bentonville, AR, USA
e-mail: amenda.Fisher@Walmart.com

© Springer Nature Switzerland AG 2021
M. Baernholdt, D. K. Boyle (eds.), *Nurses Contributions to Quality Health Outcomes*, https://doi.org/10.1007/978-3-030-69063-2_14

Healthcare Organizational Outcomes: Specific Linkages with the QHOM

The conceptual framework underlying the discussion of healthcare organizations' outcomes is based on the QHOM (Mitchell et al. 1998). Moving from Donabedian's (1966) linear structure-process-outcomes construct to a dynamic model, the QHOM depicts multiple feedback loops among the healthcare environmental context, environmental context, organizational characteristics, interventions, and organizational outcomes (Fig. 14.1). An advantage of the QHOM in relation to organizational outcomes is the ability to examine and understand macro-, meso-, and microlevel factors (Serpa and Ferreira 2019). For purposes of this chapter, macro-level factors work at the policy, regulatory, societal, and political levels. Meso-level factors span from the healthcare corporate or system level to the individual organizations (e.g., hospitals) within them. Microlevel factors are at the individual and unit levels, such as attitudes toward safety culture.

The healthcare environmental context (macro level) represents the conditions that affect both system and organizational structure, interventions, and outcomes. The environment includes healthcare policy, discussed in Chap. 2, the state of health science, and the prevailing status of population health, including social determinants of health and chronicity, discussed in Chaps. 7 and 8. The healthcare environment influences the structure of healthcare systems and individual organizations by setting physical plant and patient care requirements, conducting licensing and accreditation, and establishing reimbursement levels. Advances in health and healthcare science may result in new technology and new evidence-based practices. Environmental factors influence system organizational characteristics by

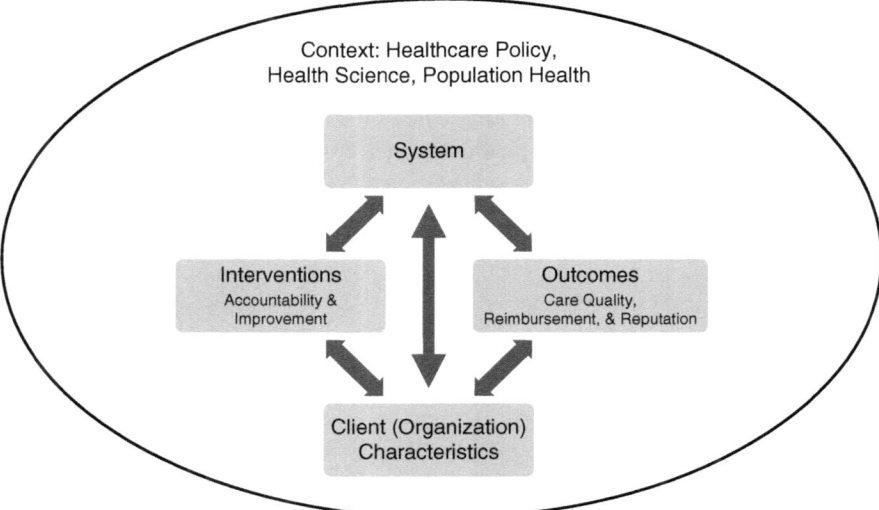

Fig. 14.1 Framework for healthcare organizational outcomes

influencing profitability, contributing to and taking advantage of new science, and meeting patient and provider populations' needs.

The focus of this chapter is primarily hospitals. Because the majority of hospitals belong to a more extensive healthcare system or corporation (AHA 2018), *the system* refers to the overall corporation, and *the client* (organization) refers to individual hospitals. Both system and client are at the meso level. Hospital organizational characteristics are descriptors such as ownership (profit, not-for-profit, public nonfederal, federal), teaching status (academic medical center, teaching, nonteaching), size (number of beds), rural or urban, critical access status, Magnet status (Magnet Recognition or not), and healthcare corporate system membership. These features reflect financial resources, professional resources, and a focus on nursing quality. Organizational characteristics may influence the healthcare environment through consideration of resources available to respond to policy change. For instance, adequately funded hospitals can financially invest in safer and cleaner environments or programs like the American Nurses Credentialing Center's (ANCC) Magnet or Pathways to Excellence (ANCC n.d.). ANCC's programs are dedicated to creating superior nurse work environments (see interventions section below and Chap. 4). Organizations with academic affiliations also influence the environment through advances in healthcare science and evidence-based practices. These attributes attract highly educated and credentialed professionals trained to focus on patient care and outcomes, thus creating the optimal environment for superior patient and organizational outcomes. In turn, organizational characteristics influence organizational outcomes in patient care quality and financial and reputational outcomes.

The healthcare environment and accountability interventions are closely linked because the interventions arise from health policy, accreditation standards, and professional guidelines in the healthcare environment (macro level). The relationship is reciprocal, as the success, or lack of success, of the interventions may lead to policy change. Accountability interventions include tracking and reporting on healthcare quality metrics and payment incentives. Generally, payment incentives are based on organizational performance on quality outcome measures. Payment incentives include nonpayment for the patient care provided as a result of an adverse event deemed to be avoidable. Payment incentives also take the form of changes to reimbursement rates, generally based on performance on patient care quality measures.

Organizational outcomes include performance on quality indicators (care quality), reputation for providing safe and high-quality care, and changes in reimbursement levels due to patient care quality. Accountability interventions work through the system and client (organization) to influence organizational outcomes. The interventions are put in place to promote the quality and efficiency of patient care. The degree to which organizations succeed in preventing adverse events and have an acceptable performance on patient outcomes constitutes part of the reimbursement calculation. Performance on some patient outcomes has reputational consequences through public reporting at federal, state, and system levels.

Outcomes provide feedback to model elements. Patient outcomes and related reputational and reimbursement outcomes influence the healthcare environment, or macro level, in that performance may stimulate healthcare quality policy changes.

In turn, policy changes may influence the specifics of accountability interventions. Finally, organizational outcomes influence system and organization (client), or meso-level, characteristics by stimulating structural changes to improve access to professional resources and to maximize revenue.

Evolution of Policies and Programs to Promote Safer Patient Care

Federal, state, and other organizations interested in healthcare outcomes have accountability policies that promote safe and high-quality patient care (see Table 14.1 for selected examples). As described in Chap. 2, policies have evolved from support for measure development for quality improvement programs to public

Table 14.1 Healthcare quality stakeholders

Stakeholder organization	Mission
Agency for Healthcare Quality and Research	To produce evidence to make healthcare safer, higher quality, more accessible, equitable, and affordable, and work within the US Department of Health and Human Services and with other partners to make sure that the evidence is understood and used
American Nurses Association	To lead the profession to shape the future of nursing and healthcare
American Nurses Credentialing Center Magnet Recognition Program Pathway to Excellence	To promote excellence in nursing and healthcare globally through credentialing programs
Centers for Disease Control	To protect America from health, safety, and security threats, both foreign and in the USA
Centers for Medicare & Medicaid Services Partnership for Patients Patient Safety Organizations	To serve Medicare and Medicaid beneficiaries
The Joint Commission	To continuously improve healthcare for the public, in collaboration with other stakeholders, by evaluating healthcare organizations and inspiring them to excel in providing safe and effective care of the highest quality and value
The Leapfrog Group	To trigger giant leaps forward in the safety, quality, and affordability of healthcare by supporting informed healthcare decisions by those who use and pay for healthcare, and promoting high-value healthcare through incentives and rewards
National Quality Forum	To scientifically assess and evaluate the quality of healthcare in various settings and create measures, or performance standards, that can be endorsed as best-practice methods to be used by healthcare facilities in the USA

reporting and recognition for quality performance, and then to financial incentives. Reputational and quality outcome measures directly influence organizational financial outcomes through payer reimbursement incentives and indirectly through consumer choice in selecting healthcare providers. This section discusses policies designed to promote safe and high-quality patient care, highlighting the reputational and reimbursement outcomes for healthcare organizations.

Quality and Safety Measurement

Recognition of escalating healthcare costs and patient safety issues in the modern era commenced with implementing capitated payment systems in the 1980s (see Chap. 2 for more details). The goal of managed care was to reduce healthcare costs. In response, many hospitals cut the number of registered nurses (RNs) in their employment. These reductions led the American Nurses Association, The Joint Commission, The Leapfrog Group, and other stakeholder organizations to be concerned about patient care quality and safety (American Nurses Association 1995; Huntington 1997). The initial responses were to develop healthcare quality and safety measures that could be used in quality improvement programs.

Importantly for nurses, the American Nurses Association began developing the National Database of Nursing Quality Indicators® (NDNQI®) in 1992, identifying measures relevant to nursing care and pilot testing them (e.g., injury falls and pressure injuries). The NDNQI database was established in 1998 to provide hospitals with unit-level quality measures for use in quality improvement programs (Montalvo 2007). NDNQI hospital reports contain unit-level data with comparison data for similar units in similar hospitals, for example. Today, more than 2000 hospitals in the USA participate in NDNQI (Press-Ganey n.d.). Table 14.2 provides an example of two NDNQI measures and how they align with the QHOM constructs of client, interventions, and outcomes.

For NDNQI® and other healthcare quality databases, quality and safety measure use was voluntary, and comparison data typically were not available. By 1999, hundreds of measures existed, and the National Quality Forum (NQF) was established to promote the adoption of standardized measures to facilitate comparisons across healthcare organizations. In 2001, the Agency for Healthcare Research and Quality (AHRQ) implemented three measurement programs: Inpatient Quality Indicators, Patient Safety Indicators, and Prevention Quality Indicators (AHRQ 2018c). AHRQ produced national comparison data for organizations to target and track quality improvement initiatives. It also provided information to federal policymakers and data for researchers. In 2005, the Centers for Medicare & Medicaid Services (CMS) implemented public reporting of a set of inpatient measures in the Hospital Compare program to promote further improvements in healthcare quality (CMS n.d.). Prospective patients were encouraged to visit the site and select hospitals with better quality and safety outcomes.

Table 14.2 NDNQI indicators organized by the QHOM concepts of client, interventions, and outcomes

Indicator	Client	Interventions	Outcomes

Pressure injuries	• Age
	• Gender
	• At risk based on last assessment
	• Physical restraints in place
		• Risk assessment on admission
		• Time since last risk assessment
		• Risk assessment scale
		• Risk assessment score
		• Prevention measures within 24 hours
		  – Skin assessment
		  – Pressure redistribution surface
		  – Routine repositioning
		  – Nutritional support
		  – Moisture management
			• Pressure injury rate
			• Stage
			  – I–IV
			  – Unstageable/unclassified
			  – Indeterminant
			  – Deep-tissue injury
			  – Kennedy terminal ulcer
			  – Healing/closed
			  – Healed
			• Origin
			  – Community
			  – Hospital
			  – Unit

Patient falls	• Age
	• Gender
	• At risk based on last assessment
	• Prior fall within last month
	• Physical restraints in place
		• Risk assessment on admission
		• Time since last risk assessment
		• Risk assessment scale
		• Risk assessment score
		• Prevention protocol in place
			• Fall rate
			• Assisted fall rate
			• Injury fall rate
			• Injury level
			  – None
			  – Minor
			  – Moderate
			  – Major
			  – Death
			• Physiological fall
			• Child/baby drop
			• Developmental fall
			• Suspected intentional fall

Quality and Safety Measure Development

Quality measures are carefully specified rates or ratios representing the structure of care, care processes (interventions), or care outcomes. Standardized measures make it possible to compare provider or organizational performance. Structural measures describe the provider organization's resources and characteristics, such as the availability of nurse staffing or the safety culture. Care process measures describe the frequency of appropriate care practices (e.g., prevention measures in place for falls or pressure injuries). Outcome measures represent the frequency of good or poor patient care, such as adverse events (e.g., injurious falls, pressure injuries, healthcare-acquired infections) or patient satisfaction with the care experience.

The development of quality measures is a multistep process, typically taking 2 years to complete (NQF 2012). Measures are based on a very detailed and specific description of data elements. Draft measures are tested for reliability and validity and then assessed for importance to improving healthcare quality. Draft measures may also be risk adjusted or stratified to promote valid comparisons across provider organizations. After initial implementation, measures are assessed for usability or the extent to which they are used in quality improvement and public reporting and as part of reimbursement formulae. Developed measures must be reevaluated every few years to ensure that they continue to represent important care concerns, remain accurately specified, capture the state of the science for each care area, are still valid and reliable, and are used by the stakeholder community.

Federal Reimbursement Accountability Initiatives

Federal and other payor reimbursement policies are based, in part, on measures of patient care quality and experience of care. In 2008, CMS implemented the Hospital-Acquired Condition (HAC) program that withheld reimbursement for care provided for 14 hospital-acquired adverse events (CMS 2018b). As part of the HAC program, the Present on Admission Program stimulated hospitals to identify whether any of the 14 conditions (e.g., pressure injuries) were "present on admission" rather than having them be identified later as a hospital-acquired condition. Reimbursement for healthcare costs was not provided for the 14 hospital-acquired conditions.

CMS implemented three additional reimbursement incentive programs between 2012 and 2014 to promote a higher quality of care for Medicare beneficiaries: Hospital Readmission Reduction Program (HRRP; CMS 2018a), Hospital Value-Based Purchasing Program (VBP; CMS 2017), and Hospital-Acquired Condition Reduction Program (HACRP; CMS 2020). These CMS programs are described in detail in Chap. 2.

AHRQ then set a national goal to reduce HACs by 20%. The goal is connected to the CMS Hospital Improvement Innovation Networks, a collaborative group of federal and private partners dedicated to improving healthcare quality by reducing HACs (AHRQ 2018a). To improve tracking and reduce HACs and adverse events, AHRQ is developing and testing the Quality and Safety Review System (AHRQ 2018b). The surveillance system automatically pulls data from electronic health records to generate HAC event rates and measure organizational performance over time.

Nonfederal Quality Improvement Initiatives

Besides federal interventions that promote healthcare quality and recognize organizations for their efforts to exceed quality standards, other stakeholder organizations have developed programs that leverage reputation to drive innovation and healthcare improvements. The American Nurses Credentialing Center, a subsidiary of the American Nurses Association, and the Leapfrog Group have been pioneers in leading changes that facilitated quality improvements. They continue to support improved organizational outcomes today.

ANCC Magnet Recognition Program

Magnet Recognition is a credentialing program designed to identify domestic and international healthcare organizations that successfully align their nursing strategy with organizational goals to optimize patient outcomes (American Nurses Credentialing Center (ANCC) n.d.). The program serves as a road map to nursing excellence. In turn, nursing excellence drives measurable improvements in organizational outcomes related to safety, quality care, and financial savings. As part of the program, Magnet organizations must measure and report nurse job satisfaction, nurse-sensitive clinical measures, and patient satisfaction (ANCC n.d.). The required reporting metrics are specific to outcomes related to each of the 14 Forces of Magnetism (e.g., nursing leadership, quality improvement, quality of care) (ANCC n.d.). See Chap. 4 for a more detailed description of the Magnet Program.

Research indicates that Magnet hospitals are associated with lower levels of burnout and turnover and greater job satisfaction in nurses (Kelly et al. 2012), which are organizational human resource outcomes associated with improved patient outcomes. A growing body of research indicates that Magnet hospitals are associated with decreased rates of central line bloodstream infections (Barnes et al. 2016), lower odds of developing hospital-acquired pressure injuries (Ma and Park 2015), reduced patient mortality (Kutney-Lee et al. 2015; Olds et al. 2017), and higher nurse-reported care quality (Stimpfel et al. 2014). Improved patient safety has also been associated with Magnet hospitals. Researchers found that patients had fewer falls in Magnet than non-Magnet hospitals (Lake et al. 2010), and Magnet hospitals demonstrated greater adoption of National Quality Forum safe practices (Jayawardhana et al. 2011).

Improved work environments for nurses, delivery of quality care, a safety culture, and better patient outcomes translate to improved healthcare organizations' revenues. According to a study commissioned by the Robert Wood Johnson Foundation, Magnet hospitals experienced an increased net patient revenue between $104.22 and $127.05 per discharge, which generated an additional $1.2 million in hospital income per year on average (Jayawardhana et al. 2014).

ANCC Pathway to Excellence Program

The ANCC Pathway to Excellence Program (PTE) is another recognition program that identifies healthcare organizations dedicated to delivering positive practice environments for nurses (ANCC n.d.). The Pathway to Excellence Program is complementary to the Magnet Recognition Program. It focuses on six standards essential for an exemplary nurse practice environment: shared decision-making, nursing leadership, safety, quality and evidence-based clinical care, practices that promote nurse well-being, and professional development (Dans et al. 2017). See Chap. 4 for more detailed information on the PTE Program.

Positive practice environments are associated with nurse job satisfaction and retention, promoting inter-professional teamwork, facilitating high-quality nurse practices, and supporting business growth of the healthcare organization (ANCC n.d.). As with the Magnet Program, the outcomes associated with the PTE designation equate to improved organizational outcomes that extend beyond the realm of nursing practice. Expenses related to human resources negatively impact an organization's profitability. On average, turnover of one bedside nurse equates to a loss of $49,500, costing hospitals between $4.4 and $7.0 million annually (Colosi 2018), and working in a suboptimal practice environment is a leading reason nurses leave their job (Park et al. 2016). Furthermore, research has shown that positive practice environments are associated with reduced staff nurse turnover (Nelson-Brantley et al. 2018).

The Leapfrog Group

The Leapfrog Group was founded in 2000 by employers and healthcare purchasers with a mission to foster safety, quality, and affordability in healthcare through performance transparency (Leapfrog n.d.). It was founded on the principle that healthcare consumers should have information about organizational and clinical outcomes and pricing to inform purchasing decisions. As large purchasers of healthcare services, employers and insurers possess significant power to affect change. Through these healthcare payors' support, the Leapfrog Group has promoted a marketplace for high-quality and high-value healthcare.

In 2001, the organization administered the first Leapfrog Hospital Survey to 496 hospitals (Leapfrog n.d.). A year later, the number of participating hospitals doubled, and Leapfrog premiered its public reporting website to promote information transparency. The initial survey was dedicated to understanding hospital performance related to quality and efficiency; however, it was expanded in 2003 to include a safety focus. The expanded hospital survey incorporated the National Quality Forum's Safe Practices for Better Healthcare, a questionnaire that examines the use of practices proven to reduce adverse healthcare events (NQF 2010).

Through the Leapfrog Hospital Survey, the organization now collects data on nearly 1900 hospitals. It provides comparable performance information specific to medication safety, never events, antibiotic stewardship, physician staffing in intensive care units, maternity care, infections, surgery volume and appropriateness, and pediatric care (Leapfrog n.d.). The survey data are also used to recognize high-performing hospitals in three Leapfrog programs: Top Hospitals, Hospital Safety Grade, and Value-Based Purchasing Program. Although similar to federal quality improvement programs, Leapfrog programs are separate and primarily serve to inform healthcare purchasers beyond the federal government.

The Leapfrog Top Hospital program identifies the best hospitals based on quality outcomes and commends these hospitals through public recognition and a hospital ranking system (Leapfrog n.d.). The organization also helps health insurance plans, employers, and other large healthcare purchasers identify the highest value hospitals in specific markets through their own Value-Based Purchasing Program. This information allows healthcare purchasers to develop benefits packages and customized provider networks that produce high-value, quality care that meets their insured populations' needs.

Rating systems that use organizational measures to identify quality outcomes are often called into question due to the lack of transparency around measurement constructs and reproducibility. Researchers praised Leapfrog's Hospital Safety Grade for measurement transparency and reproducibility of outcomes stating that Leapfrog can confidently say that their hospital safety scores represent what the organization claims to measure (Popovich et al. 2020). Researchers also compared Leapfrog's Hospital Safety Score and Magnet Designation on rates of healthcare-associated infections. They concluded that there was some evidence that the two quality initiatives were associated with lower levels of healthcare-associated infections. However, the evidence was inconsistent and highlighted the degree of difficulty in developing highly reliable quality performance indicators (Pakyz et al. 2017).

Hospital Organizational Outcomes

Improvement in Quality and Safety Measures

The federal public reporting and reimbursement incentive programs described above and in Chap. 2 were designed to improve patient care quality, as reflected in quality and safety measures, and to reduce healthcare costs. A variety of sources have reported reductions in many hospital-acquired conditions (HACs) between the early 2000s and 2018 (Bates and Singh 2018; Campanella et al. 2016; Kruse et al. 2012; Mathes et al. 2019). No single data source is available for the entire period or all outcome measures. Most sources show improvements in quality that have a loose coincidence with federal policy initiatives.

Reductions in adverse events may be related to many factors besides accountability policies, such as advancements in health sciences and care protocols combined with continuing education on best practices, implementing a safety culture, and support from hospital leadership. Absent controls for changes in health science, independent studies have provided conflicting evidence as to the effectiveness of interventions aimed at reducing HACs.

AHRQ (AHRQ 2019) is responsible for tracking 28 safety measures on behalf of the federal government. AHRQ reported that there was a 17% reduction in the number of HACs between 2010 and 2014. There were 2.1 million fewer HACs in 2014 than in 2011. Using a revised methodology, AHRQ found a further reduction in HACs between 2014 and 2017 of 13%. There were 910,000 fewer HACs in 2017 than in 2014. Between 2010 and 2017, the average annual reduction in HACs was 4.5%. The reduction rates were greatest between 2011 and 2013. This timeframe was after the nonpayment for HAC policy was implemented in 2008 and while the readmission reduction program was implemented, but before the Value-Based Purchasing Program was enacted.

In 2017, the total HAC rate was 86 HACs per 1000 discharges (AHRQ 2019). Rates varied widely across specific conditions. The highest HAC rates were for adverse drug events (24.2/1000 discharges) and pressure injuries (23.0/1000), whereas the lowest HAC rates were for central line-associated bloodstream infections (0.27/1000) and venous thromboembolism (0.7/1000). AHRQ reported that the downward trend was not the same for all HACs. Between 2014 and 2017 the

HACs with the best improvements were *Clostridium difficile* infections (−27%) and adverse drug events (−28%), whereas the pressure injury rate increased by 6%.

Lee et al. (2012) examined changes in preventable infection rates following the 2008 HAC nonpayment policy implementation and found no evidence that the policy had a measurable impact. However, other researchers measuring the effects of the HAC nonpayment policy noted reductions in central line-associated bloodstream infection (−11%) and catheter-associated urinary tract infection (−10%) rates, for which there are robust evidence-based prevention protocols (Waters et al. 2015). Waters et al. (2015) found no reductions in injurious fall rates or hospital-acquired pressure injury rates.

Independent studies have shown reductions in unplanned or avoidable readmissions following quality improvement initiatives (Baky et al. 2018; Ryan et al. 2017). In a mandated report to Congress attesting to the Hospital Readmission Reduction Program's effects, researchers showed that the program reduced hospital readmissions by 3–4% (Medicare Payment Advisory Commission 2018).

The National Database of Nursing Quality Indicators (NDNQI) has trend data on total inpatient falls and hospital-acquired pressure injuries from 2004 through 2018. Reductions in fall and pressure injury rates began in 2009 after implementing the CMS Present on Admission Program. Some improvement was due to removing community-acquired conditions from the count of hospital-acquired adverse events as required by the Present on Admission Program. However, some of the improvement was a result of hospital quality improvement initiatives.

The NDNQI trend line in the total fall rate (Fig. 14.2) shows a steady decline beginning in 2007. There was a 15% drop in the rate between 2007 and 2008, as the CMS nonpayment for HAC policy was implemented. Fall rates declined by 15% between 2011 and 2012 and by 24% between 2013 and 2014, when the CMS value-based purchasing policy went into effect.

Trends in the hospital-acquired pressure injury prevalence rate from NDNQI data are presented in Fig. 14.3. Rates were stable between 2006 and 2007. They

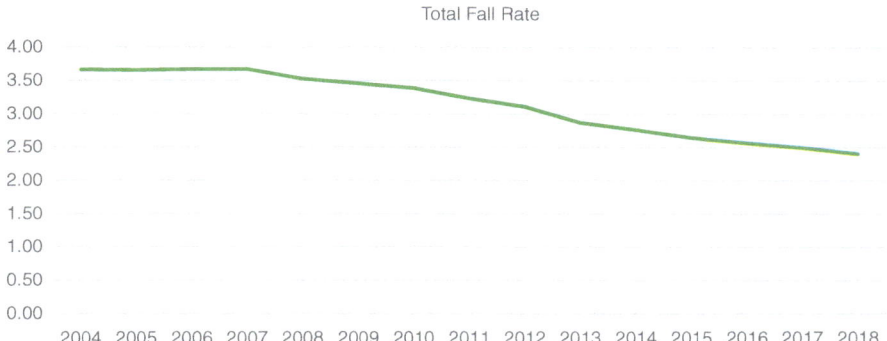

Fig. 14.2 Trends in total inpatient fall rate from 2004 to 2018. Legend: Rate is total falls per 1000 patient days

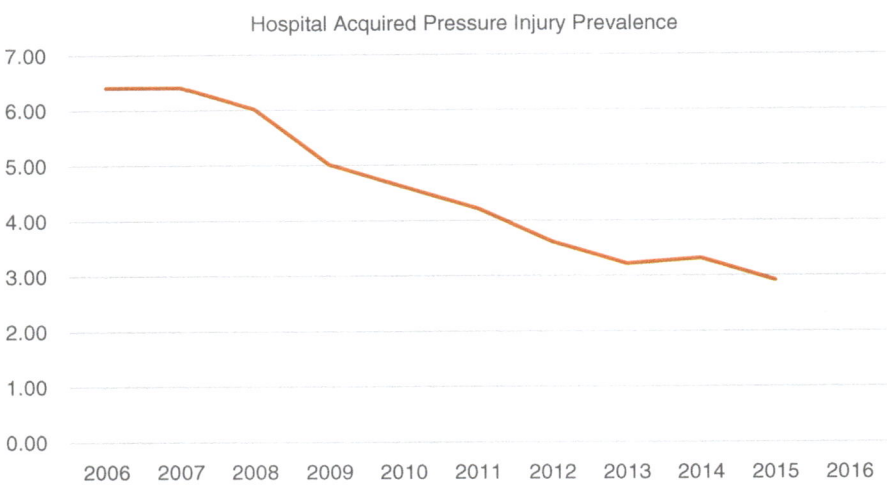

Fig. 14.3 Trends in hospital-acquired pressure injury prevalence rate from 2006 to 2016. Legend: Rate is the number of patients who acquired a pressure injury after admission to the hospital divided by the total number of patients in the population studied

declined by 6% between 2007 and 2008, and by 16% between 2008 and 2009, when the CMS nonpayment for HACs was implemented. Pressure injury rates continued to decline by 8–14% per year through 2015, except for 2013–2014 when the pressure injury rate increased.

Reimbursement Outcomes

As a result of improvement in HACs, AHRQ (2019) reported a cost saving of $19.9 billion. Between 2014 and 2017, AHRQ found that HAC reductions resulted in a $7.7 billion cost saving. Alternately, under the CMS Value-Based Purchasing Program (VBP), 751 hospitals were penalized in 2017 for safety and infection concerns. Of those hospitals penalized in 2017, over half were also penalized for underperformance in 2016 (Rau 2017). Performance varied across specific outcomes. For instance, researchers did not find significant differences in inpatient mortality between VBP hospitals and non-VBP hospitals (Figueroa et al. 2016). Similarly, the VBP program was not associated with improvements in clinical processes, patient satisfaction, or two out of three mortality measures (Ryan et al. 2017). Approximately $1.9 billion was available for VBP incentive payments in the fiscal year 2018, and 55% of participating hospitals received bonuses (CMS 2018c). In 2018, CMS reported improvement in the average Total Performance Score across all hospitals participating in VBP, indicating that healthcare quality and value in the USA had improved (CMS 2018c).

Implications and Future Directions

Interpreted through the framework of the QHOM (Fig. 14.1), healthcare policy-based accountability incentives, based on quality measures, have improved safety. Trends in improved safety are broadly coincident with the expansion of federal policy initiatives, particularly with the 2008 implementation of the CMS policy of nonpayment for HACs. Yet, hospitals' number of adverse events remains unacceptably high at 2,550,000 HACs in 2017 (AHRQ 2019). The degree to which safety has improved varies across HACs, with greater improvement in hospital-acquired infections and medication safety and limited improvement in patient falls and pressure injuries. Several studies have reported that improved patient safety has been impeded by the inconsistent implementation of evidence-based practice and the need for hospital leadership to embrace and support a culture change to a learning health system (Bates and Singh 2018).

Recent studies have found that, on balance, hospitals' reimbursement penalties are quite small relative to their operating budgets (Bazzoli et al. 2018; Kruse et al. 2012; Mathes et al. 2019). Current reimbursement policies have been subject to a variety of criticisms. Criticisms include questioning the reliability and validity of measures, especially those derived from electronic health records (EHRs); whether there is adequate risk adjustment across hospital types; the degree to which HACs are preventable; and the tendency for penalties to drive the quality improvement focus on what can be measured (Bates and Singh 2018). Moreover, reimbursement penalties for HACs may have the unintended consequence of reduced reporting by omitting the HAC from the healthcare record, coding a HAC as a different event (e.g., wound rather than pressure injury) or coding them with a level of severity that is below the policy threshold (e.g., coding a Stage 3 pressure injury as a Stage 1 or 2). Miscoded or underreported safety events may prevent a reduction in the organization's reimbursement rates and could result in invalid data upon which to assess the nation's burden of patient harm.

With the continuing need to address healthcare quality, future health policy initiatives may benefit from understanding current quality measures and incentive programs' limitations and criticisms. Members of the American Academy of Nursing's Quality Expert Panel recently published recommendations for improving quality measurement (Baernholdt et al. 2018). Issues include:

- Measure purpose: Consumer choice or quality improvement
- Meaningful measurement
- Gaps in measurement
- Importance of structural characteristics
- Validity and reliability concerns with existing measures
- Too much time devoted to measurement

Within the context of a richer data environment in EHRs, the path to safer, higher quality patient care may incorporate more complex understandings of the multiple influences on quality. These include leadership support of a learning environment, safety culture, and implementation science application in which evidence-based care protocols are widely adopted. In this environment, the capture of care processes would take on new importance. Incentives to promote safe and high-quality care may beneficially be linked to the delivery of effective care practices.

References

Agency for Healthcare Research and Quality (2018a) AHRQ national scorecard on hospital-acquired conditions: updated baseline rates and preliminary results 2014–2016. https://www.ahrq.gov/sites/default/files/wysiwyg/professionals/quality-patient-safety/pfp/natlhacratereport-rebaselining2014-2016_0.pdf

Agency for Healthcare Research and Quality (2018b) AHRQ quality and safety review system. https://www.ahrq.gov/professionals/quality-patient-safety/qsrs/index.html

Agency for Healthcare Research and Quality (2018c) AHR quality Indicators™ https://www.ahrq.gov/cpi/about/otherwebsites/qualityindicators.ahrq.gov/qualityindicators.html

Agency for Healthcare Research and Quality (2019) AHRQ scorecard on hospital-acquired conditions: updated baseline rates and preliminary results 2014–2017. https://psnet.ahrq.gov/issue/ahrq-national-scorecard-hospital-acquired-conditions-updated-baseline-rates-and-preliminary-0

American Hospital Association (2018) AHA Hospital Statistics, 2018 Edition

American Nurses Association (1995) Nursings report card for acute care. American Nurses Publishing, Washington, DC

American Nurses Credentialing Center (n.d.) Organizational programs: Magnet Recognition Program and Pathway to Excellence Program. https://www.nursingworld.org/organizational-programs/

Baernholdt M, Dunton N, Hughes R, Stone P, White K (2018) Quality measures: a stakeholder analysis. J Nurs Care Qual 33(2):149–156. https://doi.org/10.1097/NCQ.0000000000000292

Baky V, Moran D, Warwick T, George A, Williams T, McWilliams E, Marine JE (2018) Obtaining a follow-up appointment before discharge protects against readmission for patients with acute coronary syndrome and heart failure: a quality improvement project. Int J Cardiol 257:12–15. https://doi.org/10.1016/j.ijcard.2017.10.036

Barnes H, Rearden J, McHugh MD (2016) Magnet® hospital recognition linked to lower central line-associated bloodstream infection rates. Res Nurs Health 39:96–104. https://doi.org/10.1002/nur.21709

Bates DW, Singh H (2018) Two decades since to error is human: an assessment of progress and emerging priorities in patient safety. Health Aff 37(11):1736–1743. https://doi.org/10.1377/hlthaff.2018.0738

Bazzoli G, Thompson M, Waters T (2018) Medicare payment penalties and safety net hospital profitability: minimal impact on these vulnerable hospitals. Health Serv Res 53(5):3495–3506. https://doi.org/10.1111/1475-6773.12833

Bodenheimer T, Sinsky C (2014) From triple to quadruple aim: care of the patient requires care of the provider. Ann Fam Med 12(6):573–576. https://doi.org/10.1370/afm.1713

Campanella P, Vukovic V, Parente P, Sulejimani A, Ricciardi W, Specchia ML (2016) The impact of public reporting on clinical outcomes: a systematic review and meta-analysis. BMC Health Serv Res 16:296. https://doi.org/10.1186/s12913-016-1543-y

Centers for Medicare and Medicaid Services (2017) Hospital value-based purchasing. https://www.cms.gov/Outreach-and-Education/Medicare-Learning-Network-MLN/MLNProducts/downloads/Hospital_VBPurchasing_Fact_Sheet_ICN907664.pdf

Centers for Medicare and Medicaid Services (2018a) Hospital Readmissions Reduction Program (HRRP). https://www.cms.gov/medicare/medicare-fee-for-service-payment/acuteinpatientpps/readmissions-reduction-program.html

Centers for Medicare and Medicaid Services (2018b) Hospital-acquired condition reduction program fiscal year 2019 fact sheet. https://www.cms.gov/Medicare/Medicare-Fee-for-Service-Payment/AcuteInpatientPPS/Downloads/HAC-Reduction-Program-Fact-Sheet.pdf

Centers for Medicare and Medicaid Services (2018c) CMS hospital value-based purchasing program results for fiscal year 2019. https://www.cms.gov/newsroom/fact-sheets/cms-hospital-value-based-purchasing-program-results-fiscal-year-2019

Centers for Medicare and Medicaid Services (2020) CMS Hospital-Acquired Condition Reduction Program (HACRP) https://www.cms.gov/Medicare/Medicare-Fee-for-Service-Payment/AcuteInpatientPPS/HAC-Reduction-Program

Centers for Medicare and Medicaid Services (n.d.) Hospital Compare. Medicare.Gov. https://www.medicare.gov/hospitalcompare/search.html

Colosi B (2018) 2018 National healthcare retention & RN staffing report. http://www.nsinursingsolutions.com/files/assets/library/retention-institute/nationalhealthcarernretentionreport2018.pdf

Dans M, Pabico C, Tate M, Hume L (2017) Understanding the new pathway to excellence® standards. Nurse Leader 15:49–52. https://doi.org/10.1016/j.mnl.2016.09.010

Donabedian A (1966) Evaluating the quality of medical care. Milbank Memorial Fund Quart 44(part 2):166–206

Figueroa JF, Tsugawa Y, Zheng J, Orav EJ, Jha AK (2016) Association between the Value-Based Purchasing pay for performance program and patient mortality in US hospitals: observational study. BMJ 353:i2214. https://doi.org/10.1136/bmj.i2214

Huntington J (1997) Health care in chaos: will we ever see real managed care? Online J Issues Nurs 2(1):Manuscript 1. www.nursingworld.org/MainMenuCategories/ANAMarketplace/ANAPeriodicals/OJIN/TableofContents/Vol21997/No1Jan97/HealthCareinChaos.aspx

Institute of Medicine (1999) To Err Is Human: Building a Safer Health System. The National Academies Press, Washington, DC

Jayawardhana J, Welton JM, Lindrooth R (2011) Adoption of national quality forum safe practices by Magnet® hospitals. J Nurs Adm 41:350–356. https://doi.org/10.1097/NNA.0b013e31822a71a7

Jayawardhana J, Welton JM, Lindrooth RC (2014) Is there a business case for magnet hospitals? Estimates of the cost and revenue implications of becoming a magnet. Med Care 52:400–406. https://doi.org/10.1097/MLR.0000000000000092

Kelly LA, McHugh MD, Aiken LH (2012) Nurse outcomes in Magnet® and non-Magnet hospitals. J Nurs Adm 42:428–433. https://doi.org/10.1097/01.NNA.0000420394.18284.4f

Kruse GB, Polsky D, Stuart EA, Werner RM (2012) The impact of hospital pay-for-performance on hospital and Medicare costs. Health Serv Res 47(6):2118–2136. https://doi.org/10.1111/1475-6773.12003

Kutney-Lee A, Stimpfel AW, Sloane DM, Cimiotti JP, Quinn LW, Aiken LH (2015) Changes in patient and nurse outcomes associated with magnet hospital recognition. Med Care 53:550–557. https://doi.org/10.1097/MLR.0000000000000355

Lake ET, Shang J, Klaus S, Dunton NE (2010) Patient falls: association with hospital Magnet status and nursing unit staffing. Res Nurs Health 33:413–425. https://doi.org/10.1002/nur.20399

Leapfrog Group (n.d.) The Leapfrog Group: who we are. http://www.leapfroggroup.org/about

Lee GM, Kleinman K, Soumerai SB, Tse A, Cole D, Fridkin SK, Goldmann DA (2012) Effect of nonpayment for preventable infections in US hospitals. N Engl J Med 367:1428–1437. https://doi.org/10.1056/NEJMsa1202419

Ma C, Park SH (2015) Hospital magnet status, unit work environment, and pressure ulcers. J Nurs Scholarsh 47:565–573. https://doi.org/10.1111/jnu.12173

Mathes T, Pieper D, Morche J, Polus S, Jaschinski T, Eikermann M (2019) Pay for performance for hospitals. Cochrane Database Syst Rev 2019:7. https://doi.org/10.1002/14651858.CD011156.pub2

Medicare Payment Advisory Commission (2018) Report to the congress: Medicare and the health care delivery system. http://medpac.gov/docs/default-source/reports/jun18_medpacreportto-congress_sec.pdf

Mitchell PH, Ferketich S, Jennings BM (1998) Quality Health Outcomes Model. Image Natl J Nurs Scholar 30(1):43–46

Montalvo I (2007) The National Database of Nursing Quality Indicators™ (NDNQI®). OJIN: Online J Issues Nurs 12(3):Manuscript 2

National Quality Forum (2010) Safe practices for better healthcare—2010 update. https://www.qualityforum.org/Publications/2010/04/Safe_Practices_for_Better_Healthcare_%E2%80%93_2010_Update.aspx

National Quality Forum (2012) Measure evaluation criteria. http://www.qualityforum.org/Measuring_Performance/Submitting_Standards/Measure_Evaluation_Criteria.aspx

Nelson-Brantley HV, Park SH, Bergquist-Beringer S (2018) Characteristics of the nursing practice environment associated with lower unit-level RN turnover. J Nurs Adm 48:31–37. https://doi.org/10.1097/NNA.0000000000000567

Olds DM, Aiken LH, Cimiotti JP, Lake ET (2017) Association of nurse work environment and safety climate on patient mortality: a cross-sectional study. Int J Nurs Stud 74:155–161. https://doi.org/10.1016/j.ijnurstu.2017.06.004

Pakyz AL, Wang H, Ozcan YA, Edmond MB, Vogus TJ (2017) Leapfrog hospital safety score, magnet designation, and healthcare-associated infections in United States hospitals. J Pat Saf. https://doi.org/10.1097/PTS.0000000000000378

Park SH, Gass S, Boyle DK (2016) Comparison of reasons for nurse turnover in Magnet® and non-Magnet hospitals. J Nurs Adm 46:284–290

Popovich DL, Vogus TJ, Iacobucci D, Austin JM (2020) Are hospital ratings systems transparent? An examination of consumer reports and the leapfrog hospital safety grade. Health Mark Q 37:41–57

Press-Ganey (n.d.) Turn nursing quality insights into improved patient experiences. https://www.pressganey.com/docs/default-source/default-document-library/clinicalexcellence_ndnqi_solution-summary.pdf?sfvrsn=0

Rau J (2017) Medicare penalizes group of 751 hospitals for patient injuries. Kaiser Health News. https://khn.org/news/medicare-penalizes-group-of-751-hospitals-for-patient-injuries/

Ryan AM, Krinsky S, Maurer KA, Dimick JB (2017) Changes in hospital quality associated with hospital value-based purchasing. N Engl J Med 376:2358–2366. https://doi.org/10.1056/NEJMsa1613412

Serpa S, Ferreira CM (2019) Micro, meso, and macro levels of social analysis. Int J Soc Stud 7(3) https://doi.org/10.11114/ijsss.v7i3.4223

Sikka R, Moarath J, Leape L (2015) The quadruple aim: health care, cost, and meaning in work. BMJ Qual Saf:608–610

Stimpfel AW, Rosen JE, McHugh MD (2014) Understanding the role of the professional practice environment on quality of care in Magnet® and non-Magnet hospitals. J Nurs Administr 44:10–16. https://doi.org/10.1097/NNA.0000000000000015

Waters TM, Daniels MJ, Bazzoli GJ, Perencevich E, Dunton N, Staggs VS, Shorr RI (2015) Effect of Medicare's nonpayment for hospital-acquired conditions: lessons for future policy. JAMA Intern Med 175:347–354. https://doi.org/10.1001/jamainternmed.2014.5486

Part VII
Closing

The Way Forward

15

Marianne Baernholdt and Diane K. Boyle

Introduction

At the finishing of this book, the world is facing the second wave of COVID-19 pandemic. In the United States (US), there is also political and social conflict and unrest related to pandemic management and racial injustice. The complexities of both remind us that moving forward in our quest to improve healthcare quality, we have to frame our inquiries within a multilevel framework such as the QHOM (Mitchell et al. 1998). The need for understanding which factors contribute to improved quality has never been greater. In the previous chapters, these factors have been discussed using QHOM's four primary constructs: system, client, interventions, and outcomes. In this closing chapter, the quality and safety reports guiding healthcare policy and practice since the late 1990s when the QHOM was developed are revisited, including highlighting the reports focused on nurses. The last section will discuss future directions.

The QHOM in the Context of Quality and Safety Reports

The conceptualization and publication of the QHOM in 1998 occurred just before the Institute of Medicine [IOM, now the National Academy of Medicine (NAM)] released a series of reports disclosing healthcare errors as a leading cause of death in the United States. The reports also addressed the healthcare system's shortcomings and focused on making evidence-based changes moving forward. Healthcare professionals were compelled to embark on a mission to improve safety and quality.

M. Baernholdt (✉)
School of Nursing, University of North Carolina at Chapel Hill, Chapel Hill, NC, USA
e-mail: marianne_baernholdt@unc.edu

D. K. Boyle
Fay W. Whitney School of Nursing, University of Wyoming, Laramie, WY, USA

© Springer Nature Switzerland AG 2021
M. Baernholdt, D. K. Boyle (eds.), *Nurses Contributions to Quality Health Outcomes*, https://doi.org/10.1007/978-3-030-69063-2_15

The IOM/NAM and others have reports focused on nursing alone or as part of the healthcare team. All of these reports have been driving forces for nursing education, practice, and research, as well as shaping policies at the state, national, and international levels.

The Institute of Medicine

Twenty years ago, the IOM released two transformational reports on healthcare quality and safety. The first, *To Err is Human: Building a Better Health System* (2000), sent shockwaves through the healthcare industry and the public by uncovering the high frequency and broadness of healthcare errors. The report exposed healthcare errors as a leading cause of death, estimating up to 98,000 preventable deaths each year and hundreds of thousands of nonfatal injuries. Beyond human lives, other costs were the expense of additional care needed, lost income and productivity, reduced school attendance, disability, physical and psychological discomfort, lack of trust in the healthcare system, dissatisfaction, and even lower population health levels. Finally, the IOM also found that system failures, not individual failures, caused 90% of errors.

As a result, a paradigm shift occurred that was new to healthcare. The shift was not focusing on blaming individual clinicians as the cause of failures but instead assessing system-level reasons. This was a common approach in other industries, such as nuclear power plants and aviation (Reason 2000). These industries, termed high-reliability organizations, used human factors engineering to build system-level defenses to prevent errors and mitigate their effects. The second report from IOM, *Crossing the Quality Chasm: A New Health System for the Twenty-First Century*, used human factors engineering and comparisons with other high-risk industries to call for a transformational overhaul of the US healthcare system (IOM 2001). The report outlined how evidence-based system changes need to occur simultaneously in six dimensions: safety, effectiveness, patient-centeredness, timeliness, efficiency, and equity. A rationale and a framework were provided for the redesign of the healthcare system at four levels: patients' experiences; the microsystems or the nursing units/clinics that deliver the healthcare; the organizations that house and support the microsystems; and the environment of laws, rules, payment, accreditation, and professional training that shape organizational actions. These are all dimensions covered in this book's chapters, framed within the four constructs of the QHOM and the healthcare context. Specifically, Chap. 2 covers healthcare policy, Chap. 3 the nursing workforce's education, Chaps. 4 and 5 the microsystem/nursing unit, Chap. 12 the client and family experiences of care, and Chap. 14 the organizational outcomes and quality measures.

Following these two reports, the IOM/NAM has published almost yearly state of the science reports focusing on many topics important for high-quality and safe healthcare, for example rural health (IOM 2005), mental health and substance abuse (IOM 2006), improving diagnosis (NAM 2015), and clinician burnout (NAM 2019). Although these reports used global evidence, the settings they addressed were mainly in the US. However, in 2018, NAM evaluated the state of gaps in healthcare quality globally and suggested approaches to solve them. *Crossing the Global Quality Chasm: Improving Health Care Worldwide* (NAM 2018) updated the original 2001 report with a global focus and an update of the six dimensions to contemporary terms and definitions. Safety, effectiveness, efficiency, and equity remained the same with similar definitions. However, patient-centeredness was changed to person-centeredness to remind readers that circumstances beyond the clinical setting determine health. Timeliness was expanded to include accessibility and affordability (NAM 2018). Many of these aspects of healthcare are also covered in this book. In Chaps. 7 and 8, patient and population characteristics are discussed, i.e., health literacy and chronicity, while Chap. 11 covers care coordination that is important for timely healthcare.

Reports Focused on Nurses

Several reports from IOM/NAM and others, such as the World Health Organization (WHO), have focused on nursing's role in improving healthcare quality. They are described below with reference to the QHOM and chapters in this book to emphasize how pertinent the QHOM is in framing nurses' contribution to healthcare quality.

The IOM has released numerous reports focused on nurses, either solely or as part of the interprofessional team. In 2004 IOM released *Keeping Patients Safe: Transforming the Work Environment of Nurses*, which linked nurses and their work environments to patient safety and quality of care. Threats to patient safety occurred at every level and component of healthcare delivery, including work processes, workload, work hours, and nursing staff workspaces. The IOM identified that transformational leadership was needed to "assure the effective use of practices that (1) balance the tension between production efficiency and reliability (safety), (2) create and sustain trust throughout the organization, (3) actively manage the process of change, (4) involve workers in decision making about work design and workflow, and (5) use knowledge management practices to establish the organization as a 'learning organization'" (IOM 2004, p. 8). The nurse work environment is discussed in Chaps. 4 and 5.

As a follow-up to the 2004 report, the IOM, together with the Robert Wood Johnson Foundation, released *The Future of Nursing: Leading Change, Advancing Health* in 2011. The report was released concurrently as the Affordable Care Act (ACA) was passed into law (see Chap. 2). The IOM report evaluated the state of the nursing workforce and its practice, followed by recommendations. The latter was "intended to support efforts to improve the health of the US population through the contribution nurses can make to care delivery. However, they are not necessarily about achieving what is most comfortable, convenient, or easy for the nursing profession" (IOM 2011, p. S-3). Specifically, the report recommended the need for (a) ensuring that nurses can practice to the full extent of their education and training; (b) improving nurse education through seamless academic progression; (c) providing opportunities for nurses to assume leadership positions as full partners with physicians and other health professionals; and (d) improving data collection for policymaking and workforce planning. Chaps. 2, 3, 4, and 10 discuss the policy, workforce, nurse work environment, and interprofessional collaboration that the Future of Nursing report recommends.

A follow-up report is planned for 2020 to include lessons learned since the previous report and recommendations regarding nurses' role in the COVID-19 pandemic. The overall goals remain to "chart a path for the nursing profession to help our nation create a culture of health, reduce health disparities, and improve the health and well-being of the US population in the twenty-first century" (NAM 2020).

A final NAM report focused on nurses is *Taking Action Against Clinician Burnout: A Systems Approach to Professional Well-Being* from 2019. This report addresses the dual objective of clinician burnout and well-being and improving patient care. Similar to work using the QHOM, the report is guided by a multilevel systems model—frontline care delivery, healthcare organization, and external environment that influence each other. The report recommends that healthcare organizations (a) create positive work environments for clinicians, (b) create positive learning environments for health professions education and training, (c) reduce administrative burden, (d) enable technology solutions, (e) provide mental health support to clinicians and learners, and (f) invest in research on clinician well-being. All of these recommendations are addressed in Chaps. 4, 5, 6, 10, and 13 of this book in topics that include the work environment, workflow, turbulence, and cognitive complexity in nurses' work; the use of health information technology; nurses as part of the interprofessional team; and nurse outcomes.

In 2020, the World Health Organization (WHO) published the *State of the World's Nursing 2020* report in partnership with the International Council of Nurses (ICN) and the Nursing Now campaign. ICN is a federation of more than 130 national nurses' associations representing more than 27 million nurses worldwide. ICN was founded in 1899 and is the world's oldest and largest international organization for health professionals (ICN 2020). The Nursing Now 3-year campaign (Nursing Now n.d.) was launched in 2018 to respond to the *Triple Impact of Nursing* report from the All-Party Parliamentary Group on Global Health in Britain (2016). The Triple Impact report concluded that to ensure that everyone in the world has access to healthcare, nursing has to be strengthened globally. The Nursing Now campaign focuses on five areas:

1. Ensuring that nurses and midwives have a more prominent voice in health policymaking
2. Encouraging greater investment in the nursing workforce
3. Advocating for more nurses in leadership positions
4. Encouraging research that helps determine where nurses can have the greatest impact
5. Sharing examples of best nursing practice (https://www.nursingnow.org/who-we-are/)

The WHO report has similar goals. After assessing the evidence in the 152 countries (out of the world's 157 countries) that provided data on nursing education, scope of practice, nursing regulation (licensing), working conditions, and role in policy, the report concluded:

"No global health agenda can be realized without concerted and sustained efforts to maximize the contributions of the nursing workforce and their roles within interprofessional health teams. To do so requires policy interventions that enable them to have maximum impact and effectiveness by optimizing nurses' scope and leadership, alongside accelerated investment in their education, skills and jobs" (WHO 2020b, p. xii). This much-anticipated report was published in the year the World Health Assembly designated the International Year of the Nurse and the Midwife (WHO 2020a). The year coincides with the 200-year birthday of Florence Nightingale, who is heralded as the founder of the nursing profession. Florence and her writings have inspired many nurse scholars, including the two authors of this book. However, as nurse scientists, we have to evaluate all the evidence about Florence's contribution to nursing. Besides being a forward-thinking nurse leader, it has recently come to light that she also held racist views (Stake-Doucet 2020). She considered indigenous people inferior and promoted colonization in the British Empire. In fact, because of her role as advisor to the Governor of New Zealand during the Maori-anti-colonial uprisings in 1861–1868, the New Zealand Nurses' Organization has decided not to partake in the year of the nurse campaign.

Future Directions

Since the publication of the QHOM and the IOM landmark study (IOM 2000), few would dispute that the healthcare industry still faces significant and compelling healthcare quality challenges. In a 2016 analysis for the *BMJ*, Makary and Daniel found that the mean number of deaths from preventable medical errors was about 250,000 per year in the US and therefore it was the third leading cause of death. In a more recent systematic review and meta-analysis, Panagioti et al. (2019) reported that 1 in 20 patients is still exposed to preventable harm in healthcare. In the world, between 5.7 and 8.4 million patients in low- and middle-income countries die because of poor-quality healthcare (NAM 2018), which is the equivalent of 15% of overall deaths in these countries. Although healthcare quality has improved since 1998 when the QHOM was published—for example, in the US, overall hospital-acquired conditions have improved (AHRQ 2019)—there is no doubt that healthcare quality remains a significant problem.

The way healthcare has changed since the publication of the QHOM in 1998 is enormous. The development of technology has catapulted the healthcare environment into new ways of delivering, reporting, studying, and regulating. With the healthcare quality improvements in the first two decades of this century, the development and implementation of healthcare technology brought unintended consequences. For example, the toll that increased electronic documentation burden has taken on clinicians (NAM 2019). The QHOM can guide implementations to address these problems and the problems on the horizon, for example, the emergence of artificial intelligence (AI) as a tool to improve healthcare quality. AI is not one technology, but rather a collection of them. One is machine learning, where statistical algorithms applied to a large quantity of data can produce predictions for clinicians on what treatment protocols are likely to be best for an individual patient (Davenport and Kalakota 2019). Since AI's successful predictions require population-representative datasets, so as not to create biased results, the NAM special publication from 2019, *Artificial Intelligence in Health Care: The Hope, the Hype, the Promise, the Peril*, (Matheny et al. 2019) stresses the need to prioritize equity and inclusivity in the data used. Otherwise, the existing inequities in health outcomes caused by individual and organizational biases can become much larger using AI on biased data. However, AI can offer unparalleled opportunities to improve patient and clinical team outcomes, reduce costs, and impact population health.

The COVID-19 pandemic is another example of a complex problem where the QHOM can be applied to plan, implement, and evaluate solutions. Healthcare systems or organizations had to shift operations to accommodate changes in supply chains and patient healthcare needs (Short and Mammen 2020). The well-known personal protective equipment (PPE) shortage across all healthcare organizations, from nursing homes to acute care hospitals, placed tremendous stress on organizations and healthcare workers. So did the many examples of peers becoming infected and dying of COVID-19 (Shaw et al. 2020). Further, healthcare workers worried about exposing their families to COVID-19, which added extra pressure. Thus healthcare workers are faced with responsibility to their family and obligations to their patients (Sasangohar et al. 2020). Finally, as experts develop vaccine guidelines at the Centers for Disease Control and Prevention and NAM, both with nurses at the table, the success of deployment and implementation will, in no small degree, depend on healthcare workers, including nurses (Schwartz 2020).

As we stated in Chap. 1, nurses play a significant role in delivering and coordinating care activities within and across healthcare teams. Consequently, few healthcare elements do not pass through nurses' hands, and few outcomes are not influenced in some way by nursing care. Using the QHOM as a framework nurses in practice, education, research, and policy will lead changes to improve quality and safety, remembering that:

> For us who Nurse, our Nursing is a thing, which, unless in it we are making progress every year, every month, every week, take my word for it we are going back. The more experience we gain, the more progress we can make.
> Florence Nightingale, 1872 (Baly, 1997)

References

Agency for Healthcare Research and Quality (2019) Analysis finds hospital-acquired conditions declined by nearly 1 million from 2014–2017. https://www.ahrq.gov/news/newsroom/press-releases/hac-rates-declined.html

All-Party Parliamentary Group on Global Health (2016) Triple impact—how developing nursing will improve health, promote gender equality and support economic growth. http://www.appg. globalhealth.org.uk/

Baly M (1997) As miss nightingale said .... Bailliere Tindall. Published in Association with the Royal College of Nursing, London, England

Davenport T, Kalakota R (2019) The potential for artificial intelligence in healthcare. Future Healthc J 6(2):94–98. https://doi.org/10.7861/futurehosp.6-2-94

Institute of Medicine (2000) To err is human: building a safer health system. The National Academies Press, Washington, DC

Institute of Medicine (2001) Crossing the quality chasm: a new health system for the 21st century. The National Academies Press, Washington, DC

Institute of Medicine (2004) Keeping patients safe: transforming the work environment of nurses. National Academies Press, Washington, DC

Institute of Medicine (2005) Quality through collaboration: the future of rural health. National Academies Press, Washington, DC

Institute of Medicine (2006) Improving the quality of health care for mental and substance-use conditions: quality chasm series. National Academies Press, Washington, DC

Institute of Medicine. Committee on the Robert Wood Johnson Foundation Initiative on the Future of Nursing, at the Institute of Medicine (2011) The future of nursing: leading change, advancing health. National Academies Press, Washington, DC

Makary MA, Daniel M (2016) Medical error—the third leading cause of death in the US. BMJ 353:i2139. https://doi.org/10.1136/bmj.i2139

Matheny M, Thadaney SI, Ahmed M, Whicher D (2019) Artificial intelligence in health care: the hope, the hype, the promise, the Peril. NAM Special Publication. National Academy of Medicine, Washington, DC

Mitchell PH, Ferketich S, Jennings BM (1998) Quality health outcomes model. Image Natl J Nurs Scholar 30(1):43–46. https://doi.org/10.1111/j.1547-5069.1998.tb01234.x

National Academies of Sciences, Engineering, and Medicine (2015) Improving diagnosis in health care. The National Academies Press, Washington, DC

National Academies of Sciences, Engineering, and Medicine (2018) Crossing the global quality chasm: improving health care worldwide. The National Academies Press, Washington, DC

National Academies of Sciences, Engineering, and Medicine (2019) Taking action against clinician burnout: a systems approach to professional well-being. The National Academies Press, Washington, DC

National Academies of Sciences, Engineering, and Medicine (2020) The future of nursing 2020–2030. A Consensus Study from the National Academy of Medicine. https://nam.edu/publications/the-future-of-nursing-2020-2030/

Nursing Now (n.d.) Who we are. https://www.nursingnow.org/who-we-are/

Panagioti M, Khan K, Keers RN, Abuzour A, Phipps D, Kontopantelis E, Bower P, Campbell S, Razaan H, Avery AJ, Darren MA (2019) Prevalence, severity, and nature of preventable patient harm across medical settings: a systematic review and meta-analysis. BMJ 366:l4185. https://doi.org/10.1136/bmj.l4185

Reason J (2000) Human error: models and management. BMJ (Clin Res Ed) 320(7237):768–770. https://doi.org/10.1136/bmj.320.7237.768

Sasangohar F, Jones SL, Masud FN, Vahidy FS, Kash BA (2020) Provider burnout and fatigue during the COVID-19 pandemic: lessons learned from a high-volume intensive care unit. Anesth Analg 131(1):106–111. https://doi.org/10.1213/ANE.0000000000004866

Schwartz JL (2020) Evaluating and deploying Covid-19 vaccines—the importance of transparency, scientific Integrity, and public trust. N Engl J Med 383:1703–1705. https://doi.org/10.1056/NEJMp2026393

Shaw A, Flott K, Fontana G, Durkin M, Darzi A (2020) No patient safety without health worker safety. Lancet 396(10262):1541–1543. https://doi.org/10.1016/S0140-6736(20)31949-8

Short JB, Mammen AA (2020) Pandemic application of creative destruction in healthcare. Front Health Serv Manag 37(1):4–9. https://doi.org/10.1097/HAP.0000000000000093

Stake-Doucet N (2020) The Racist lady with the lamp. Nursing Clio. https://nursingclio. org/2020/11/05/the-racist-lady-with-the-lamp/

The International Council of Nurses (ICN) (2020) Who we are. https://www.icn.ch/who-we-are

The World Health Organization (2020a) Year of the nurse and the midwife 2020. https://www.who. int/campaigns/year-of-the-nurse-and-the-midwife-2020

The World Health Organization (2020b) State of the world's nursing 2020. Investing in education, jobs and leadership. ISBN: 978-92-4-000327-9

Batch number: 10091879

Printed by Printforce, the Netherlands